STUTTER'S CASEBOOK

A JUNIOR HOSPITAL DOCTOR
1839–1841

STUTTER'S CASEBOOK

A JUNIOR HOSPITAL DOCTOR
1839–1841

Edited by

E. E. COCKAYNE and N. J. STOW

General Editor

DAVID DYMOND

The Boydell Press

Suffolk Records Society
VOLUME XLVIII

A Suffolk Records Society publication
First published 2005
The Boydell Press, Woodbridge

ISBN 1 84383 113 9

Issued to subscribing members for the year 2004–2005

The Boydell Press is an imprint of Boydell & Brewer Ltd
PO Box 9, Woodbridge, Suffolk IP12 3DF, UK
and of Boydell & Brewer Inc.
668 Mt Hope Avenue, Rochester, NY 14620, USA
website: www.boydellandbrewer.com

A CIP catalogue record for this book is available
from the British Library

This publication is printed on acid-free paper

Printed in Great Britain by
St. Edmundsbury Press, Bury St. Edmunds, Suffolk

CONTENTS

List of illustrations   vi

Acknowledgements   ix

Abbreviations   x

General introduction   xi

Pharmaceutical introduction   xxxiii

Editorial methods   xli

Index of patients   xliii

W.G. STUTTER'S CASEBOOK   1

Appendices

I. Biographies of doctors and nurses   91

II. Diseases   106

III. Diagnostic methods   118

IV. Physical treatments   121

V. Drugs and chemicals   129

Bibliography   161

Indexes:
    People and Places   163
    General and Medical Subjects   168
    Pharmaceutical Materials and Methods   174

ILLUSTRATIONS

1. The hospital, Bury St Edmunds, 1852   xii
2. Plowman Young's house, Bury St Edmunds, 2001   xiii
3. Market place, Bury St Edmunds, 1930s   xix
4. 'Elaboratory' of John Bell & Co. in London, in   xxxiv
    the 1840s
5. Stutter's Casebook, pages 66 and 67 (part of), relating   42
    to Kezia Atkins
6. Stethoscope of the Laennec type   118
7. Drawing of a Laennec-type stethoscope   119
8. Surgeon bleeding young woman's arm, 1784   121
9. Cupping glasses   122
10. Automatic scarifier showing spring mechanism   123
11. Automatic scarifier showing blades   123
12. Leech   125
13. Trocar and cannula   126
14. Vapour bath   127
15. Vertical section through capsule of an opium poppy   129
16. Transverse section through calumba root   133
17. Spanish fly or blistering beetle   134
18. Castor oil plant   136
19. Bark of *Cinchona* tree   136
20. Corm of meadow saffron, *Colchicum*   137
21. Leaves and seeds of *Croton* tree   138
22. Foxglove, *Digitalis*   139
23. Rye contaminated by ergot fungus   140
24. Roots of ginger   141
25. Hemlock plant   142
26. Leaves and flowering tops of henbane   143
27. Jalap roots, *Ipomoea purga*   144
28. Seed from *Nux vomica* tree   145
29. Spearmint   146
30. Rhubarb rhizomes   147
31. Squill bulb   149
32. Valerian plant   150

Illustrations 1, 3, 4 and 5 are reproduced by permission of the Suffolk Record
Office; illustrations 6 and 8–11 are reproduced by permission of the Wellcome

Library, London; illustrations 12, 13, 15–17, 20–23, 25–30 and 32 are reproduced from J. Harter, *Images of Medicine*; whilst images 19, 24 and 31 come from T.E. Wallis, *Textbook of Pharmacognosy.*

Figures

1.	Numbers of inpatients and outpatients, 1839	xxvii
2.	Methods of administering drugs orally	xxxviii
3.	Methods of applying medications externally	xxxviii

Tables

1.	Hospital admission details for all patients in Stutter's casebook	xxiv–vi
2.	Occupation and marital status of Stutter's patients as mentioned in his casebook	xxviii
3.	Drugs and chemicals prescribed by Stutter: their frequency of use	131

The two editors first met when they occupied adjacent beds in the orthopaedic ward of the West Suffolk General Hospital in 1974. It therefore seems appropriate to dedicate this book to the patients of that institution, both past and present.

ACKNOWLEDGEMENTS

Many friends, relatives and associates have assisted with this book and we would like to thank them most sincerely. They include Dr Pat Murrell, who first suggested the project; Dr David Dymond, our patient general editor; Mr Peter Northeast, who helped with the Latin; Dr Melvin Earles of Eltham, who knew about Ferri persessquinitrate; Bryony Kelly of the Royal Pharmaceutical Society, who identified the picture of Bell's pharmacy; Dr Walter Sneadon of the Department of Pharmaceutical Sciences, University of Strythclyde, who helped with the 1lb symbol; Michael Stow of Thurlow Design, who fashioned the apothecary fonts etc., and Frances Ridsdill Smith who drew the diagram of Laennec's stethoscope. The Medical Photographic Library of the Wellcome Trust provided most of the photographs that illustrate the appendices whilst Dr Sarah Cockayne, consultant dermatologist, Sheffield, commented on some of Stutter's dermatological patients. Angela Sharpe, photographer, did a splendid job on the cartoon which adorns the cover. And last but not least, we must mention the staff of the Bury St Edmunds and Ipswich Record Offices, who supported us for many months and provided us with an extremely pleasant environment in which to do our research.

ABBREVIATIONS

BPC	*British Pharmaceutical Codex*, London, 1934
Consp.	A.T. Thomson, *A Conspectus of the Pharmacopœias*, 3rd edn, London, 1820
Cullum	Letters of T.G. Cullum: SROB E2/21/2
Extra	W. Martindale, *The Extra Pharmacopœia*, 22nd edn, vol. II, London, 1943
Guide	R. Farquharson, *A Guide to Therapeutics*, London, 1877
Herbal	C. Newall, L. Anderson and D. Phillipson, *Herbal Medicines: A Guide for Health-care Professionals*, London, 1996
London	A.T. Thomson, *The London Dispensatory*, 5th edn, London, 1830
Medical	R. Reece, *The Medical Guide*, 11th edn, London, 1814
Nunn	Prescription Books of Nunn, Hinnell & Co.: SROB 2195
Barnardiston	Medicinal Recipes of Sophia Barnardiston: SROB 613/779
SROB	Suffolk Record Office, Bury St Edmunds
SROI	Suffolk Record Office, Ipswich
Translation	R. Phillips, *A Translation of the Pharmacopœia of the Royal College of Physicians of London, 1836*, London, 1848
Wallis	T.E. Wallis, *Textbook of Pharmacognosy*, London, 1946

GENERAL INTRODUCTION

Partridges

It is said that the famous historian W.G. Hoskins once read an article in *The Times* which was entitled 'A Bad Year for Partridges'. In the text of the article he learned that very many fewer partridges had been shot that year than was usually the case, and from this he concluded that it had been a rather good year if you happened to be a partridge. There and then he determined that henceforth he would try to write history from the point of view of the partridges. That is, those people who are normally shot at and reviled and thought to be of no account whatsoever. This book is in that tradition.

Aims

For most of his professional career W.G. Stutter (1815–1887) was a respected general medical practitioner in the village of Wickhambrook in Suffolk. When he was a young man, however, he worked as House Apothecary and House Surgeon to the Suffolk General Hospital from 1839 to 1841. His casebook for part of that period in his life has survived, and as such it is a fairly rare document, because the author was a veritable partridge of the medical profession, a junior doctor in a small provincial hospital. The book itself does not look very impressive. It measures 14½ inches by 5 inches and is just 2 inches thick. The binding of cardboard covered with lambskin is unfortunately beginning to fall apart, but happily the inner pages are still in reasonable condition.

In editing the casebook we have had three aims in mind. The first is that the edited version should act as a kind of 'Rosetta stone' to those who attempt to read the original document. This is because it is very difficult for the modern reader to make any sense of the pharmaceutical terms and dog-Latin employed by early nineteenth-century doctors without some sort of guidance, and the hope is that what follows will help the reader to translate both the document in question and others of the same ilk.

When he moved to Wickhambrook in 1842, Stutter began to make entries in visiting and account books, and it seems that he continued to do this for the next thirty-two years. A cache of Stutter's books, including the first 'hospital' casebook, was discovered by some workmen in the attic of Brooke House, Wickhambrook, in the late 1970s. This had been Stutter's residence until his death in 1887. Like many of us, he had apparently dumped all his junk under the eaves and left it there. Some of the books are still in private hands, but many of them have been deposited in the Suffolk Record Office.[1] As far as we can ascertain, however, none of these further volumes is equal in detail to the book that he kept as a junior hospital doctor.

A subsidiary aim in editing Stutter's casebook has been to try to throw light upon the treatments that were commonly employed in a run-of-the-mill medical

---

[1]   Stutter's visiting and account books: SROB HC 517/2–18.

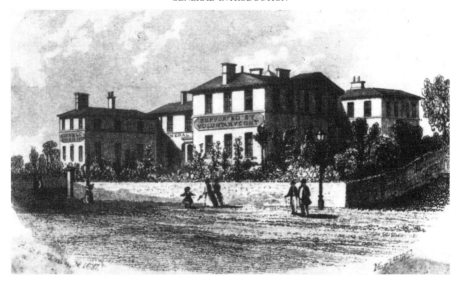

1. This is a copy of an etching of the hospital, Bury St Edmunds, done in 1852. Reproduced by permission of SROB.

establishment in the late 1830s and early 1840s. And, last but not least, we have attempted to illustrate something of the life of a provincial general hospital in the first half of the nineteenth century.

Unfortunately, apart from the word 'pragmatic' scrawled three times on the front page, the casebook itself does not tell us what Stutter thought of what he was doing, or how he interacted with the physicians and surgeons, nurses and patients in the Suffolk General Hospital. Perhaps in his doodle he was telling himself to be pragmatic, as most doctors find they have to be if they are to cope. But although the book is bereft of personal comment, it does record patients' clinical histories, sometimes the diagnoses that were made, and invariably the treatments given. And when these records are married with the knowledge gleaned from the minutes of the Hospital Committee Meetings and brief references in local newspapers, we gain an impression of what it must have been like to be a doctor, nurse or patient in the Suffolk General Hospital in the years 1839–1841.

Stutter is appointed

William Gaskoin Stutter LSA, MRCS, was appointed as House Apothecary and House Surgeon at The Suffolk General Hospital, Bury St Edmunds, at a Special General Meeting of the Governors held on 27 February 1839.[2] According to his casebook he had already been working in that capacity since 12 February 1839, so it seems that he most probably spent the first two weeks as a *locum tenens*. His predecessor, Mr Ward, had resigned, giving the required three months' notice on 8 December 1838,[3] and the job had been advertised in the local press.[4] The person

---

2   Minute books of Committee and Board Meetings of the Suffolk General Hospital: SROB ID 503/5.
3   *Ibid.*: ID 503/5.
4   *Bury and Norwich Post*, 2 Jan. 1839, p. 3, col. 5.

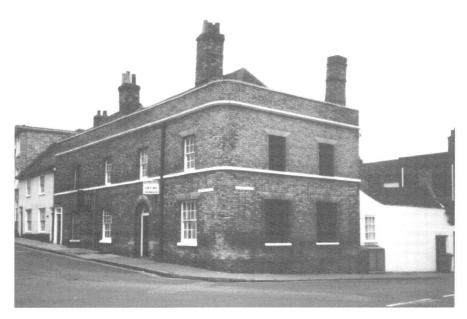

2. This photograph of Plowman Young's old house in Bury St Edmunds was taken in 2001.

sought had to be over twenty-one years of age and a Licentiate of the Society of Apothecaries. There had been two other applicants,[5] but Stutter was the only local man and the others had withdrawn their names before the governors met. Stutter, born in Flempton, Suffolk, in 1815,[6] had been an apprentice to a local surgeon, Plowman Young,[7] and no doubt his old master strongly supported his ex-pupil's application for the job at the hospital. Young had originally practised in Norton,[8] a village nine miles to the east of Bury St Edmunds, but he had moved to the town two years before Stutter had joined him as an apprentice in 1832.

The training of doctors

At that time in East Anglia an apprenticeship to a general practitioner (who was both a surgeon and apothecary but usually styled himself 'surgeon'), was still the commonest way for a boy from a modest middle-class background to enter the medical profession. For a fee he would join the master's household, usually between the ages of fourteen and twenty, and be instructed in the mysteries of the craft for the next five years. Afterwards, he would usually go to London to attend lectures at a teaching hospital or dispensary for another fifteen to eighteen months. Then, provided that he was aged twenty-one or more, the apprentice would take an exami-

5   *Ibid.*
6   The van Zwanenberg papers: SROI q s 614.
7   D. van Zwanenberg, 'The Training and Careers of those Apprenticed to Apothecaries in Suffolk 1815–1858', *Medical History* 27,1983, pp. 139–150.
8   The van Zwanenberg papers: SROI q s 614.

nation at Apothecaries' Hall. If he passed, he became a Licenciate of The Society of Apothecaries (LSA), and was licensed to practise. The LSA examination had been introduced by the Apothecaries' Act of 1815, and was the first examination specifically designed for aspiring general medical practitioners.

Those who wanted to demonstrate a more rounded education also took the examination of the College of Surgeons and became Members of the Royal College of Surgeons (MRCS). By Stutter's time it was becoming accepted that passing through 'College and Hall' was the proper way to enter general practice. In fact, after 1837 68 per cent of prospective entrants were so qualified, but the LSA on its own remained the basic requirement. In 1839 there were still many practitioners who had no qualifications other than a previous seven-year apprenticeship and/or a spell served as a ship's surgeon before the year 1815, when the Apothecaries' Act was passed. This was a source of irritation to some of those who had run the full course and passed the relevant examinations, and so-called 'irregular practitioners' were the whipping boys of the more militant medical politicians of the time.[9] The situation did not begin to be resolved until the Medical Register was introduced in 1858, when it was found that in fact a third of practising medical practitioners did not have any degree or diploma!

Wealthier parents would perhaps send their sons to Oxford, Cambridge or Edinburgh to obtain degrees in medicine that would make them acceptable as physicians in the larger towns and cities, dealing with the better sort of patients. The physicians had long regarded themselves as the aristocrats of the medical profession and looked down on surgeons and apothecaries. In the bigger centres, surgery was itself becoming more of a specialty and it was common for those who were aiming for the top posts to become apprenticed to the men with the best reputations. Nepotism was rife and it was difficult to break into the system if you had not got the right connections. It was easier to rise in the provinces. John Green Crosse,[10] who was born at Great Finborough in 1790, did his apprenticeship in nearby Stowmarket. His master was Thomas Bayly, who had four daughters. After further study in London, Paris and Dublin, Crosse married Bayly's daughter Dorothy and went on to become a noted senior surgeon at the Norfolk and Norwich Hospital.[11] He specialised in the removal of bladder stones, which were very common at the time, especially in children.[12]

But on the whole, the tripartite division of the medical profession into physicians, surgeons and general practitioners did not have much relevance in the small towns and villages of East Anglia, where nearly all doctors were general practitioners to a greater or lesser extent. Certainly this is true even of John Green Crosse, who had a large medical, surgical and midwifery practice throughout his professional career.

The apprenticeship system had been in place for centuries, and although by the 1830s its value was being challenged, at least it gave young men an idea of the life they would be likely to lead when they finished their studies. John Steggall

---

[9] See E. Cockayne, 'The Misfortune of John Steggall (1789–1881)', *Journal of the Royal Society of Medicine* 92, Feb. 1999, 91–93.

[10] See Appendix I.

[11] V. Mary Crosse, *A Surgeon in the Early 19th Century*, Edinburgh and London, 1968.

[12] The frequency of bladder stones has been attributed to factors such as deficiency of milk in the diet of children and a general lack of vitamin A. The incidence declined rapidly in the early twentieth century and this has been explained by a change in East Anglia to mixed farming instead of the limited crop farming of previous generations. See John A. Shepherd, 'William Jeaffreson (1790–1865): Surgical Pioneer', *British Medical Journal* 119 (Nov. 1965), pp. 1119–1120.

(1789–1881), who was apprenticed to a surgeon in Bacton at Suffolk wrote that his job as an apprentice was to 'mix up medicines, hold men's heads and arms and bind up wounds. Limbs were set, teeth drawn, pills made and of course swallowed, and many cured of various complaints; but nervous disorders and rich fat farmers and their wives and daughters were all our best subjects in the Esculapian [*sic*] profession'.[13] Some found it all rather tedious, as did Sir James Paget who was apprenticed to a surgeon in Great Yarmouth from 1830 to 1835.[14] For apprentices too much time was probably spent in writing out the bills, keeping the shop clean and dispensing medicines. Formal education seems to have been a bit haphazard, and living conditions cramped. In about 1771 John Crabbe the poet was an apprentice at Wickhambrook (where Stutter ended up in practice seventy-two years later). His master was a farmer, and Crabbe had to help out with work on the farm as well as sleep in the same room as the ploughboy. This did not suit the aspiring poet, who after about three years successfully pleaded with his father to let him change masters. He moved from Wickhambrook to Woodbridge to conclude his training with a Mr Page.[15]

The apprentice in Norton, where Stutter's master Plowman Young had been apprentice and later master when he took over from Benjamin Clayton in 1819, slept in a tiny room above the surgery reached by a stepladder through a trapdoor. The apprentices whiled away their time as best they could, looking forward to fairs and other entertainments. Some twenty-four young men passed through the Norton practice between the years 1793 and 1856.[16] It is difficult to see why Norton had so many apprentices, but perhaps the explanation is to do with money. In those days country practitioners needed a sideline. Some surgeons were part-time farmers and others were part-time medical teachers. The village of Norton was never very populous (879 in the 1841 census) and the surgeon probably found that the apprentice provided a useful source of income, especially since the house had long been set up prepared to receive its young guests. But having vigorous and sometimes bored young men about did sometimes have unwelcome side effects.

Woodward Mudd, who was Benjamin Clayton's apprentice from 1801 to 1805, entered a relationship with a young woman called Susan Barrell. She became pregnant and had his child. On 24 May 1803 Woodward appeared before two justices on a charge of bastardy. He did not deny his paternity and so he was ordered to pay six shillings to the parish of Norton for lying-in costs, plus one shilling and sixpence a week thereafter. The child's mother, Susan Barrell was herself ordered to pay sixpence a week to the parish.[17] This episode does not seem to have diminished Mudd's libido. Three years later he was charged again, this time for begetting a child on the body of a Mary Leech.[18] None of the above seems to have affected Woodward Mudd's professional career. On 3 April 1811 he was elected a member of the Suffolk Medical Benevolent Society.[19]

---

[13] R. Cobbold (ed.), *John Steggall: A Real History of a Suffolk Man*, London, 1857. See also Appendix I.

[14] D. van Zwanenberg, 'Training and Careers', pp. 139–150.

[15] *Life of George Crabbe by his son*, 1834; reprinted London, 1957.

[16] This knowledge is partially gleaned from Dr van Zwanenberg's article mentioned above, but also by viewing signatures on some dispensary drawers owned by the present (2003) inhabitants of Stanton House in Norton, Mr and Mrs McBrien. It was obviously a custom for the apprentices to sign the backs of the drawers in the dispensary.

[17] Bastardy bond: SROB 54612/7/34/1 and FL 612/7/33/2.

[18] *Ibid.*: SROB FL 612/9/2/1.

[19] *Ipswich Journal*, 20 April 1811.

It is worth noting in passing that seduction could also be used as a weapon to extract oneself from an uncongenial apprenticeship. In London back in 1777 an apprentice to the noted Percival Pott (1714–1788) complained that the teaching he received from his master was completely obsolete, but he was released from his contract when 'a courtship of one fortnight terminated the virginity of Miss Pott [Percival's daughter]'.[20] This quickly resulted in the apprentice being discharged!

In 1819, Plowman Young's liason with his master's daughter ended more romantically. He married Ann Maria Clayton, and took over the Norton practice when his father-in-law Benjamin died of tuberculosis that same year.[21] Young moved to Bury in 1830 and Stutter was his apprentice from 1832 to 1837. Following his apprenticeship with Plowman Young, Stutter spent fifteen months walking the wards at St George's Hospital. After Bury St Edmunds (population 12,538 in 1841),[22] London must have seemed a very busy place. It was probably not to Stutter's taste, because as soon as he could he applied for a job back in Suffolk. He was to spend the whole of the rest of his working life in the county. When he left his hospital job in 1841 he joined Dr Dunthorn[23] in partnership in Wickhambrook, and it was there that he died, much lamented, at the age of seventy-one on 9 March 1887.[24]

The paid staff of the hospital

Of course, in this volume we are solely concerned with Stutter's time at the Suffolk General Hospital, where, in 1839 at a salary of £70 per annum, he was the only paid doctor. It seems that there was no limit on the length of time a House Apothecary and Surgeon could remain in post. Doctors sometimes just did the job until something better turned up. For instance, Francis Charles Pyman, a previous incumbent, had resigned on 14 November 1833 after five years service in order to join the East India Company.[25] Like Stutter, most went into general practice, but for some the 'something better' never turned up. The medical market was overcrowded and jobs were scarce. Some young doctors became pretty desperate. On 28 March 1840 an advertisement appeared in the *Ipswich Journal*, put there by a Robert Lloyd, who had originally been apprenticed to William Hamilton of Ipswich. Lloyd explained that he had 'expended all his resources in obtaining a medical education'. He now had a wife and three children to support and 'wished to procure any employment, however menial, which could keep him from parochial relief'.[26] Although it was unusual, his cry for help is a good indication of the state of the prevailing job market, and it is no wonder that young medical men often remained in junior hospital posts for several years. Later in the century, a doctor by the name of Harry Fuller (1835–1900) was granted a pension when he retired from the Suffolk General Hospital in 1892 after having served as House Surgeon for no less than thirty-three years.[27]

In 1839 the rest of the employed clinical staff at the hospital consisted of the matron, Mrs Woodroffe, who received £35 per annum (with a £5 Christmas bonus),

---

20 T.N.B. Bonner, *Becoming a Physician*, Oxford, 1995.
21 van Zwanenberg: SROI q s 614.
22 Census, 1841.
23 See Appendix I.
24 *Bury and Norwich Post*, 19 March 1887, p. 8, col. 7.
25 Hospital minute books: SROB ID 503/3.
26 The plea may have worked because Lloyd is recorded as practising in Ipswich in 1844: W. White, *History, Gazetteer and Directory of Suffolk*,1st edn, Sheffield, 1844, p. 114.
27 J.W.E. Cory, *A Short History of the Suffolk General Hospital*, printed by W.W. Hawes, Elmswell, 1973, p. 23.

three senior nurses named Pentney, Smith and Buckle, who were paid £10 10s per annum each, a junior nurse, Arbon, who was paid £6 6s per annum and a 'girl assisting' who received £4 4s per annum. The support team consisted of cooks, a kitchen girl (on £4 4s per annum), a housemaid (on £8 per annum), a laundry maid and a porter (on £5 16s per annum).[28]

The hospital

The hospital itself was a converted ordnance depot (presumably left over from the Napoleonic Wars). The conversion had been a happy one and the building looked attractive and was well fitted out with water closets and baths[29] fed with running water pumped from a well.[30] In 1839 oil lamps were used for lighting. Gas was not used for illuminating the wards until 1847.[31] The institution had opened in 1826, replacing a Dispensary that had existed since 1789.[32] It was the first general hospital in Suffolk. The East Suffolk Hospital in Ipswich did not open its doors until ten years later. The intention of such hospitals was to care for the deserving poor who could not obtain medical attention in any other way. The rich paid for their own physicians or surgeons, and it had long been accepted that the more fortunate members of society would also pay for a doctor to care for their servants.[33] Some artisans would be members of a Friendly Society or Box Club that had appointed a doctor to look after its sick members.[34] These societies had flourished in Suffolk for some time.[35] For a small weekly fee, club members could insure themselves against the possibility of sickness and injury.

After the Poor Law Reform Act of 1834 unions appointed their own surgeons. They were contracted to treat the paupers, and so, paradoxically, the very poor may sometimes have fared better than the servant class, because the union surgeon was obliged to see and treat those on his books, whereas servants had to await their master's or mistress's goodwill (or at least sense of obligation).

Admission policy

The hospital was able to house fifty-three patients when full to capacity.[36] Only certain categories of cases were admitted. Those patients suffering from smallpox were definitely refused, as were known cases of phthisis (tuberculosis) and anyone thought to be dying of cancer, dropsy, venereal diseases or chronic leg ulcers. Children under seven were not admitted except for surgical emergencies and maternity cases were not taken in at all.[37] When cholera was sweeping England in 1832,

---

28 Hospital minute books: SROB ID 503/6.
29 Plans of the Suffolk General Hospital: SROB ID 503/41.
30 Hospital minute books: SROB ID 503/5.
31 *Ibid.*: ID 503/8.
32 J.W.E. Cory, *Short History of Suffolk General Hospital*, p. 10.
33 The custom took a long time to die in Suffolk. One of the authors remembers a member of the landed gentry paying for his farm-worker to have a hip replacement done privately in the 1990s.
34 Joan Lane, *A Social History of Medicine*, London, 2001.
35 Norman Scarfe, *A Frenchman's Year in Suffolk: French Impressions of Suffolk Life in 1784*, Suffolk Record Society 30, Woodbridge, 1988, p. 190.
36 *Bury and Norwich Post*, Wed. 5 Feb. 1840, p. 2, col. 3.
37 Perhaps in retrospect this was an entirely good thing, in view of the frequency with which erysipelas struck the hospital. Any woman admitted for childbirth would have been at considerable risk of death from childbed fever. See *The Tragedy of Childbed Fever* by Irvine Loudon, Oxford University Press, 2000.

nity cases were not taken in at all.[37] When cholera was sweeping England in 1832, the Committee discussed the problem on 26 July 1832. The result was a letter to the aldermen of Bury to 'respectfully inquire if the town of Bury be provided with a Cholera Hospital in order that if any patients here [i.e. in the hospital] be attacked with the malady the Committee may know where they be sent without delay'. The aldermen replied that the Feoffment Trust had consented to give the use of the Spital Houses in Risbygate Street provided that the previous occupants could be provided for. In the event cholera did not strike the hospital and the cottages were not needed. When smallpox was prevalent in the area in 1835 the hospital administration behaved in a more proactive fashion. On 16 June 1835 the Committee agreed that the poor could be vaccinated free of charge on application to the hospital on Wednesdays and Saturdays from 8 to 10 a.m. One suspects that this was another job for the House Apothecary.

In view of the general attitude towards illnesses like smallpox and cholera it was interesting to find that in 1844 a Mr Kemp petitioned the committee to allow his daughter to be admitted as a paying patient because she had leprosy.[38] The committee acceded to his request and she came in as a paying patient for ten shillings per week. She stayed for fifteen weeks.

Subscribers

When patients were admitted they generally had to be recommended by a subscriber to the hospital. An annual subscriber of two guineas was allowed to recommend two outpatients and one inpatient each year.[39] The letter of recommendation for an inpatient entitled the patient to six weeks in hospital[40] and it was woe betide a subscriber who tried to send in more than his or her quota of patients. The Committee had no compunction in refusing admission to those sufferers whose benefactor had already referred his or her allocation for that year.[41] Medical men who had not paid their subscriptions had no automatic admitting rights either. At a committee meeting on 12 April 1836, a patient by the name of James Clark was recommended by Mr Smith, a surgeon of Clare. But the admission was refused because Mr Smith was not entitled to admit a patient.[42]

On completion of his or her stay in hospital the patient was expected to write (or get someone else to write) to the subscriber to thank them for their generosity. They were also expected to attend the chapel to thank God for their cure. And one has to say that, given the state of medical science at the time, God probably had more of a hand in their cures than did the doctors.

Patients were 'admitted' or 'discharged' at the weekly committee meeting on a Tuesday. This was to enable the carriers to take discharged patients back to their home villages by cart on Wednesday, that day being the day on which the market was (and is still) held in Bury St Edmunds.

---

[38] Hospital minute books: SROB ID 503/7.
[39] *Ibid.* See also Appendix II.
[40] Interestingly, the level of subscription remained much the same for many years. In 1925, the annual donation of two guineas still allowed the donor one inpatient letter a year, but the outpatient quota had been reduced from two to one. See *The Suffolk County Handbook and Official Directory*, 1925.
[41] J.W.E. Cory, *Short History of Suffolk General Hospital*, pp. 13–14.
[42] Hospital minute books: SROB ID 503/6.

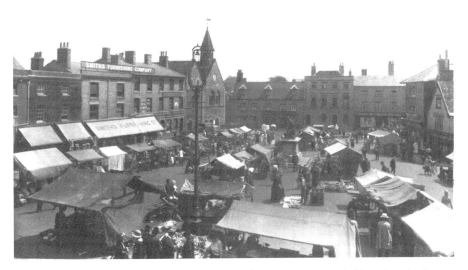

3. This photograph of Bury St Edmunds market place was probably taken in the late 1920s or early 1930s. Reproduced by permission of SROI.

The consultants

The two (later three) physicians and three surgeons (plus one 'consulting' surgeon) who served the hospital, were elected by the Board. The consultants were not paid for their work, the assumption being that they would be able to live quite well on their income from private practice. This was certainly true of F.G. Probart MD, who in his first year in Bury (1827) earned £898 4s 0d gross.[43] Presumably, the attraction of the job to the consultants was that on the Hospital Board and Committee meetings, which the duty surgeon and the duty physician attended weekly, the doctors would have the opportunity to mix with the great and the good in local society. Certainly Probart seems to have made a point of doing so. He was out to dinner two or three times a week and assiduously noted the names of his fellow diners in his diary. Unfortunately, he did not write down much about his medical work, but he did record important matters such as when he had the house painted, brewed beer or arranged for hay to be cut in his meadow. He also carefully noted when he hired and fired servants. Cooks in particular seemed to last only a short time in the Probart household![44]

The Bury and Suffolk Medical Book Club

Stutter's name appears in Probart's diary only once, on 27 February 1839, the day he was appointed at the hospital. It seems that the Physician did not make it a practice to invite his House Apothecary to dinner, but he did perhaps encourage him to join the Medical Book Club of which Probart was secretary. The fee at joining was three

---

43 Dr F.G. Probart's account books: SROB 2753/4/21.
44 Diaries of Dr F.G. Probart: SROB 2752/4/20.

guineas. Thereafter, each member subscribed one guinea annually with a fine of sixpence for overdue books. Since 1833 the club had held its quarterly meetings at the hospital,[45] but there was also an annual general meeting for which a penalty of five shillings was levied on those who did not attend. Later on, when he was living and working in Wickhambrook, Stutter was to pay this fine on several occasions over the next ten years.[46] The annual general meeting of the Book Club usually took place on the third Monday afternoon in September at The Angel Hotel in Bury St Edmunds, with dinner served at 4 p.m. It sounds a convivial affair but one can forgive those rural practitioners who found it difficult to attend. It would mean leaving the practice area and might also involve making a twenty-mile or more round trip on horseback.[47]

Matron

As both House Apothecary and House Surgeon, Stutter was something of a one-man band. He had to please several masters, and no doubt Mrs Woodroffe, the Matron, had to be kept happy too. Stutter's successor, Mr Newham,[48] obviously fell foul of Mrs Woodroffe's successor Mrs Lawrence, who was elected from an original shortlist of nine applicants at a General Meeting of the Governors on 21 August 1844.[49]

Mrs Lawrence was soon putting her foot down. It sounds as if Newham and the pupils were sometimes late for their meals. The matron obviously complained about this behaviour, because on 4 March 1845 the Committee ordered that the House Apothecary and pupils take breakfast, dinner and supper with Mrs Lawrence in her room at fixed hours. The Committee also felt that it was desirable that they should take tea with the matron 'when not inconvenient to them to do so'. The fixed hours were: breakfast 8.30 a.m., dinner 2 p.m., tea 6 p.m. and supper 9 p.m.

Although this is the first time that mealtimes were mentioned in the Committee's minutes it is likely that the House Apothecary had always taken his meals with matron. This may have had some benefits from time to time, but it may also have created difficulties on both sides if the pair of them did not see eye to eye.

Previous House Apothecaries

In 1826, Mrs Goodchild, the then matron, accused Mr Mornement, who was the first House Apothecary and Surgeon to the hospital, of 'certain improprieties' with one of the nurses. Unfortunately, the page in the hospital minute book that probably

---

[45] Hospital minute books: SROB ID 503/3.

[46] Medical Book Club accounts: SROB 2753/4/25.

[47] Not that they would think this exceptional. Rural doctors spent many hours on their horses, and, as an editorial in *The Lancet* rather ponderously put it in 1841, 'the country doctor's horse is as indispensably necessary as himself in the pursuit of his practice': *The Lancet*, 1841–42, ii. 95.

[48] See Appendix I.

[49] Few of the applicants appear to have had any nursing experience whatsoever. They were: Mrs Bellamy, aged forty-seven, sixteen years Matron of the Deaf and Dumb Asylum, Edgbaston; Mrs Brewin, aged fifty, Matron of the Clergy Orphan School, St John's Wood; Mrs Collins, aged fifty-five, postmistress at Workington; Mrs Cooper, aged forty-five, housekeeper in a family; Mrs Cronin, aged forty, keeping a school; Mrs Lancellas, aged forty-eight, fifteen years Matron of Clerkenwell Union; Mrs Mc Auliffe, aged forty-five, Assistant Superintendent at East London Union; Mrs Lawrence, aged forty-six, housekeeper; Mrs Snow, frequently an attendant at Guy's Hospital. The list was evidently pared down to two, and in the final vote Mrs Lawrence easily beat Mrs Cronin by 382 votes to 87.

contained the meat of these accusations has been torn out, but we do know that Mrs Goodchild resigned shortly afterwards.[50] Although the committee found the accusations against Mr Mornement not proven, he did not fare very well. He became ill and sent for his mother, who, with the committee's permission, stayed in the hospital for several weeks to look after him. On 1 March 1827 she attended the weekly Committee Meeting to hand in her son's resignation. Mr Mornement died at his parents' house on 26 June 1827, aged twenty-three.[51] There is no doubt that the job of House Apothecary was stressful and risky because of the ever-present danger of infection, especially from tuberculosis. The second incumbent, Mr George Catton, also became ill and resigned due to ill health on 25 September 1828.[52] He died on the 2 June 1829.[53]

When Mr Mornement had been appointed he also had to act as the hospital Secretary and he found this very onerous. Eventually, help did come. Mr Nathaniel Warren was appointed Assistant Secretary at a salary of £20 per annum in January 1829,[54] but it was pointed out that as a consequence of this appointment the House Apothecary should have more time 'for compounding medicines and also for visiting in their own houses those outpatients as are unable to attend personally at the Hospital'. In addition the House Apothecary, by then Mr Pyman, was also encouraged to take a pupil or pupils. They were to be articled to him for five years, three of which should be in the hospital. Two thirds of the premium would be paid to the hospital, but the remaining one third would be paid to the House Apothecary, spread out over the three years.[55]

The pupils

There were two pupils in residence when Stutter arrived. They were Mr Barrington Mudd and Mr Henry Jardine. Stutter received £7 10s per half-year for teaching the former and £10 per half-year for the latter.[56] Just how good he was as a teacher we will never know, but he was at least being paid. Modern Senior House Officers and Registrars might be somewhat envious of this, because they usually have to teach their juniors for nothing.

The work

On 12 February 1839, which was an admission day, six patients were taken in but five patients were refused 'for want of room'. The next week, 19 February 1839, ten patients were admitted but six had to be put off for lack of beds. Fifty-one patients remained in the hospital.[57] By 26 February 1839, although there were fifteen discharges, there was only one admission (presumably an urgent case) and five patients were put off for the very simple reason that erysipelas[58] had broken out in the hospital. There were no more admissions until 19 March 1839 when the backlog

50 Hospital minute books: SROB ID 503/1.
51 *Bury and Norwich Post*, 4 July 1827, p. 2, col. 1.
52 Hospital minute books: SROB ID 503/2.
53 van Zwanenberg: SROI q s 614.
54 Hospital minute books: SROB ID 503/2.
55 *Ibid.*
56 *Ibid.*: ID 503/6.
57 *Bury and Norwich Post*, 27 Feb. 1839, p. 2, col. 4.
58 See Appendix II.

was taken up.[59] Erysipelas was to strike again in April 1839 and March 1841 so Stutter would become accustomed to the disease. And, in a perverse way, he may have welcomed this first outbreak because it would have given him a chance to make himself familiar with the remaining patients and the hospital dispensary. It is not clear how much work he was able to delegate to the pupils, although from time to time the House Apothecary was able to take a few days off with the permission of the committee.[60] But this was the exception rather than the rule. The apothecary was normally resident and was required to be available at any hour of the day or night.[61] He did, however, as mentioned above, have to visit some patients who were unable to attend the hospital as outpatients, and this was one of the duties that Stutter found irksome.[62] Throughout the year of 1839 the average number of outpatients at any one time was 161.[63] When he was later asked to present statistics it transpired that Stutter had visited two thirds of these outpatients in their own homes.[64]

Consultant resignations

In February 1839 one of the Physicians, Dr Bayne, had just resigned. Dr Andrew Ross had replaced him on 6 February 1839[65] but some of Dr Bayne's former patients were still in the hospital. Against the names of six of the patients mentioned in Stutter's casebook is written 'from Dr Bayne's book'. As a matter of fact, the physicians seem to have been in a state of turmoil throughout Stutter's time as House Apothecary. Only Dr Probart stayed the course. Dr Ross resigned on 16 June 1840 to be replaced by Dr Hake. Dr Jackson was elected as a third physician on 11 March 1839 but resigned on 24 March 1840, being replaced by Dr Ranking on 22 April 1840. It all smells of discontent and possibly personality clashes.

Surgery

Unfortunately Stutter's casebook is incomplete because it only covers the period from February 1839 to June 1840, whereas he did not resign his post until 2 August 1841.[66] In addition it seems to relate solely to medical cases (which ties in with the takeover from Dr Bayne, who was a physician). There is no doubt, however, that the surgeons were also active in the hospital. The Annual Report for 1839 stated that 'the number of casualties has been unusually large (there being in the House at the same time Seven Patients with fractured limbs from riding on waggons. Very few of these terminated fatally)'.[67]

Surgeons of the time were well able to suture wounds, operate for hare lip, deal with strangulated hernias, lance abscesses, catheterise bladders, reduce dislocations, set fractures and amputate limbs. Compound fractures were usually treated by

---

[59] Hospital minute books: SROB ID 503/6.

[60] *Ibid.*

[61] His bedroom was on the upper storey of the hospital and measured 17ft 6in. by 13ft – the same size as the matron's. See the Plans of the Suffolk General Hospital: SROB ID 503/41.

[62] Hospital minute books: SROB ID 503/6.

[63] Statistics collected from figures given weekly in the *Bury and Norwich Post*, 1839.

[64] Hospital minute books: SROB ID 503/6.

[65] *Ibid.*

[66] *Ibid.*

[67] Annual reports of the Suffolk General Hospital: SROB ID 503/26.

amputation and these operations were often successful, despite the risks of bleeding and infection. Statistics of amputations carried out at University College Hospital, London, between 1835 and 1841 showed that fifty-six out of sixty-six of the operations succeeded.[68]

From the early days of the hospital there are records of the purchase of lithotomy[69] and other instruments, but the abdominal cavity was still regarded as forbidden territory and it is doubtful if any of the surgeons at the Suffolk General Hospital would have risked going there. The American surgeon Ephraim McDowell (1771–1830) of Kentucky had done a successful ovariotomy (removal of an ovarian cyst) on a Mrs Jane Todd in 1809. The patient apparently sang hymns all the way through the operation, and she lived to tell the tale for another thirty years. William Jeaffreson (1790–1865) of Framlingham did the first ovariotomy in Suffolk on 8 May 1836.[70] It is said that Jeaffreson was unaware of Ephraim Mc Dowell's work. He operated with the assistance of his friend Mr Robert Carew King (1781–1842) who came from Saxmundham.[71] Jeaffreson made a midline suprapubic[72] incision about an inch and a half in length, withdrew 12 pints of fluid and then extracted the collapsed ovarian cyst. The pedicle of the tumour was tied and the ends of the ligature cut short, the skin being closed by two sutures (the deeper layers not being included). It is not recorded whether or not the patient sang during the operation, but she had recovered completely by the fifteenth day. The case was recorded in the *Transactions of the Provincial Medical and Surgical Association* in 1837. It provoked considerable debate and some sharp criticism from the London surgeons. There is no doubt that resourceful and independently minded country surgeons like McDowell and Jeaffreson had the advantage of those who worked in hospitals, because they operated in either their own or their patients' houses, where infection rates were bound to be lower than in any institution.

Although it is unlikely that any of the surgeons at the Suffolk General Hospital were as brave as William Jeaffreson, many of their treatments were no doubt effective, although unfortunately they did not record much of what they did. From time to time the Committee complained about this,[73] and requested that the House Apothecary and Surgeon should keep a prescription book to carry with him from ward to ward.[74] Unfortunately, this book (if it ever existed) has not survived among Stutter's papers in the Suffolk Record Office.

Medical patients

The table below lists Stutter's patients as taken from his casebook and cross-referenced with the minute books of committee meetings of the Suffolk General Hospital to confirm dates of admission and discharge.

Where the patient was admitted twice, two entries have been made. Only two definite deaths are recorded, that of James Clark, aged thirty-six (p. 86), who had

---

[68] P. Hunting, *The History of the Royal Society of Medicine*, London, 2002, p. 86.

[69] Lithotomy is the word used to describe the removal of bladder stones – a very painful procedure before general anaesthesia became available in 1847.

[70] J.A. Shepherd, 'William Jeaffreson (1790–1865): Surgical Pioneer', *British Medical Journal*, 6 Nov. 1965, pp. 1119–20. See also Appendix I.

[71] See Appendix I.

[72] Just above the pubic bone.

[73] Hospital minute books: SROB ID 503/5.

[74] Hospital minute books: SROB ID 503/6.

pneumonia (he was admitted and died on the same day), and Mary Willingham, aged thirty-five (p. 132), who had tuberculosis. In the hospital minute books deaths are covered by the euphemism 'discharged', and for the real truth of the weekly death rate for both medical and surgical cases it is often necessary to consult local newspapers. However, cumulative figures were published in the hospital's Annual Reports. Twenty inpatient deaths occurred in 1839, fourteen in 1840 and eleven in 1841.[75] The *Bury and Norwich Post* published weekly statistics of the number of patients admitted, discharged and who died. Bearing in mind that the hospital was very selective in its admission policy, it is no wonder that deaths did not seem to occur very often in the medical wards. Fatalities on the surgical side may have been more numerous because, as mentioned above, there were certainly a lot of accidents. Of course the governors wanted to show that the benefactors' money was being put to good use and so statistics were expressed in terms of those 'cured', and if not cured, 'relieved' or even 'much relieved'.

Table 1. Hospital admission details for all patients in Stutter's casebook

Name	Age	Diagnosis	Admitted	Discharged	Days in hospital
Arnold, James	68	Hypertrophia cordis	19-2-1839	26-2-1839	7
Atkins, Keziah	20		12-11-1839	21-1-1840	70
Baker, Frances	34		14-1-1840	5-5-1840	112
Banham, Susan		Eczema	1-1-1839	5-3-1839	63
Brame, George			3-12-1839	14-1-1840	42
Bird, Morris	37		1-1-1839	4-6-1839	154
Bryant, Sarah	25		14-1-1840	4-2-1840	21
Bullass, Mary	19		4-6-1839	25-6-1839	21
Burman, Samuel	20	Phthisis	22-10-1839	26-11-1839	35
Canham, Elizabeth	42	Leucorrhoea and gastralgia	26-3-1839	23-4-1839	28
Carter, Isaac	76	Hepatitis chronica	9-4-1839	30-4-1839	21
Carter, James			22-10-1839	17-12-1839	57
Channell, George	16		1-10-1839	22-10-1839	21
Chinery, John	45	Hypertrophy of heart	18-6-1839	16-7-1839	28
Chinery, Samuel			4-6-1839	27-8-1839	84
Clark, James	36	Pneumonia (died)	10-12-1839	10-12-1839	1
Clarke, Caroline	19	Chlorosis	19-3-1839	30-4-1839	42
Cocksedge, John	39		26-11-1839	21-1-1840	57
Cook, Mary			14-1-1840	31-3-1840	77
Copping, Ann	30		12-11-1839	17-12-1839	36
Cousins, Maria	16	Chorea	9-4-1839	11-6-1839	63
Cross, Leah	22		9-7-1839	17-9-1839	70

---

[75] Hospital annual reports: SROB ID 503/26.

Death, Mary	41	Chronic rheumatic hepatitis	17-3-1840	21-4-1840	35
Downey, William	23	Bubo post ulcus venerum	18-12-1838	26-2-1839	70
Fane (Fen), James	10		31-12-1839	21-4--1840	112
Ford, Sarah	18		12-11-1839	31-12-1839	50
Gladwell, Robert		Neuralgic affliction of V [sic]	30-7-1839	27-8-1839	28
Gladwell, Robert			22-10-1839	10-12-1839	50
Haywood, Sarah			12-2-1839	26-2-1839	14
Horrex, Phoebe	28		14-1-1840	18-2-1840	35
Isaacson, Esther	19		1-10-1839	22-10-1839	21
Jackson, Susan	57		18-12-1838	9-4-1839	112
Leech, William	38		9-6-1840	18-8-1840	70
Lifley, Martin	46		19-3-1839	30-4-1839	42
Ling, Minter	45		20-8-1839	10-9-1839	21
Math/Malt, William	20	Paraplegia	1-1-1839	19-3-1839	77
Matthews, Elizabeth			30-7-1839	5-11-1839	98
Motte, Mary	15	Opthalmia scrofulosa	9-4-1839	30-4-1839	21
Mulley, William	46	Rheumatism	19-2-1839	23-4-1839	63
Nelson, Robert	60	Bronchitis	14-4-1840	19-5-1840	35
Nelson, William	47	? Infected finger	26-3-1839	23-4-1839	28
Nelson, William	47		29-10-1839	7-1-1840	71
Nunn, Isaac			4-6-1839	18-6-1839	14
Orris, Abraham	43	Psoriasis	19-2-1839	23-4-1839	63
Pawsey, Elizabeth	22		20-8-1839	5-11-1839	77
Payne, Elizabeth	12	Chorea	17-3-1840	31-3-1840	14
Plumbe/Plume, Susan	19		1-10-1839	3-3-1840	153
Pratt, Hannah	58		14-4-1840	9-6-1840	54
Rands, Ann(e)	28	Abscess L pectoral region	12-2-1839	26-2-1839	14
Rands, Ann(e)	28		19-3-1839	23-4-1839	35
Reeve, Susan	23		4-2-1840	21-4-1840	77
Ruddock, Thomas	41		10-12-1839	28-1-1840	49
Rumble, Matilda	11	Chorea	9-4-1839	30-4-1839	21
Savage, James	17	Epilepsia	1-1-1839	5-3-1839	63
Scarff, Harriet	24	Anaemia	14-4-1840	19-5-1840	35
Scott, John	25	Purpura and urticaria	22-10-1839	26-11-1839	35
Scott, Samuel	44		14-1-1840	25-2-1840	42
Scott, Thomas	19		4-2-1840	10-3-1840	35
Sharpe, James	42		28-4-1840	19-5-1840	21
Sharpe, John			19-5-1840	23-6-1840	35
Sharpe, Susan	18		1-10-1839	26-11-1839	56
Shepherd, Wm			2-4-1839	30-4-1839	28
Shepherd, Wm			24-12-1839	3-3-1840	70
Sindell, Matthew	40		31-3-1840	19-5-1840	49
Smith, Charlotte	25		20-8-1839	10-9-1839	21

Steggles, Frances	25		14-4-1840	9-6-1840	56
Sturgeon, Jonathan			31-12-1839	7-4-1840	98
Talbot, George	58	Hypertrophy of right side	18-6-1839	13-8-1839	56
Tweed, David	40		17-3-1840	21-4-1840	35
Wade, Mary	63		30-7-1839	3-9-1839	35
Warren, Susan	15	Disease of ovary	30-7-1839	15-10-1839	77
Warren, Susan	15	(?died)	18-2-1840	10-3-1840	21
Wingfield, Caroline	19		19-5-1840	15-6-1840	27
Welch, Susan	18		20-8-1839	29-10-1839	70
Wilkinson, Wm	12	Epilepsy	14-1-1840	2-4-1840	79
Willingham, Mary	35	(died)	28-4-1840	19-5-1840	21

Average stay in hospital   48.76 days

The first thing that strikes the modern reader about the above list is the relative youth of patients, with an average of thirty-two years for those whose ages are recorded. The oldest was Isaac Carter, aged seventy-six (p. 28) and the youngest James Fane (p. 118), who was aged ten. Of the seventy-seven admissions, thirty-nine were male and thirty-eight female. The length of time patients stayed in hospital is also interesting. By the rules they were allowed forty-two days, but in our sample the average length of stay is forty-nine days (in round figures). Quite a few people had to have their recommendations renewed. The only acute medical admission seems to have been James Clark, who, as mentioned above, was admitted with pneumonia and died on the same day.

Taking histories and examining people

It seems that Stutter was a conscientious doctor. He normally took histories from his patients and examined them when they first arrived in hospital. The treatment he prescribed was entered in his book and any subsequent changes carefully noted. There is no indication as to whether these changes were at the recommendation of a consultant physician, but presumably they often were. His history taking seems to lack structure and occasionally scathing remarks creep in, such as in the record of Mary Death, aged forty-one (p. 114), who had 'lost all her teeth due to excessive salivation thirteen years ago'. This was undoubtedly due to the overuse of mercury. Or the delicate Sarah Bryant, aged twenty-five (p. 96), who had been 'seized about four months ago with what was called inflammation of the chest (for which she was blistered and had nauseating medicine)'. Most modern doctors would recognise this as the 'St Elsewhere syndrome', i.e. 'all sorts of terrible things happened to the patient before being admitted to our care. But we can do better.'

He examined the patient's skin, pulse, tongue, heart, chest and abdomen. Sometimes the specific gravity of the urine and the presence or absence of albumen in the urine was noted too.[76] On occasions he recorded more. Phoebe Horrex, aged twenty-eight (p. 98), had had an impediment in her speech since childhood. It was, however, confined to the first syllable, after which she talked fluently. Sarah Bryant's appearance was delicate with hectic flushing of the cheek and emaciation.

---

[76] See Appendix III.

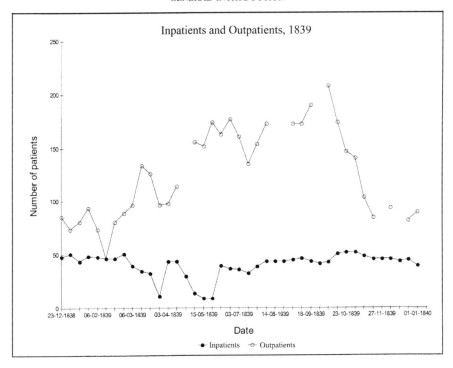

Fig 1. This shows the number of inpatients and outpatients for the year 1839, taken from the weekly figures published in the *Bury and Norwich Post*. The upper peaked graph represents outpatients. The dip in the number of inpatients in April and May was almost certainly due to erysipelas.

She had nightly perspirations and despite the fact that on admission there was a clear sound on percussion over the whole chest, three weeks later she was discharged incurable with signs of a cavity at the summit of the right lung. She undoubtedly had tuberculosis. Matthew Sindell, aged forty (p. 122), had muffled heart sounds, and 'the heart's action was not in accordance with the pulse at the wrist, being much stronger in proportion'. Susan Plumbe, aged nineteen (p. 68), had a pulse rate of 130 and had 'dullness on percussion on the praecordium extending from half an inch to the right of the miscal [middle] line of the sternum as far as the left nipple, [with a] very distinct bellows sound in the region of the cartilage of the sixth rib which disappears towards the centre and apex of the heart'. Stutter was presumably using a wooden Laennec-type stethoscope to listen to the heart and chest.

In the case of Susan Warren, aged fifteen (p. 47), who almost certainly had a cancer of the ovary, he recorded abdominal girth before and after paracentesis abdominis (tapping of fluid from the abdomen).[77] On 4 October 1839 she had nineteen pints of fluid withdrawn. Another twenty-four pints were taken off on 26 February 1840. Ominously, his last note is 'tumour (ovarian?) again distinctly felt'. In the case of Frances Baker, aged thirty-four (p. 100), he recorded the girth of each side of the chest as well as the results of percussion. On the left side respiration was

---

[77] See Appendix IV.

inaudible except at the summit, with 'distinct egophony in the region of the angle of the left scapula'. It sounds as if she too had tuberculosis, although Stutter has recorded no diagnosis against her name. Even when the case may have warranted it, as with Susan Warren (see above), there is no record of any rectal or vaginal examinations.

The class and physical condition of patients

Interesting social pointers and the ravages of previous diseases can be culled from his notes. Susan Reeve, aged twenty-three (p. 108), was extremely tall – nearly six feet. It was a family trait. Both her parents, however, had died of phthisis. She was deficient in the sight of the left eye due to measles when she was eleven. Ann Copping, aged thirty (p. 62), had had four children but they had all died before the age of four months. Matthew Sindell (p. 122) was a waterman between Bury St Edmunds and King's Lynn.[78] Susan Sharpe, aged eighteen (p. 64), a servant to a washerwoman, 'had a hard place of work'.

Table 2. Patients whose occupation or marital status is mentioned in Stutter's casebook

Samuel Burman, aged 20, Shoemaker.
George Channell, aged 16, Baker's boy.
Ann Copping, Married.
William Malt, aged 20, Labourer.
John Scott, aged 25, Carpenter.
Thomas Scott, aged 19, Tailor.
John Sharpe, Carpenter.
Susan Sharpe, aged 18, Servant to a washerwoman.
Matthew Sindell, aged 40, Waterman.
Mary Willingham, aged 35, Married.
Esther Isaacson, aged 19, In service.
Morris Bird, aged 37, Basketmaker.
Phoebe Horrex, aged 28, Married.

The hospital regime

Firm emphasis was placed on diet. According to the recommendations of the Hospital Committee these were split into the categories of full, middle, common, low and milk, depending on the disease from which the patient was thought to be suffering. The tenders put out every three months for the supply of groceries contain a long list of bread, milk, meat, suet, rice, cheese, tea and sugar. Matron bought potatoes at the weekly market, where one suspects she might have bought other vegetables as well. In 1840 the annual accounts include the sum of £18 4s 4d for vegetables, £10 10s 3d for eggs, £32 9s 6d for milk and £9 5s 10d for the garden and seeds.[79] On 1 December 1835 the Committee ordered that patients were to have no

[78] This would have been using the River Lark, which is no longer navigable.
[79] Hospital annual reports: SROB ID 503/26.

more than a pound of meat a day.[80] Beer, porter and wine were also provided and prescribed by Stutter with the same care as he did the medicine. It is interesting to note that this included the children. On 10 April 1840 Stutter ordered that ten-year-old James Fane (p. 118), who suffered from epilepsy, should omit the wine and have a pint of beer a day.

Not much can be gleaned about exercise, but males and females were strictly segregated, the latter being allowed to walk in the grounds from 11.00 a.m. to 12.30 p.m. and 2 p.m. to 3.30 p.m. each day. During these times the men had to stay in their own wards. Visiting times were restricted. Only relatives were allowed entry, and the Matron and House Apothecary strictly controlled the numbers. Visitors from both town and country were allowed to see their relations between 2 p.m. and 4 p.m. on Wednesday afternoons. But for country patients there was a further special dispensation. Their loved ones were allowed in between 9 a.m. and 10 a.m. on Sundays too.[81]

Treatments

The medical therapies available to patients were those of the day. Bleeding, cupping, purging and the application of emplasters and leeches were the standard treatments for many conditions.[82] It was still thought that most diseases were caused by inner poisons that had to be forced out of the body by these various means. To the modern reader the treatments seem futile, often amusing and sometimes downright dangerous. But it does not do to be too complacent. All experienced doctors know that today's dogma is tomorrow's curiosity. In the student textbook *The Elements of the Practice of Medicine* jointly written by the Guy's physicians Bright and Addison, and published in 1839, students were exhorted to learn how to give succour, anticipate recovery or render peace as death approached. Looking after people meant learning how to take pressure off protruding bones by rubbing in lead ointment, by positioning cushions or using water pillows. It also meant learning how to treat a bedsore and knowing how diluted brandy or laudanum would stimulate healing. The student needed to know that nitric acid with distilled water would clear pus and that linseed poultices would remove scabs. Although the diagnostic methods and treatments can sometimes seem primitive to the modern observer, the best nineteenth-century doctors would have done their utmost to try to discover what was ailing their patients. And even if they failed in this task, at the very least they would try to make those in their care as comfortable as they possibly could.

The most useful drugs were possibly opium, mercury, quinine, colchicine and digitalis. Thomas Scott, aged nineteen (p. 110), had pain and swelling in his left foot. He was treated with colchicine, digitalis and the application of twelve leeches, which relieved him greatly. He was discharged cured. Frances Baker (p. 100), who probably had tuberculosis of the left lung, had twenty leeches applied to that side of the chest. Two days after that she was bled and 15 ounces of blood were removed. Later she had an emplaster of Lytta (cantharides – a blistering agent) applied to the chest. Mary Willingham, aged thirty-five (p. 132), whom Stutter records as suffering from chronic peritonitis and pulmonary tubercles, was given Tincture of Opium (as well as a quarter of a pint of beer a day) when she was in a terminal state.

---

[80] Hospital minute books: SROB ID 503/4.
[81] Hospital minute books: SROB ID 503/5.
[82] See Appendix IV.

Chest conditions were treated with camphor mixtures and there was a range of tonics among which valerian was probably the foremost.

In addition the doctor could order sulphur vapour baths (installed at the instigation of the Reverend Colvile in 1837).[83] And for diseases of the nervous system there were two 'galvanic troughs' that had been bought at the recommendation of Dr Bayne in 1834.[84] An iron mixture was given to cases of anaemia such as Harriet Scarff, aged twenty-four (p. 128). Caroline Clarke, aged nineteen (p. 24), who was diagnosed as having chlorosis, was also treated with iron, but in addition she had ten ounces of blood removed from the region of the left hypochondrium by wet cupping. If one accepts that chlorosis was probably a form of iron-deficiency anaemia the treatment seems illogical. But nevertheless the patient was cured.

With the benefit of hindsight it would seem that the chief good the patients would derive from the hospital would be from being admitted to a place where they would receive an adequate diet and be kept clean, warm and dry for six weeks or so. Inevitably, some patients did die, but they were not admitted for terminal care. Quite the contrary; admission was usually refused if the patient was obviously close to death.[85]

Money worries

The doctors and benefactors of the hospital firmly believed in the usefulness of medical treatment. The Annual Report for 1839 complained that 'in some instances, it is to be feared, Patients have been recommended to whom good food was quite as necessary as medicine, and some caution should be used in this respect; for although it is right that inpatients should be supplied fully and liberally with all they need, an Hospital is not to be considered as a refuge to supply the destitute with subsistence, but for the relief of sickness and disease'. The same report mentioned the increasing expenditure on medicines and leeches as well as the amount of time the House Apothecary had to spend in visiting those outpatients who could not get to the hospital. Subscribers were asked to think very hard before making a referral.[86] On 19 November 1839 a drug bill of £158 11s 0d from Apothecaries' Hall was put off until after 1 January 1840. A sub-committee was set up to review drug expenditure. This sub-committee continued to meet and report gloomily on the expense of drugs. In March 1846, it proposed that a Suffolk General Hospital pharmacopoeia should be constructed. This was to be modeled on those already existing at Guy's and St George's although the doctors serving the hospital were asked to contribute to its pages.[87] All this has modern reverberations, as does the shortage of beds, which usually became acute in January each year. But the institution was a laudable attempt to ease the suffering of those who could not afford medical help at a time when they sorely needed it. As a business the house ran efficiently, with almost everything under the control of matron, who was in turn beholden to the Committee. In July 1830 the matron of the time was given five days' paid leave to visit Addenbrooke's Hospital in Cambridge to see if she could pick up any ideas. She came back with the notion (adopted on 31 July 1830) that the Suffolk hospital could save £30 per annum by insisting that patients should arrange for their own linen to

[83] Hospital minute books: SROB ID 503/6.
[84] Hospital minute books: SROB ID 503/3.
[85] Ibid.
[86] Hospital annual reports: SROB ID 503/26.
[87] Hospital minute books: SROB ID 503/8.

be washed![88] But by 1840 this may have changed again because a washing machine was purchased on 21 July 1840.[89]

House visitors and dealing with complaints

Each week house visitors were appointed whose job it was to report any complaints back to the Committee. This they did, as did some of the subscribers who had recommended patients. For instance John Worledge of Ingham attended the Committee Meeting on Tuesday 13 March 1838 to complain that James Balls, a patient recommended by him, had not been seen by Mr Dalton from his admission on 6 March 1838 until the13 March. To cap it all, James Balls had not received any medical or surgical treatment whatever. Mr Dalton attended the Committee Meeting a week later to give his reasons. On hearing them the Committee took no further action. But the problem persisted and several years later, on 6 May 1843, Dalton resigned as surgeon to the hospital following a complaint by the Hospital Visiting Committee that he had not visited the wards for a week.[90] On 12 February 1839 a patient called Isaac Hanslip wrote to say that he had been an inpatient under Mr Creed[91] for eight weeks but had only seen him eight times. The next week Mr Creed attended the Committee Meeting. He seems to have explained himself satisfactorily because no further action was taken.[92]

Reading between the lines of all this, it seems that the consultants were difficult to control.[93] As mentioned above, their note keeping was perceived to be poor, and this applied especially to the surgeons. On 29 August 1837 the Committee was moved to write to each of the surgeons calling to their attention 'the expediency of a fuller entry in their books of the cases under their care'.[94] But when taxed about their deficiencies the consultants were always at pains to point out that they were giving their services free of charge.

The House Apothecary is overworked

The thing that seemed to irritate the lay members of the Committee most was that the physicians in particular were dilatory in visiting outpatients in their own homes (because they were presumably spending most of their time visiting their fee-paying patients). This was a long-running saga and there was no resolution of the problem while Stutter was in post.[95] But it was no doubt partly because of this heavy visiting list that the House Apothecary felt that he was overworked. Barrington Mudd, one of the pupils, departed in August 1839, and there is no mention of the other pupil, Mr Henry Jardine, after September 1839 (although his father paid his premium for 1840).[96] So it seems that he must have left sometime in 1840, leaving the House Apothecary on his own. On 29 December 1840 the Committee asked the medical men to meet to discuss Mr Stutter's request for assistance for three hours daily in the

---

[88] Hospital minute books: SROB ID 503/2.
[89] Hospital minute books: SROB ID 503/6.
[90] Hospital minute books: SROB ID 503/7.
[91] See Appendix I for a short biography of Mr Creed.
[92] Hospital minute books: SROB ID 503/5.
[93] *Ibid.*
[94] *Ibid.*
[95] Hospital minute books: SROB ID 503/6.
[96] Hospital annual reports: SROB ID 503/26.

dispensary. They were also asked to deliberate upon the terms which should be given to any future apprentice.[97]

On 12 January 1841 Foster Stedman was appointed as assistant to Mr Stutter for six months. In consideration Foster was to receive his board and lodging.[98] He was undoubtedly a useful pair of hands. Then twenty-three years old, he had done an apprenticeship at Thetford in Norfolk followed by fifteen months at Guy's.[99] But for Stutter, Foster's arrival must have been tempered by the resignation due to ill-health of the Secretary, Mr Warren, on 26 January 1841. Fortunately, on 20 April 1841, a Mr Hubbard[100] was engaged as Dispenser and Secretary until 29 September 1841.

Resignation

Stutter himself resigned on 2 August 1841, giving three months notice.[101] His next existing daybook starts on 1 January 1842 when he was in practice in Wickham-brook. On that day he saw eleven patients, seven of them on visits. One of the patients he visited, a Mr Frost of Hawkedon Hall, was catheterised. Another, Mrs Ingram of Chedburgh, was an obstetric case.[102] The daily grind had started, but Stutter no doubt relished the more independent atmosphere of general practice, where he was able to act upon his own decisions and use the knowledge and experience that he had gained in his long training.

His life as a village doctor would still be hard and not particularly lucrative. Country practice was noted for its long journeys and short fees. But at least he would no longer have to play the diplomat between the various hospital consultants and do their home visits for them when they were busy with their private practices. Nor would he have to take his meals with matron. He could even start looking for a wife.

---

97 At the same meeting Mr Creed was asked to see outpatients at the hospital and not at his own home, which he had been doing: hospital minute books: SROB ID 503/6.
98 *Ibid.*
99 van Zwanenberg: SROI q s 614.
100 This was probably George Prettyman Hubbard (1822–72). See Appendix I.
101 Hospital minute books: SROB ID 503/6.
102 W.G. Stutter's day-books: SROB HC 517/2.

PHARMACEUTICAL INTRODUCTION

Prescriptions were traditionally written in Latin. Stutter followed the tradition, and all the prescriptions in the casebook are written in that language. Many words that were used frequently were abbreviated, for example *infusum* (an infusion) was routinely written as *inf.* or *infus.* whilst *fiat* (let it be made) almost invariably appeared as *ft*. Prescriptions generally followed a recognised format consisting of four parts, the first, known as the *Superscription*, contained the symbol 'R⟩' from the Latin verb *Recipio* to take;[1] hence the origin of the term 'recipe'. The second part or body of the prescription, the *Inscription*, was the most important and included the names of the substances to be administered with their quantities, using the apothecary's system of symbols, weights and measures (which is described below). The *Subscription* followed; it contained directions for the guidance of the dispenser, for example, 'mix and make a draught'. Finally came the *Signature*, which contained directions or instructions for the benefit of the patient, for example, 'one tablespoonful to be taken three times a day'. A typical example of a nineteenth-century prescription written by Stutter in his casebook appears below:

Mary Cook	
R⟩	Take
Quinine Disulphate gr xii	12 grains Quinine Disulphate,
Infus Rosæ ℥viii	8 ounces Infusion of Rose,
Acid Sulph Dil ʒſs	½ drachm Dilute Sulphuric Acid.
M ft mist	Mix, make a mixture.
cochlear iii magna ter in die	Three tablespoonfuls to be taken three times a day.

The apothecary's system of weights and measures was in universal use until the mandatory change to the metric system in the second half of the twentieth century. Solids were given as follows:

gr, *granum*	grain		
℈, *scrupulus*	scruple	20 grains	
ʒ, *drachma*	drachm	3 scruples	or 60 grains
℥, *uncia*	ounce	8 drachms	or 480 grains[2]
℔,[3] *libra*	pound	12 ounces	

Apothecary's measures of volume were similar, except that it was not customary to use a scruple for liquid measurements:

---

1 French physicians commenced their prescriptions with P, from *prenez*, take.
2 An apothecary's ounce of 480 grains was very slightly larger than the imperial ounce of 437.5 grains.
3 The use of this symbol had become uncommon by the 1830s, although it occurs on several occasions in Stutter's casebook.

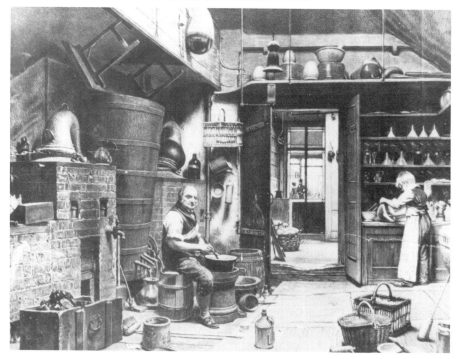

4. The 'elaboratory' of John Bell & Co. at 38 Oxford St, London, in the 1840s, in which large numbers of extracts, infusions, tinctures, etc. were prepared for use in the dispensary. The seated figure is John Simmonds who had been Bell's laboratory man since 1798. (Photograph of mezzotint after a watercolour of W.H. Hunt; photographed by H. & J. Kiddy.)

℔, *minimum*	minim	
ℨ, *drachma*	drachm	60 minims
℥, *uncia*	ounce	8 drachms or 480 minims
℔, *libra*	pound	12 fluid ounces
O, *octarius*	pint	20 fluid ounces
C, *congius*	gallon	8 pints

Patients were directed to take medicines by the spoonful (*cochleare*), the approximate equivalents being:

A teaspoonful (*c. minimum* or *parvum*)	one fluid drachm
A dessertspoonful (*c. modicum*)	two fluid drachms
A tablespoonful (*c. amplum* or *magnum*)	four fluid drachms or half a fluid ounce

More potent medicines were prescribed in drops, one drop usually being considered to have the same volume as a minim. This was not strictly accurate, since the size and shape of the bottle, as well as the type of fluid, influenced the size of the drop.

An examination of prescriptions in the casebook reveals that the ingredients included tinctures, decoctions, extracts, infusions, syrups, vinegars, etc. Most frequently used (sixty-two times) were **tinctures**, prepared by mixing the coarsely powdered drug with alcohol, then leaving it to stand, usually for seven to ten days (a process known as **maceration**), after which the liquor was strained off. Tinctures were particularly useful where the active ingredient was not soluble in water or was unstable at high temperatures. Later in the nineteenth century **percolation** replaced maceration. This was a process in which alcohol slowly percolated through the raw material packed in cylindrical or conical vessels. **Wines**, for example Ipecacuanha Wine, were made in a similar way to tinctures, the proof spirit being replaced by Spanish White Wine or Sherry. In general, tinctures had better keeping properties than **infusions**, which were made by pouring hot water on to the raw drug and allowing it to stand in a covered vessel. In most cases the standing time was two hours, although this could be as little as fifteen minutes for orange infusions or as much as four hours in the case of digitalis. The liquid when strained was ready for use. The whole process was the same as making a pot of tea in the home, but fortunately infusions of tea are ready to drink in minutes rather than hours. Infusions appear thirty-six times in the casebook.

Decoctions, dispensed on nineteen occasions, were prepared by boiling the drug with water and then straining. A simple decoction, like that of chamomile, was soon made. Chamomile flowers with caraway and fennel seeds were boiled in water for just fifteen minutes. Other drugs, for example, sarsaparilla, needed a longer process: in 1820 the instructions for its preparation were 'Macerate 4 ounces of the sliced root in 4 pints of hot water for four hours near the fire, in a slightly covered vessel; then bruise the root, and macerate again for two hours; then boil to 2 pints and strain.'[4] Stutter used this decoction and also that of aloes, which also had a lengthy production time; it is probable that both these preparations would have been bought ready-prepared.[5]

Extracts were preparations containing the active principles of a drug in a concentrated form containing a minimum amount of inert matter. Many were obtained by simply evaporating the excess water from a decoction; in most cases the evaporation was continued until a semi-solid soft extract was obtained, especially if the extracts were to be dispensed in pill form, which was the case in all but one of the total of forty-six occasions on which Stutter prescribed extracts. **Vinegar**, or **acetic acid**, is capable of dissolving the water-insoluble active principles of some plants and was especially useful as a means of extracting the alkaloids of squill and colchicum. Vinegar of Squill, made by macerating the squill bulb with vinegar for twenty-four hours, was the most frequently used vinegar and it was popular for coughs, especially when mixed with honey, when it was known as **Oxymel** of Squill. **Syrup**, made by dissolving sugar in hot water, was used to sweeten mixtures. Syrup of Orange, containing orange peel, was a popular flavouring, and was used to mask the unpleasant taste of some drugs. Stutter used it for this purpose when he prescribed cinchona bark, quinine and iron.

Prescription dispensing

Mixtures were the most popular means of administering medication by mouth. Nearly 40 per cent of the prescriptions that Stutter wrote were for mixtures and draughts.[6] Mixtures usually contained several ingredients – mostly two, three or

---

4   *Consp.*, p. 36.
5   From Apothecaries Hall or Barron & Co of London.
6   Mixtures containing only one or two doses frequently, but not exclusively, were prescribed as a sleeping or purgative draught.

four. One of these would be the vehicle in which the others were dissolved or suspended if heavy insoluble powders were present. The vehicle frequently provided a pleasant flavour; in fifty of Stutter's prescriptions, Camphor Mixture served this purpose. Where unpleasant-tasting ingredients were present, the prescription might contain infusions of orange peel or rose petals in an attempt to mask the taste; plain syrup or syrup of oranges were also often added. In some cases peppermint or spearmint waters replaced the camphor mixture. The vast majority of these mixtures would have had to be prepared individually for each patient, although to lessen the work of the dispenser, in many hospitals it became the practice to keep certain stock recipes ready for use. The Bristol Royal Infirmary began doing this as early as 1779. In 1846, the University College Hospital, London, had the *U.C.H. Pharmacopœia*, which contained formulae such as that of the Domestic Purge, containing senna, epsom salts and ginger. At a Suffolk General Hospital Committee Meeting in 1846 it was decided to send a copy of Guy's and St George's pharmacopœias to each medical officer with a request to indicate any formula which they wished be included in a proposed 'Suffolk General Hospital Pharmacopœia'.[7] Camphor Mixture, which was so frequently used, may have been kept ready prepared or possibly have been bought from one of the sources mentioned above. Before the nineteenth century **juleps** were used. These consisted of the active ingredient mixed with sweet syrup, flavouring and water; for example Camphor Julep of the *London Pharmacopœia* (1746) consisted of camphor, sugar, water and gum arabic, the latter substance serving to suspend the insoluble camphor. Stutter's casebook contains no mention of a julep (not to be confused with the drug jalap – see p. 144).

By Stutter's time it had become common practice to administer medicines internally in the solid dose form. No less than 75 per cent of Stutter's prescriptions were for mixtures, **pills** or **powders**. As with mixtures, nearly all the pills and powders would have been made by hand. To make pills the ingredients were first mixed together in a mortar and pestle. Next the 'mass', had to be prepared. This was achieved by adding a small quantity of a binding liquid to the mixed powders – confection of rose was frequently used in Stutter's day. The ingredients were then worked together using a small long-handled pestle in a mortar small enough to be firmly grasped in the left hand; by vigorous manipulation heat was produced, softening the mass and making it easier to work. A properly prepared mass would leave the mortar cleanly and not stick to the pestle. The mass was then worked by hand and rolled like a piece of pastry into a 'pipe' before being divided into sections and finally rounded into a spherical shape. Hopefully each pill would be of identical size but inevitably some pills contained more active constituents than others. Newcomers to the art of 'pill rolling' soon found that pressure from the pestle produced a painful blister on the palm of the hand.

Ready-prepared masses for popular pills were obtainable from drug wholesalers; these saved much time and effort. A piece of mass of the required weight was either rolled into pills directly or other ingredients could be incorporated into the mass prior to rolling. Mercury pill mass is one that would almost certainly have been bought ready prepared. If a pill was bitter to the taste, or found to be difficult to swallow, it might be given an outer coating of varnish, which also protected ingredients that might otherwise oxidise. A **bolus** was much larger than a pill, the drugs being compressed into a ball or cylindrical shape. Willis, in his seventeenth-century casebook, frequently mentions the use of these, for example on 14 August

---

[7] SROB, ID 503/8, 17 March 1846.

1650 he gave 'rhubarb ½ drachm in a bolus of conserve of red roses'.[8] By the nineteenth century the term bolus or ball had become almost entirely restricted to veterinary pharmacy.

During the early 1840s an artist, William Brockeden, infuriated by the fact that he could not obtain drawing pencils free from grit, had the idea of compressing pure powdered graphite in a die between two punches. Realising that his invention could have other uses, in 1844 he took out a patent for a device for 'Shaping of pills, lozenges and black lead by pressure in a die'. The new product was named a **tablet**, which was destined to become the most important single influence in the foundation of the pharmaceutical industry. In spite of the introduction of the tablet, the art of pill-making remained an essential skill for the pharmacist and his apprentices for another hundred years. Proprietary medicine-makers continued to advertise and sell pills well into the twentieth century; probably the most famous were Beecham's Pills, reputed by the manufacturers 'to be worth a guinea a box'.

Powders were dispensed either by providing a quantity from which the patient measured a specific dose (for example, a teaspoonful), or several individual doses were supplied, each separately wrapped in white paper. The prescription dispensed on 30 April 1840, for Mary Willingham (p. 133), is a typical example where six powders had to be prepared, each containing half a grain of mercury and chalk powder with five grains of compound ipecacuanha powder. Every four hours Mary would have unwrapped the powder and carefully stirred the few grains into a little milk or water before swallowing it. This method of administering medicaments had the advantage of providing accurate dosage in a stable form and was suitable where small amounts of drugs were being employed. Where larger quantities had to be used in doses of, for example, one or two teaspoonfuls, then prescribing the powder in bulk was a better proposition. In either case the preliminary preparation of the powder was the same. The final product had to be finely powdered, usually with a mortar and pestle, to a condition known as an 'impalpable' powder, that is, one that is not gritty to the palate.

Electuaries were mixtures of drugs of vegetable origin or light chemical powders sweetened with honey or syrup and formed into a mass of moderate consistence. They were originally meant to be licked off the spoon by a patient,[9] but were usually given in the form of a bolus, or the patient was instructed to take a small amount, for example a piece the size of a nutmeg. Electuaries were only suitable for substances whose taste could be masked by honey or syrup. They were considered to be more active than **confections** in which fresh vegetable material was beaten into a uniform mass with sugar. For example, to prepare Confection of Rose Petals the *London Pharmacopœia* directed that a pound of petals should be beaten in a stone mortar, then three pounds of sugar added and the whole well beaten. It was hoped that by this means the properties of the fresh material would be preserved and decomposition prevented. This process was only successful for a few materials, because almost all lost potency in storage. Although it was directed that confections should be kept in 'closely covered jars to preserve a proper degree of moisture' this frequently did not happen. Fortunately the London College of Physicians said that if they became hard from long keeping they could be moistened with water. Senna confection was popular; it was prepared by mixing senna leaves with caraway, coriander, tamarind,

---

8   K. Dewhurst, *Willis's Oxford Casebook 1650–1652*, London, 1981, p. 130.
9   The word *electuary* is derived from a Greek word meaning *to lick up*.

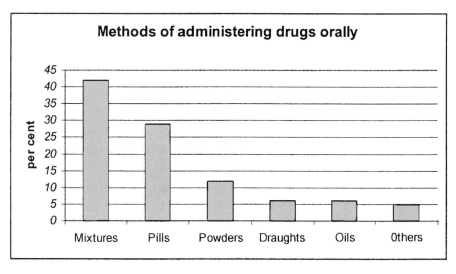

Fig. 2. Showing the relative use of mixtures, pills etc. as prescribed by Stutter.

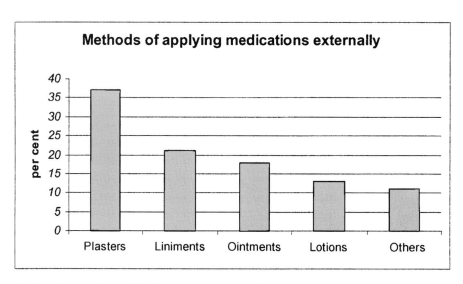

Fig. 3. Plasters headed the list of external applications.

prunes, figs, liquorice, sugar and water. Confections and electuaries were also known as **conserves**.[10]

The most frequently used method of applying drugs externally was by using a **plaster**, also known as an emplaster or plaister. Stutter used plasters on twenty-seven occasions, seventeen of them being for the blistering plaster of cantharides or Emplastrum Lyttae, prepared by melting together lard, beeswax, resin and suet. While it was cooling, powdered cantharides was stirred in.[11] This mass was then spread on a piece of leather of the required size. Normally a hot spatula or plaster iron would be used, but heat was said to destroy the blistering properties of the cantharides and the recommendation was to spread it using the thumb. It is very likely that the plaster base would have been bought ready prepared from one of the drug wholesalers mentioned above.

A **cerate** was defined as 'an unctuous[12] preparation for external use, consisting of wax or resin or spermaceti mixed with oil, lard, and medicinal ingredients'. Such mixtures were meant to be of intermediate firmnesses between that of plasters and of ointments. Cantharides cerate was used to promote a discharge from a blistered surface without causing much irritation. In this aim they were not always successful; a case was reported of a blister on the scalp being dressed for four days with this cerate, 'causing the head to swell to an alarming size with erysipelas covering the face as well as the scalp and closing up the eyes'.[13] Although there were formulæ for eight cerates in the *London Pharmacopœia*, none appear in the casebook. **Ointments**,[14] also referred to as salves, were defined as preparations made with a fatty base and intended for external application. Sometimes they were required to exert a soothing emollient action, in which case no medication was added. Usually the fatty base served as a vehicle for some medicament required to exert a local surface action on the skin. Sulphur ointment is an example of this use; flowers of sulphur were incorporated in a base of lard and applied to the body in cases of 'itch' or scabies. In addition, beeswax, resin, suet and spermaceti were used in bases of **ointments**. Stutter also employed **poultices** (Cataplasma) on several occasions, but only once[15] specified the ingredient – yeast – which was mixed with flour and water and left in a warm place to rise before being applied to the affected area.

Sinapism was the use of a mustard plaster or poultice; the latter contained powdered mustard seed, linseed and warm vinegar. It was recommended that sinapisms should be applied to the soles of the feet in the delirium and coma of typhus fever, and to the affected part in rheumatism.[16] Poultices were commonly used to promote suppuration (that is, bring abscesses to a head); as late as the second half of the twentieth century kaolin poultices were still very much in demand for this purpose. Poultices were frequently made in the home from barley meal, mashed turnip or even bread and milk. A mixture of rye meal, yeast and almond oil, which was then applied as hot as possible, made an eighteenth-century Suffolk remedy considered to be 'An Excellent Remedy for Gout'.[17] **Liniments** were liquid

---

[10] From the Latin *conservare*, to preserve, keep.
[11] See Appendix V for a description of cantharides.
[12] *Unctus*, Latin for anointing.
[13] *London*, p. 970.
[14] The Latin for ointment is *unguentum* (from *unguere*, to anoint).
[15] For Matthew Sindall (p. 122).
[16] *Consp.*, p. 24.
[17] Barnardiston.

or semi-liquid preparations functioning as rubefacients[18] or counter-irritants when applied to the skin, usually by friction with the hand, or less frequently on lint. Liniments containing oils emulsified with water were often known as **embrocations**. A **lotion** was an aqueous solution applied to the skin soaked in lint or dabbed on with cotton wool. Stutter prescribed lotions of lead for sprains and bruises and one of dilute nitric acid, which was considered to be a good astringent, for sores. Silver nitrate was dissolved in water for use as an **eye drop** and Susan Plumbe was given a solution of common salt to use as a **gargle**.

---

[18] Causing redness of the skin.

EDITORIAL METHODS

The original document is a long thin book which has already been described (p. xi above). At the front of the book is an alphabetical index in which Stutter has made an (incomplete) entry of his patients' names and the page number on which each sufferer's record starts. On each opening, a person's medical history was usually entered on the left page, and his or her treatment on the right. Between pages 56 and 72 a slight modification was made. The history was still recorded on the left hand page but the right hand page was divided into three pencilled columns respectively headed 'date', 'treatment' and 'diet'. Stutter probably abandoned this system later in the book because he realised that it took up too much space.

The case-histories are often badly punctuated and are sometimes vague, while the treatments are written in Latin and in a highly abbreviated medical-cum-phar- maceutical shorthand. To present this technical and difficult document in an acces- sible form, the following editorial decisions were made.

First, at the head of each case the editors have inserted their own comments and assessments in the light of modern knowledge and practice. Secondly, as the tech- nical language of the treatments is illegible to most modern readers, and indeed to most of today's medical profession, it was decided to transcribe them as they stand, in abbreviated Latin, but with an English translation in a parallel column.

Entries in the original casebook were sometimes written in pencil, and we have made a note where this happened. Deletions have been indicated with strike- through, but ink stains, broader crossings-out and numerous ticks have been omitted. The ticks were normally made next to prescriptions, and probably mean that this particular medicine had been dispensed and given to the patient. Long dashes appearing in prescriptions mean 'ditto'. Queries are indicated by ques- tion-marks immediately preceding the doubtful word, e.g. ?aloes. All editorial inser- tions appear in italics and within square brackets, e.g. [*sic*].

Although Stutter allocated to every sick person at least two pages of his case- book, sometimes leaves were left blank or only half filled. In this transcription, to save space, all the texts have been run on, though always with a careful note of the original page-numbers. Sometimes this means that three or four original pages appear on one in this volume. The layout of Stutter's book has been largely retained. The only exception is where, in a few cases, he ran out of space and continued the record by jumping to later pages. For ease of reading, the later treatments have been shifted back to the main entry, and the effect on pagination carefully noted.

The English case-histories appear as written, though modern punctuation has been introduced to help readers, and the use of capital letters has also been modern- ised. In the second half of the book, the case-histories grow distinctly longer. The reason may be that, when he started as House Apothecary at the hospital, Stutter took over a group of patients from his predecessor, and did not feel it necessary to record their clinical details in full.

In recording treatments Stutter was inconsistent in his punctuation. We have therefore taken the decision to remove all punctuation from the abbreviated Latin column, but have retained capital letters for chemical compounds and medicines. Among the most common abbreviations in the Latin prescriptions are the following:

Acet (for *Acetum*, vinegar)
Conf (for *Confectio*, confection)
Decoct (for *Decoctum*, decoction)
Emp *or* Emplast (for *Emplastrum*, plaster)
Ext (for *Extractum*, extract)
Inf or Infus (for *Infusum*, infusion)
Liq (for *Liquor*, solution)
Mist (for *Mistura*, mixture)
Ol (for *Oleum*, oil)

Pil (for *Pilula*, pill)
Pulv (for *Pulveris*, powder)
Solut (for *Solutio*, solution)
Sp (for *Spiritus*, spirit)
Syr (for *Syrupus*, syrup)
Tinct (for *Tinctura*, tincture)
Ung (for *Unguentum*, ointment)
Vin (for *Vinum*, wine)

The names of drugs were routinely shortened, for example *Hydrargyrum* (mercury) was abbreviated to *Hydrarg* or simply *Hyd*. Similarly *Colocynthidis* (colocynth) appeared as *Colocynth* or *Col*. A single 'C' appearing after the name of a drug indicated that the compound was required: thus Compound Extract of Colocynth was frequently written as *Ext Col C*, which was far quicker than using the full title of *Extractum Colocynthidis Compositum*. An 'M' in the prescription stands for *misce* (mix). It is frequently followed by 'f' or 'ft', which are shorthand for *fiat* (make).

In the casebook the following symbols or abbreviations of Apothecary weights and measures were used (see also Pharmaceutical Introduction, pp. xxxiii–iv above), and have been reproduced in the transcription:

℥   ounce   ℳ   minim   Q   octarius, pint
℈   drachm   gr   grain   C   congius, gallon
℈   scruple   ℔   pound

A 'half' was indicated in the original by 'ſs' (a long 's' followed by a short 's'), representing the Latin *semis, -issis*. This convention has been retained in the transcription. Thus, ℥ſs stands for 'half an ounce'. The symbol ℞ at the beginning of each prescription represents the Latin *Recipe* (take). It was an instruction to select and measure or weigh the various drugs that follow.

INDEX OF PATIENTS IN STUTTER'S CASEBOOK

Page numbers refer to those in the original casebook.

Arnold, James   15
Atkins, Kezia   66–7, 91
Baker, Frances   100–01
Banham, Susan   7
Bird, Morris   9
Brame, George   84–5
Bryant, Sarah   97–8
Bullas, Mary   33
Burman, Samuel   76–7
Canham, Elizabeth   26
Carter, Isaac   28
Carter, James   80–1
Channell, George   72–3
Chinery, John   38
Chinery, Samuel   35–6
Clark, James   86–7
Clarke, Caroline   24
Cocksedge, John   82
Cook, Mary   102–3
Copping, Ann   62–3
Cousins, Maria   32
Cross, Leah   41–2
Death, Mary   114–15
Downey, William   8
Fane, James   118
Ford, Sarah   78–9
Gladwell, Robert   45
Hayward, Sarah   1
Horrex, Phoebe   98–9
Isaacson, Esther   60–1
Jackson, Susan   11
Leech, W   140–1
Lifley, Martin   21
Ling, Minter   52–3
Malt, William   5

Matthews, Elizabeth   49
Motte, Mary   34
Mulley, William   19–20
Nelson, Robert   130–1
Nelson, William   22
Nunn, Isaac   38
Orris, Abraham   17–18
Pawsey, Elizabeth   50–1
Payne, Elizabeth   112–13
Plumbe, Susan   70–1
Pratt, Hannah   126–7
Rands, Anne   13
Reeve, Susan,   108–9
Ruddock, Thomas   88–9
Rumble, Matilda   30
Savage, James   3
Scarf, Harriet   128–9
Scott, Samuel   104–5
Scott, John   74–5
Scott, Thomas   110–11
Sharpe, James   134–5
Sharpe, John   138–9
Sharpe, Susan   64–5
Shepherd, William   93
Sindell, Matthew   122–3
Smith, Charlotte   54–5
Steggles, Frances   124–5
Talbot, George   40
Tweed, David   116–17
Wade, Mary   43
Warren, Susan   47–8
Wayfield, Caroline   136–7
Welch, Susan   56–9
Wilkinson, William   106–7
Willingham, Mary   132–3

W.G. STUTTER'S CASEBOOK

HC 517/1

Suffolk Record Office (Bury St Edmunds)

[p.1]

Sarah Haywood [*age not recorded*]

[*Nineteenth-century doctors were ever ready to prescribe laxatives, as this case fully demonstrates. On 12 February 1839 Sarah Haywood was given mercury and colocynth pills, followed by a draught of senna and magnesia. The next morning she had a draught of castor oil and more mercury and colocynth pills. There followed a break of five days before she was prescribed decoction of aloes which was to be taken each morning. On 22 February it was ordained that she should take it in the evening as well, should this be necessary. There is no case history for Sarah and it is only possible to guess at a diagnosis. Apart from laxatives, her only other medication was for mixtures containing respectively valerian and iron. At the time both these medicines were used in the treatment of amenorrhoea (absence of menstrual periods). Galbanum, included in the mercury pills, was reputed to be of value in hysteria accompanying cases of deficient menstruation.*]

1839		[*1839*]
Feb 12	R Pil Hydrarg gr iii Ext Colocynth C gr vi M[3] divide in pilul ii st sd	*Feb 12. Take[1] 3 grains of Mercury Pill,[2] 6 grains Compound Extract of Colocynth. Mix. Divide into two pills. To be taken at once.*
	R Infus Sennæ ʒiſs Magnes ʒii M ft Haust post horas quatuor sumendum	*Take 1½ fluid ounces Infusion of Senna, 2 drachms Magnesia. Mix. Make a draught. To be taken after four hours.*
13	R Hyd c Creta gr i Pulv Ipecac gr i Pil Galbani C gr v ft pilula bis die sumenda	*Feb 13. Take 1 grain Mercury with Chalk,[4] 1 grain Ipecacuanha Powder, 5 grains Compound Galbanum Pill. Make a pill. To be taken twice a day.*
	R Ol Ricini ʒvi Mane sumend si alvus non soluta fuerit	*Take 6 drachms Castor Oil. To be taken in the morning if the bowels have not been opened.*
	R Ext Colocynth C gr vii Hyd Submur[5] gr iii divde [*sic*] in pilulæ ii	*Take 7 grains Compound Extract of Colocynth, 3 grains Mercurous Chloride. Divide into two pills.*

---

[1] The symbol R occurring at the beginning of all prescriptions is from the Latin imperative *recipe* meaning 'take'. It is an instruction, originally to the apothecary, now the pharmacist, to select and measure or weigh the various drugs that are written after the symbol. The last section of prescriptions contains directions or instructions for the benefit of the patient. Where medicines are to be administered internally the words 'to be taken' (Latin *sumend*) tell the patient, for example, that two tablespoonfuls are to be taken three times a day. (See pp. xxxiii–iv in the Pharmaceutical Introduction above.)

[2] Making mercury pills was a time-consuming process involving mixing mercury with rose confection, in a pestle and mortar, until the globules disappeared, then adding liquorice powder and beating the whole into a uniform mass. Ready prepared masses were available from manufacturing chemists. The hospital's minute books show that drug purchases were made from Apothecaries Hall and Barron & Co. of London; it is most likely that these purchases would have included commonly used pill masses.

[3] Abbreviation for Latin *misce* meaning 'mix'.

[4] Prepared by mixing mercury and chalk, using a pestle and mortar, until the powder had a uniformly grey colour.

[5] The submuriate of mercury, later renamed mercurous chloride. Hydrochloric acid was originally named muriatic acid; hence chlorides were known as muriates.

15	Contin^r Pil Galbani &c Rep^r Pil Colocynth c Hyd Subm si opus fuerit	*Feb 15. Continue the Galbanum etc pills.* *Repeat the Colocynth and Mercurous Chloride* *pills if needed.*
	℞ Ung Hyd Nit ʒſs capiti	*Take ½ ounce of Mercury Nitrate Ointment.* *[Apply] to the head.*
18	℞ Tinct Valerian ʒi Tinct Valerian Comp ʒi Sodie Sesquicarb ʒſs Mist Camph ʒvi M Sign^r cochlear ii magna ter die Continuentur cetera	*Feb 18. Take 1 drachm Tincture of Valerian,* *1 drachm Compound Tincture of Valerian,* *½ drachm of Sodium Bicarbonate,* *6 ounces of Camphor Mixture.[6] Mix.* *To be labelled: two tablespoonfuls [to be taken]* *three times a day.* *Continue [with] the rest.*
20	℞ Decoct Aloes C ʒiſs sing auroris sumend. Contin^r pill Galbani &c Diæta commun Omissis oleribus	*Feb 20. Take 1½ ounces Compound Decoction* *of Aloes.* *To be taken every morning.* *The Galbanum etc. pills to be continued.* *Common diet.* *Vegetables left out.*
22	Rep^r Haust ?Aloes vespere si opus fuerit habeat cerevisiam cras [Overwritten] Cured Discharged	*Feb 22. The Aloes draught to be repeated* *in the evening if required.* *Let her have beer tomorrow.* *[Overwritten] Cured.* *Discharged.*
26	℞ Mist Ferri C ʒv Aquæ Menth Pip ʒſs Syr Aurantii ʒſs M Cochlear i magnam ter die [in margin] omitte pilulas	*Feb 26. Take 5 ounces Compound Iron Mixture,* *½ ounce Peppermint Water,* *½ ounce Syrup of Orange. Mix.* *One tablespoonful [to be taken] three times a* *day.[7]* *Leave off [taking] the pills.*

[p.2, *blank*]

[p.3]

recommended by[8]	*recommended by*
1839 **James Savage** æt 17	*1839 James Savage, age 17*
from Dr Bayne's Book[9]	*from Dr Bayne's Book*
(Epilepsia?)	*[A possible diagnosis of epilepsy had been made]*

---

6   Camphor mixture was particularly favoured as a convenient and pleasant vehicle for other drugs. Stutter used it in fifty-one of his prescriptions (see Appendix V).
7   This mixture was prescribed four days after the patient had been discharged; possibly she returned as an outpatient.
8   Stutter omitted to write who had recommended this patient.
9   Dr Bayne was a previous consultant at the hospital (see Appendix I).

[James had a brief stay in the hospital, possibly because he had had a fit. He was prescribed asafoetida mixture and discharged relieved. The mixture may have been given as a placebo[10] or maybe as it was considered useful in hysteria.]

1839		*1839*
Feb 15	℞ Tinct Assæfoetid ʒiii Mist Camph ʒxii M bibatur pars quarta bis die	*Feb 15. Take 3 drachms Tincture of Asafoetida,* *12 ounces Camphor Mixture. Mix.* *A fourth part to be drunk* *twice a day.*
	Discharged relieved	*Discharged relieved.*

[p.4, *blank*]

[p.5] Recomd by Revd White	*Recommended by Reverend White.*
1839 **William Malt** Æt 20, labourer	*1839 William Malt, age 20, labourer.*
From Dr Bayne's Book	*From Dr Bayne's Book*

[William had lost the use of his legs, but we have no means of knowing how this had come about (see Appendix II under Paraplegia). It seems likely that this admission was due to a separate problem, since a cure of paraplegia would be unlikely.
Stutter repeated a cantharides plaster that had presumably been prescribed on some other occasion by his predecessor. Both potassium nitrate and solution of ammonium acetate were commonly used to reduce fever. The quinine draught may have been given for the same reason, or it may simply have been used as a tonic. No doubt the beer was also prescribed as a 'pick me up'.]

Jan 3	(Paraplegia)	*Jan 3. (Paraplegic)*
Feb 15	Rep^r Emplast Lyttæ sacro applicandum	*Feb 15. Repeat the Cantharides Plaster.* *To be applied to the sacrum.[11]*
18	℞ Potaſs Nit ʒi Tinct ~~Digit ʒiss~~ Valerian ʒſs Liquor Ammon Acet ʒſs Syrupi ʒiii Mist Camphor ʒxi M cochlear ii magn ter die	*Feb 18. Take 1 drachm Potassium Nitrate,* *~~1½ drachms Tincture of Digitalis~~* *½ ounce Tincture of Valerian,* *½ ounce Solution of Ammonium Acetate,* *3 drachms Syrup,* *11 ounces Camphor Mixture. Mix.* *Two tablespoonfuls [to be taken] three times a day.*
Martii 5	Contin^r Mistura habeat cerevisiam	*Mar 5. Continue [taking] the mixture.* *Let him have beer.*
8	℞ Quinae Disulphat gr i Syr Aurantii ʒi Infus Rosæ C ʒi M ft haust bis die sumend	*Mar 8. Take 1 grain Quinine Disulphate,[12]* *1 drachm Syrup of Orange,* *1 ounce Compound Infusion of Rose. Mix.* *Make a draught. To be taken twice a day.*

---

10 A medicine which is given for merely psychological reasons.
11 The sacrum lies at the base of the spine.
12 Later renamed quinine bisulphate.

Cured   *Cured.*

[p.6, *blank*]

[p.7]

Susan Banham [*age not recorded*]

[*Here we have a clear diagnosis and some logical prescribing. In the nineteenth century both potash and sarsaparilla were used for skin conditions. Diluted hydrocyanic acid was much used to relieve irritation, and the lead acetate solution would have served as an ideal vehicle for the acid as well as being a favoured lotion. Sulphur ointment had a long tradition of usefulness in a wide variety of dermatological complaints, including eczema, scabies and psoriasis (see Appendix II). Despite all this, Susan did not escape without having to take laxative pills of mercury and colocynth.*]

1839 from Dr Baynes book.
       (Eczema)

	℞ Liquoris Potassæ ℥i	*Take 1 drachm Solution of Potassium,*
	Decocti Sarzæ ℥viii M	*8 ounces Decoction of Sarsaparilla. Mix.*
	bibat misturam quotidie	*Let her drink the mixture daily.*
	Diæta media rejectis oleribus	*Medium diet, leaving out vegetables*
	ac cerevisiam	*and beer.*
15	℞ Ext Colocynth C gr vi	*Jan 15. Take 6 grains Compound Extract of Colocynth,*
	Hyd Chlorid gr iii M	*3 grains Mercurous Chloride. Mix.*
	ft Pil altera quaque nocte	*Make pills. [To be taken] every other night.*
18	Rep^r pil ℞ Liq Plumbi Diacet	*Jan 18. Repeat pills. Take 1 pint Dilute Solution*
	diluti Oi Acid Hydrocyan	*of Lead Diacetate,[13] Hydrocyanic Acid[14]*
	℥ſs M ft lotio ter die utend	*½ drachm. Mix. Make a lotion. To be used three times a day.*
20	℞ Ung Sulphuris C ℥ii	*Jan 20. Take 2 ounces Compound Sulphur Ointment.*
	bis die applicand	*To be applied twice a day.*
26	Rep^r frictiones	*Jan 26. Repeat the rubs.[15]*
	Cured	*Cured.*

[p.8]

William Downey Aet 23   *William Downey, age 23.*

[*Sarsaparilla was a popular treatment for venereal disease (see Appendix II under Bubo post ulcus venerum) as well as for skin conditions. Dilute nitric acid was sometimes used to stop the irritation caused by mercury; William took this drug in the form of a nightly pill.*]

---

13 Later renamed lead subacetate.
14 The *London Pharmacopœia* of 1836 contained only dilute hydrocyanic acid (see Appendix V).
15 Presumably of the lead lotion prescribed two days earlier.

1839	from Dr Bayne's book	*1839 from Dr Bayne's book.*
	(Bubo post ulcus venereum)	*(Gland resulting from a venereal ulcer.)*
	℞ Decocti Sarzæ ℥viii	*Take 8 ounces Decoction of Sarsaparilla,*
	Acidi N dil ʒi	*1 drachm Dilute Nitric Acid,*
	Syrup ʒii M	*2 drachms Syrup. Mix.*
	bibat misturam quotidie	*Let him drink the mixture daily.*
22	℞ Pil Hyd Iodid gr v	*Jan 22. Take 5 grains Mercury Iodide Pill.*
	omni nocte sumendæ	*To be taken every night.*
	Continuetur mistura	*Continue [taking] the mixture.*
	habeat cerevisiam	*To have beer.*
	Cured	*Cured.*

[p.9]

	recom^d by Mr Sabine	*Recommended by Mr Sabine.*

Morris Bird Aet 37 Basketmaker
1839 from Dr Bayne's Book

Morris Bird, age 37. Basketmaker.

[*Blood taking, purging and blistering formed a major part of this patient's treatment. The first four prescriptions were all laxative in operation – senna confection, colocynth pills, magnesium sulphate mixture and mercury pills. Ten ounces of blood were taken from his lower back by wet cupping, and a blistering plaster of cantharides applied. Camphor liniment was used to relieve pain, particularly that of rheumatism. There is no indication as to why he was given sulphur fumigation every other day, but sulphur was commonly used to eradicate scabies from the body (see Appendix II).*

~~Jan~~			~~Jan~~
Feb 12			*Feb 12.*
13	~~℞ Confect Sennæ ʒiii~~		*Feb 13. ~~Take 3 drachms of Confection of Senna,~~*
	~~hora somni sumend~~		*~~To be taken at bedtime.~~*
	℞ Ext Col C gr viii		*Take 8 grains Compound Extract of Colocynth,*
	Ext Hyos gr iii M		*3 grains Extract of Henbane. Mix.*
	ft pil ii st sd		*Make two pills, to be taken immediately.*
15	℞ Infus: Rosæ C ℥vi		*Feb 15. Take 6 ounces Compound Infusion of Rose,*
	Magnes Sulphatis ℥iſs M		*1½ ounces Magnesium Sulphate. Mix.*
	bibatur pars quarta		*A fourth part to be drunk*
	omni mane		*every morning.*
20	℞ Hyd Chlorid gr iii		*Feb 20. Take 3 grains Mercurous Chloride,*
	Ext Hyos gr iii M		*3 grains Extract of Henbane. Mix.*
	ft pil hac nocte sd		*Make a pill. To be taken tonight.*
26	℞ Liniment Camph C		*Feb 26. Take 2 ounces Compound Liniment of*
	℥ii nocte maneque applic		*Camphor. To be applied night and morning.*
28	Full diet with beer		*Feb 28. Full diet with beer.*
	balneum tepidum		*[To have a] warm bath.*
Martii 12 Ommitte cerevisiam			*Mar 12. Leave off the beer.*

	Mitte sanguinis ℥x e lumbis per cucurbitulas	Extract 10 ounces of blood from the back using wet cups.
14	Applicitur Emplast Lyttæ sacro	Mar 14. Cantharides Plaster to be applied to the sacrum.
15	habeat fumigationem Sulph alternis diebus	Mar 15. Let him have Sulphur Fumigation every other day.
Maii 14	applicatio Emplast Lyttæ parvi lumbis	May 15. Apply a small Cantharides Plaster to the back.
	curetur quotidie c Strychniæ gr ½	Let him be treated daily with half a grain of Strychnine.[16]
	Relieved	Relieved.

[p.10, *blank*]

[p.11]

Susan Jackson Aged 57

[*The cinchona and guaiacum mixture suggests that this patient may have been suffering from rheumatism. The warm footbath at night was possibly used to help relieve painful feet and ankles. Susan was taking small doses of strychnine regularly; this was considered to be a very good tonic which helped to increase the appetite. A purging draught completed her medication.*]

from Dr Bayne's books

1839		1839
Feb 12	℞ Decocti Cinchonæ Misturæ Guiaici aa ℥iii	Feb 12. Take 3 ounces of each Decoction of Cinchona and Guaiacum Mixture,
	T Cinchonæ C ℥i M	1 ounce Compound Tincture of Cinchona. Mix.
	capiat coch	Let her take a spoonful.
26	~~Continue galvanism~~ [17]	Feb 26. ~~Continue Galvanism.~~
28	℞ Strychiæ gr ii Aceti Distil ℥ii solve	Feb 28. Take 2 grains Strychnine. Dissolve in 2 drachms of Distilled Vinegar.
	℞ solutionis ♏ vi-ix Infus Aurantii ℥iſs M ft haust ter die bibend	Take six to nine minims [*of this*] solution,[18] 1½ ounces Infusion of Orange. Mix. Make a draught. To be drunk three times a day.
	ommittatur Mist Cinchon	The Cinchona Mixture to be stopped.

---

[16] No scale was available to weigh half a grain; one way to obtain this amount would have been to weigh two grains of strychnine, mix thoroughly with ten grains of an inert powder, e.g. finely powdered sugar. Three grains of the resulting mixture would then contain half a grain of strychnine.

[17] See Appendix IV.

[18] Strychnine was prescribed in very small doses, in this case starting with one tenth of a grain, far too small a quantity to be weighed on any available scale. Consequently 2 grains were weighed and dissolved in 2 drachms (120 minims) of vinegar; 6 minims of this solution would then contain the required one tenth of a grain.

Martii 5	Contin^r Mist adde Strych solution ℩i dosibus singulis	*Mar. 5. Continue the mixture adding one minim of [the] strychnine solution to each dose.*
8	Haust Purgans ss	*Mar 8. Purging draught.[19] To be taken at once.*
12	Continuentur medicamenta habeat pediluvium tepid nocte	*Mar 12. The medicines to be continued. Let her have a warm footbath at night.*
19	℞ Tinct Cinch C ℥i Infus Aurantii ℥v Syrupi ʒii M cochlear ii magna bis die	*Mar 19. Take 1 ounce Compound Tincture of Cinchona,* *5 ounces Infusion of Orange,* *2 drachms Syrup. Mix.* *Two tablespoonfuls [to be taken]* *twice a day.*
26	℞ Strychniæ gr ii Micæ panis qs ut fiant pilulæ xlviiii quarum capiat duas ter die Relieved	*Mar 26. Take 2 grains Strychnine,* *a quantity of breadcrumbs[20] sufficient* *to make 48 pills.[21]* *Of which let her take two three times a day.* *Relieved.*

[p.12, *blank*]

[p.13]

Anne Rands age 28 (tumour)

[*The 'tumour' seems to have developed into an abscess in the left upper chest.*]

[*Leeches, lead lotion and ointments were applied to the tumour and then poultices. A draught of morphine was given at night to relieve pain and aid sleep, as well as a tonic mixture of quinine flavoured with infusion of rose petals. These all seem sensible measures in the light of contemporary medical knowledge.*]

Feb 1	Applicantur Hirudines iv loco dolenti	*Feb 1. Let four leeches be applied to the painful area.*
	℞ Liq Plumbi Diacet Dil ℥vi pro lotione assidue applicand	*Take 6 ounces Dilute Solution Lead Diacetate. To be applied continuously as a lotion.[22]*
20	Applicantur Hirudines vi alternis diebus tumori	*Feb 20. Let six leeches be applied every other day to the tumour.*
	Diæta communis c cerevisia	*Common diet with beer.*
26	℞ Ung \Plumbi/ Iodid ∈ ℥ſs tumori applicand nocte maneque	*Feb 26. Take ½ ounce ~~Compound~~ Lead Iodide Ointment.* *To be applied to the tumour night and morning.*

---

19 Purging draughts typically contained laxatives such as aloes, senna, magnesium sulphate; the hospital probably had its own formula.

20 It was essential that the strychnine should be spread evenly throughout the pill mass; using a light excipient such as dry breadcrumbs made this easier to achieve.

21 Each pill would have contained one twenty-fourth of a grain of strychnine.

22 Commonly known as Lead Lotion.

Discharged. Made out-patient	*Discharged. Made outpatient.*

Martii 26 Readmitted as in patient with abscess in the region of the left pectoral muscle, to apply poultices.	*Mar 26. Readmitted as [an] inpatient with abscess in the region of the left pectoral muscle. To apply poultices.*

28 ℞ Morphiæ Hydrochlorid gr ½ Mist Camph ℥iſs solve ft haust nocte sd	*Mar 28. Take ½ grain Morphine Hydrochloride. Dissolve in 1½ ounces of Camphor Mixture. Make a draught. To be taken at night.*

Aprilis 5 ℞ Quinæ Disulph: gr v Infus Rosæ C ℥vi cochlear 2 magna 4^tis horis	*Apr 5. Take 5 grains Quinine Disulphate, 6 ounces Compound Infusion of Rose. Two tablespoonfuls [to be taken] every four hours.*

Cured	*Cured.*

[p.14, *blank*]

[p.15]

James Arnold [*age*] 68

[*The enlarged heart would have resulted in poor circulation which in turn caused fluid retention in the body. Digitalis, by making the heart muscles work more efficiently, improves circulation by allowing the kidneys to excrete more urine. The potassium nitrate and spirit of nitric
ether included in the digitalis mixture also had diuretic properties as did the mercury and
squill pills. Venesection (or bleeding) was very much in accord with contemporary practice
and it may well have been beneficial to this patient (see Appendix IV).*]

Hypertrophia cordis	*Enlarged heart.*

Feb 20 V S ad ℥ x	*Feb 20. Venesection;[23] 10 ounces of blood withdrawn.*

℞ Pil Hyd gr vi Pil Scillæ C gr x M divide in pil iv quarum capiatur una 4^tis horis	*Take 6 grains Mercury Pill, 10 grains Compound Squill Pill. Mix. Divide into 4 pills, of which let one be taken every 4 hours.*

℞ Potass Nit ℈ſs Sp Æther Nit ℈iſs Tinct Digit ♏ xl Aquæ Menth Virid ℥vi sign^r cochlear ii magna ter die	*Take ½ drachm Potassium Nitrate, 1½ drachms Spirit of Nitrous Ether, 40 minims Tincture of Digitalis, 6 ounces Spearmint Water. Label. Two tablespoonfuls [to be taken] three times a day.*

Diæta commun	*Common diet.*

Left the Hospital by his [*illeg.*]	*Left the hospital by his [illeg.]*

[p.16, *blank*]

---

23 Surgical blood-letting by opening a vein (see Appendix IV).

[p.17]

Abraham Orris [*age*] 43

[*Stutter treated this skin condition with external applications of a very dilute solution of nitric acid, elderflower ointment containing a small amount of hydrocyanic acid, lead lotion, and a decoction of mallow with chamomile. The latter was soothing whilst the lotions helped to allay irritation. A lotion of silver nitrate was also prescribed, but it is not clear why it was used in this case. The arsenic solution that Abraham had been taking internally was replaced by a decoction of elm bark; both drugs were considered to be useful for psoriasis. Once again sarsaparilla, in combination with elm bark or mercury, was prescribed for a skin condition. A pleasant effervescing drink flavoured with orange peel was made from tartaric acid and potassium bicarbonate. All the ingredients of the powder prescribed had laxative properties to a greater or lesser degree.*]

	Psoriasis	*Psoriasis*
Feb 20	R̵ Ext Col. C. gr viii	*Feb 20. Take 8 grains Compound Extract of Colocynth,*
	Hyd Chlorid gr v ft pil ii nocte s^d	*5 grains Mercurous Chloride. Make two pills. To be taken at night.*
	R̵ Liq Potass Arsenit ℳ xxviii Decoct Ulmi ℥vi M ¼ ter die bibend	*Take 28 minims of Potassium Arsenite Solution, 6 ounces Decoction of Elm Bark. Mix. [Of which] a fourth part to be drunk three times a day.*
	Omittatur interim [*in margin*]24	*Meanwhile to be omitted.*
	R̵ Ung Zinci ℥i pubi applicand	*Take 1 ounce of Zinc Ointment. To be applied to the pubis.*
	Diæta communis	*Common diet.*
21	R̵ Magnes Sulphat ʒii Sodie Sulphat ʒi Potass Bitart ʒſs ~~Potass Sulphuret~~ gr v M Potass Sulphatis gr x Sulphuris gr viii ft pulv singulis auroris in ℥xii aquæ tepidæ sum	*Feb 21. Take 2 drachms Magnesium Sulphate, 1 drachm Sodium Sulphate, ½ drachm Potassium Bitartrate, 5 grains ~~Sulphuret of Potassium~~ 25 5 grains Potassium Sulphate, 8 grains Sulphur. Make a powder. To be taken each morning in 12 ounces of warm water.*
26	R̵ Ext Col C gr v	*Feb 26. Take 5 grains Compound Extract of Colocynth,*
	Hyd Chlorid gr iii M nocte sd	*3 grains Mercurous Chloride 3 grains. Mix. To be taken at night.*26
28	Bibat mist quotidie	*Feb 28. Let him drink the mixture*

---

24 The significance of this instruction is not clear.

25 This was a compound of potassium and sulphur. Stutter, having initially included it in the prescription, decided instead to prescribe potassium sulphate and sulphur separately.

26 There is no indication of the way these two drugs were to be given; probably the two powders were simply mixed together and swallowed with a drink of water or milk.

	c Liquor Potass Arsenitis	*with Solution of Potassium Arsenite* [27] *daily.*
	habeat balneum tepidum ter in hebdomada	*Let him have a warm bath* *three times a week.*
Martii 5	Continᴿ medicamenta	*Mar 5. Let the medications be continued.*
12	℞ Acid Nitrici ʒii Aquæ ℥xii M ft lotio ter die utend	*Mar 12. Take 2 drachms [Dilute] Nitric Acid,* *12 ounces Water. Mix.* *Make a lotion. To be used three times a day.*
	ommitte unguent continuentur cetera	*Leave off [using] the ointment.* *Let the rest be continued.*
19	Omittatur lotio	*Mar 19. Leave off the lotion.*
	℞ ~~lotionu~~ Liq Plumbi Dil	*Take 6 ounces of Dilute Solution of Lead* *[Diacetate].*
	℥vi ?pilatur pro lotione	*To be used as a lotion.*
26	℞ Potass Bicarb ℈iv Aquæ ℥vi Syr Aurantii ʒii M ft mist cujus capiatur pars 4ᵗᵃ ter die cum ℞ Acid Tart gr x	*Mar 26. Take 4 scruples Potassium Bicarbonate,* *6 ounces Water,* *2 drachms Syrup of Orange.* *Mix. Make a mixture. Of which let a fourth part* *be taken three times a day [mixed] with [blank].* *Take 10 grains Tartaric Acid.* [28]
28	℞ Decoct Malvæ C ℥xii	*Mar 28. Take 12 ounces Compound Decoction* *of Mallow.* [29]
	ft fotus sæpe utendus	*Make a fomentation, to be used frequently.*
Aprilis 9	℞ Argenti Nitratis gr xv Aquæ ℥i M ft lotio	*Aprl 9. Take 15 grains Silver Nitrate,* *1 ounce Water. Mix. Make a lotion.*

[p.18]

Aprilis 13	℞ Liquoris Hyd Bichlorid ʒiſs	*Apr 13. Take 1½ drachms Solution of Mercuric* *Chloride.* [30]
	Decoct Sarzæ ℥ſs M ft haust bis die sd	*½ ounce Decoction of Sarsaparilla. Mix.* *Make a draught. To be taken twice a day.*
Maii 10	℞ Tinct Canthar ~~Mf~~ ℳL	*May 10. Take 50 minims Tincture of* *Cantharides,* [31]
	Decoct Ulmi ℥xiv Syr Sarzæ ℥ii	*14 ounces Decoction of Elm Bark,* *2 ounces Syrup of Sarsaparilla.*

---

[27] Given internally, arsenic was considered to be a tonic. As late as the 1950s mixtures containing solution of arsenic continued to be prescribed.

[28] Adding the tartaric acid powder to the bicarbonate mixture would cause effervescence (see 'Effervescing mixtures' in Appendix V).

[29] Contained mallow and chamomile flowers.

[30] Mercuric chloride (as distinct from *mercurous* chloride) was a dangerous poison with a dose of half to one grain. By using the solution very small doses of mercury could be given; in this instance the patient would receive approximately one tenth of a grain.

[31] Cantharides was rarely given internally; a contemporary indication for/of its use was in gleet (chronic inflammation of the urethra in gonorrhoea): Ballieres's *Nurses' Dictionary*, 21st edn, London 1990, p. 206.

cap coch ii magna bis die	*Let him take two tablespoonfuls twice a day.*
R̸ Ung Sambuci ʒi Acidi Hydrocy ♏x ft ung app^d pubi nocte maneque	*Take 1 ounce Elder Ointment,[32]* *10 minims of [dilute] Hydrocyanic Acid.* *Make an ointment. Apply to the pubis night and* *morning.*
Omitt^r vapo balneum	*Let the vapour bath[33] be omitted*
Bottle	*Bottle.*
Relieved.	*Relieved.*

[p.19]

William Mulley [*age*] 46

[*On 20 February 1839 pills containing mercury and colchicum were prescribed; the combination of these two drugs was recommended in cases of rheumatism. The mixtures with potassium iodide, cinchona and guaiacum as ingredients were used for the same condition. Antimony and potassium tartrate was employed to promote sweating in cases of fever, although nothing suggests that William had a fever, except possibly the fact that he was ordered to have a light diet on the same day. Colocynth and mercury pills were prescribed on 1 and 4 March. Was their purgative effect too great, resulting in diarrhoea and the need for ipecacuanha and opium powder on 28 March? The quinine mixture of 11 April may have been intended as a tonic, and the final prescription again contains ipecacuanha and opium powder and compound chalk powder, both of which were used in diarrhoea, as was the other ingredient, calumba.*]

	Rheumatism	*Rheumatism.*
Feb 20	R̸ Ext Col C gr viii	*Feb. Take 8 grains Compound Extract of* *Colocynth,*
	Ext Colchici Acet gr ii	*2 grains Acetic Extract of Colchicum,[34]*
	Pil Hydr ~~Chlorid~~ gr iii	*3 grains Mercury ~~Chloride~~ Pill*
	ft ?utatur in pill ii nocte s^d	*Make into pills. Two to be taken at night.*
	R̸ Liq Ammon Acet ʒii Vin Ant Pot Tart ʒii	*Take 2 ounces Solution of Ammonium Acetate,* *2 drachms Antimony and Potassium Tartrate* *Wine,*
	Aquæ ʒiiiſs Syrupi ʒii M cochlear ii magna 4^tis horis	*3½ ounces Water,* *2 drachms Syrup. Mix.* *Two tablespoonfuls [to be taken] every four* *hours.*
	Diæta tenuis	*Light diet.*
26	Rep^r pilulæ nocte sumendæ	*Feb 26. Repeat the pills, to be taken at night.*

---

32 Made from the flowers of the elder tree.

33 The installation of medical vapour baths had been approved by the Medical Committee of the hospital in March 1837. See Appendix IV ('Vapour baths').

34 Acetic acid was used to extract the active principle (identified later in the century as the alkaloid colchicine) from the colchicum (meadow saffron) bulb.

Martii 1	Ext Col C gr viii Hyd Chlorid gr iv M ft pil ii nocte s^d	*Mar 1. Take 8 grains Compound Extract of Colocynth, 4 grains Mercurous Chloride. Mix Make two pills, to be taken at night.*
3	℞ Pulv Opii gr i Conf Rosæ q s f pil	*Mar 3. Take 1 grain Powdered Opium, a sufficient quantity of Confection of Rose to make a pill.*
5	℞ Potass ~~Hy~~ Iodid Əi Mist Camphor ʒviii solv cochlear iii ter die	*Mar 5. Take 1 scruple Potassium Iodide. Dissolve in 8 ounces of Camphor Mixture. Three spoonfuls[35] [to be taken] three times a day.*
12	Common diet	*Mar 12. Common diet.*
14	℞ Ext Col C gr x Hyd Chlorid gr v M ft pil ii nocte s^d	*Mar 14. Take 10 grains Compound Extract of Colocynth, 5 grains Mercurous Chloride. Mix. Make two pills. To be taken at night.*
19	℞ Tinct Cinchonæ ʒi Tinct Guaiaci ʒſs Mist Acaciæ ʒi Infus Aurantii ʒiiiſs cochlear i magn ter die	*Mar 19. Take 1 ounce Tincture of Cinchona, ½ ounce Tincture of Guaiacum, 1 ounce Acacia Mixture, 3½ ounces Infusion of Orange. One tablespoonful [to be taken] three times a day.*
	Omittantur cetera	*Let the rest be omitted.*
28	℞ Pulv Ipecac C gr x st sd si diarrhea ~~perst~~ perstituit	*Mar 28. Take 10 grains Compound Ipecacuanha Powder. To be taken at once if the diarrhoea persists.*
Aprillis 11	℞ Quininæ Disulphat gr ii Tinct Capsici ♏ viii Infus Rosæ C ʒiſs M ft haust ter die s^d	*Apr 11. Take 2 grains Quinine Disulphate, 8 minims Tincture of Capsicum, 1½ ounces Compound Infusion of Rose. Mix. Make a draught. To be taken three times a day.*
16	Habeat balneum vapor sulph alternis diebus	*Apr 16. Let him have a Sulphur Vapour Bath[36] on alternate days.*

[p.20]

Maii 12	℞ Pulv Columbæ gr x Pulv Ipecac C gr vi Pulv Cretæ C Əi M ft pulv bis die sumend in aquæ cyatho[37] mitte xii	*May 12. Take 10 grains Calumba powder, 6 grains Compound Ipecacuanha Powder, 1 scruple Compound Chalk Powder. Mix. Make powders. To be taken twice a day in a glass of water. Send 12.*
	To be out-patient	*To be outpatient.*

---

[35] Three tablespoonfuls were probably intended.

[36] Sulphur vapour baths had been fitted at the hospital in 1837 (see Appendix IV).

[37] Cyathus was originally a liquid measure equivalent to one twelfth of a pint (approximately one and three quarter ounces). In medicine it became interpreted as a glass; more frequently the abbreviation *cyath vinos* (wine glass). was used.

[p.21]

Martin Lifley [*age*] 46

[*There is no diagnosis for this patient and the drug record gives few clues, although the digitalis mixture might indicate that he had a heart condition. Thirty-two ounces of blood were withdrawn by wet cupping and bleeding. Syrup of poppies, used mainly in coughs and to aid sleep, was prescribed three times. Mercury and colocynth pills were taken twice a day, their purgative action being reinforced by a laxative draught.*]

Martii 22	℞ Tinct Digitalis ʒii	*Mar 22. Take 2 drachms Tincture of Digitalis,*
	Sp Æther Nit ʒiii	*3 drachms Spirit of Nitrous Ether,*
	Potass Nit ʒiii	*3 drachms Potassium Nitrate,*
	Syrupi ~~Althæa~~ Papav ʒſs	*½ drachm Syrup of ~~Marsh Mallow~~ Poppies,*
	Mist Camph ʒxi M	*11 ounces Camphor Mixture. Mix.*
	cohlear [*sic*] i magn ter die	*One tablespoonful [to be taken] three times a day.*
26	Common diet	*Common diet.*
26	V S ad ʒviii	*Mar 26. Let 8 ounces of blood be withdrawn.*
Aprilis 5ti	℞ Pil Hyd Ɔi	*Apr 5. Take 1 scruple Mercury Pill,*
	Ext Col Ɔii M	*2 scruples Extract of Colocynth. Mix.*
	divide in pil xii quarum	*Divide into 12 pills of which*
	sumatur una bis die	*one to be taken twice a day.*
11	Continuentur pilulæ	*Apr 11. The pills are to be continued.*
	℞ Sodie Sesquicarb gr x	*Take 10 grains Sodium Bicarbonate,*
	Tinct Hyosciam ♏ xv	*15 minims Tincture of Henbane,*
	Mist Camph ʒiſs M	*1½ ounces Camphor Mixture. Mix.*
	ft haust bis die	*Make a Draught. [To be taken] twice a day.*
13	℞ Sp Æther Nit ʒſs	*Apr 13. Take ½ drachm Spirit of Nitrous Ether,*
	Sp Ammon Ar ♏xx	*20 minims Aromatic Spirit of Ammonia,*
	Mist Camph ʒiſs M	*1½ ounces Camphor Mixture. Mix.*
	ft haust ter die sd	*Make a Draught. To be taken three times a day.*
	℞ Haust Aper	*Take Aperient Draught.*
16	Continua	*Apr 16. Continue.*
22	℞ Infus Rosæ ʒi	*Apr 22. Take 1 ounce Infusion of Rose,*
	Syr Papav ʒi M	*1 drachm Syrup of Poppies. Mix.*
	ft haust ter die sd	*Make a Draught. To be taken three times a day*
25	Ditrahantur [*sic*] ʒxii sangunis per curcubitulas	*Apr 25. Let 12 ounces of blood be withdrawn by wet cups.*
	Relieved	*Relieved.*

13

[p.22]

William Nelson [*age*] 47

[*A straightforward case of an injury or infection of a finger, to which thirteen leeches, lead lotion and tincture of iodine were applied. Two tablespoonfuls of a colchicum mixture were taken twice a day, probably as an analgesic.*]

Marti 28	Applicentur Hirudines iv digito indici manus sinistræ	*Mar 28. Let four leeches be applied to the index finger of the left hand.*
	℞ Liq Plumbi Diacetat. Dil ℥vi ft lotio assidue applicand	*Take 6 ounces Dilute Lead Diacetate Solution. Make a lotion, to be applied continuously.*
Aprilis 1	℞ Vin Colchici ʒii Mist Camphor ℥vi M Syrupi ʒii cochlear ii magna bis die	*Apr 1. Take 2 drachms Colchicum Wine, 6 ounces Camphor Mixture. Mix. 2 drachms Syrup Two tablespoonfuls [to be taken] twice a day.*
3	Applicentur Hirud v digito indici sinistro	*Apr 3. Let five leeches be applied to the left index finger.*
13	Applicatio Tinct Iodin	*Apr 13. Application of Tincture of Iodine.*
16	Reapplicatio ejusdem	*Apr 16. Reapplication of the same.*
22	Applica Hirundines iv digito	*Apr 22. Apply four leeches to the finger.*
	Cured	*Cured.*

[p.23, *blank*]

[p.24]

Caroline Clark [*age*] 19

Chlorosis	*Chlorosis [See Appendix II.]*

[*Decoction of aloes was basically a purge but was also recommended for chlorosis; it was given to Caroline to take each night. Chlorosis is thought to have been due to iron deficiency anaemia and it was common in young females. There was, therefore, a sound pharmacological reason to prescribe the iron mixture. The patient apparently had a high temperature since a fever-reducing mixture was prescribed; the combinations of jalap, mercury and rhubarb would have had quite a strong purgative action. A painful area of her upper abdomen was treated by the removal of ten ounces of blood by wet cupping.*]

Martii 28	℞ Decoct Aloes C ℥iʃs omni nocte sumend	*Mar 28. Take 1½ ounces Compound Decoction of Aloes. To be taken each night.*
Aprilis 3	℞ Mist Ferri Mist Camphor aa ʒvi ft haust ter die s^d	*Apr 3. Take 6 drachms each of Iron Mixture [and] Camphor Mixture. Make a draught. To be taken three times a day.*
9	℞ Pulv Jalap gr x Pulv Rhei gr v	*Apr 9. Take 10 grains Jalap Powder, 5 grains Rhubarb Powder,*

14

	Hydr Chlorid gr iv M ft pulv st s^d	*4 grains Mercurous Chloride. Mix.* *Make a powder. To be taken immediately.*
11	Applia Emplast Picis hypochondrio sinistro	*Apr 11. Apply a Pitch Plaster* *to the left abdomen.*
13	℞ Hyd Chlorid gr iv Jalapæ Contrit gr xi M ft pulv st sd	*Apr 13. Take 4 grains Mercurous Chloride,* *11 grains pounded Jalap. Mix.* *Make a powder. To be taken immediately.*
14	℞ Mist Febrifug[38] ʒi 4^tis horis	*Apr 14. Take 1 ounce[39] Fever Reducing mixture* *every four hours.*
25	℞ Infus Rhei ℥iſs Tinct Rhei ʒi Liq Potass ♏v M ft haust ter die	*Apr 25. Take 1½ ounces Infusion of Rhubarb,* *1 drachm Tincture of Rhubarb,* *5 minims Solution of Potassium. Mix.* *Make a Draught. [To be taken] three times a* *day.*
	Omitte cetera	*Leave off the rest.*
27	Applicantaur cucurbitulæ ?venentæ ut ditrahantur sanguinis ℥x hypochondrio dolenti	*Apr 27. Let cupping glasses be applied to* *vein* *and withdraw 10 ounces of blood* *from the painful upper abdomen.*
	Cured	*Cured.*

[p.25, *blank*]

[p.26]

Elizabeth Canham [*age*] 42

Leucorrhoea et Gastralgia   *Vaginal discharge and pain in the stomach.*

[*It is difficult to imagine that the pills and mixture prescribed would have been of any more benefit than the ½ pint of porter. See Appendix II for a discussion of leucorrhoea and gastralgia.*]

Martii 28	℞ Bismuth Trisnitrat Əii Ext Lupuli[41] ʒſs M divide in pilulas xii quarum sumantur ~~una~~ duæ ter die	*Mar 28. Take 2 scruples Bismuth Trinitrate,[40]* *½ drachm Extract of Hops. Mix.* *Divide into 12 pills, of which let* *~~one~~ two be taken three times a day.*
	~~℞ Mist Gentian C ℥iſs~~ ~~Potass Nit gr x~~ ~~singulis auroris s^d~~	*~~Take 1½ ounces Compound Gentian Mixture,~~* *~~10 grains Potassium nitrate,~~* *~~to be taken every morning.~~*

---

38 A mixture to reduce fever.
39 An ounce was approximately two tablespoonfuls.
40 Also known as bismuth oxynitrate.
41 The Latin name of hops is *Lupulus humulus*; the English synonyms were Hops, Humulus, and Lupuli. Stutter prescribed hops on five occasions, twice referring to it as Humulus and three times as Lupuli.

Aprilis 13 ℞ Infus Calumbæ ʒi	*Apr 13. Take 1 ounce Infusion of Calumba,*
[*deletion*] Sodie Sesquicarb ʒſs	*½ drachm Sodium Bicarbonate,*
Sodie Sulphat Ɔii	*2 scruples Sodium Sulphate,*
Tinct Gentian ʒſs M	*½ drachm Tincture of Gentian. Mix.*
ft haust ter die s^d	*Make a draught. To be taken three times a day.*
To have ½ pint of porter[42]	*To have ½ pint of porter.*
To be out patient	*To be outpatient.*

[p.27, *blank*]

[p.28]

Isaac Carter [*age*] 76

[*The only medication this patient received was a mildly laxative draught and some purging pills containing mercury and rhubarb. See Appendix II for a discussion of hepatitis.*]

1839	Hepatitis chronica	*Chronic Hepatitis.*
Aprilis 11 Diæta communis		*Apr 11. Common diet.*
13	℞ Pil Hyd gr ii	*Apr 13. Take 2 grains Mercury Pill,*
	Pil Rhei C gr iii M	*3 grains Compound Rhubarb Pill. Mix.*
	ft pil bis die sd	*Make a pill. [One] to be taken twice a day.*
16	Continuentur pilulæ	*Apr 16. Let the pills be continued.*
	℞ Sodæ Sesquicarb Ɔi	*Take 1 scruple Sodium Bicarbonate,*
	Sodæ Sulphat Ɔii	*2 scruples Sodium Sulphate,*
	Infus ~~Gentian~~ [*illeg.*] ʒiſs	*1½ ounces Infusion of ~~Gentiam~~ [illeg].*
	ft haust bis die	*Make a draught. [To be taken] twice a day.*
	Relieved[43]	*Relieved.*

[p.29, *blank*]

[p.30]

Matilda Rumble [*age*] 11

[*The only reason for using a combination of castor oil and turpentine was because it effectively expelled tape worms from the intestines, and we assume this is why the eleven-year-old was prescribed the unpleasant draught. Two nights later Matilda was given laxative pills of aloes possibly to ensure that the tape worm had been completely expelled. Strychnine is a stimulant to the central nervous system and was widely used as a 'nerve tonic'. The decoction of barley in the draught taken every three hours was perhaps given for its nutritive value.*]

1839 Chorea	*1839 Chorea [See Appendix II.]*

---

[42] A heavy dark-brown beer brewed from browned or charred malt. The hospital's minute books record a gallon of porter being purchased from Mr Greene in 1841 at a cost of one shilling: SROB ID 503/6 14 Dec. 1841.
[43] This page contains entries in pencil, confusingly overwritten in ink.

April 11	℞ Ol Ricini ʒiii Ol Terebinth ʒv M st sumend	*Apr 11. Take 3 drachms Castor Oil,* *5 drachms Oil of Turpentine. Mix.* *To be taken immediately.*
13	Pil Aloes C gr x divide in pil duas singulis noctibus sumendas	*Apr 13. Take 10 grains Compound Aloes Pill.* *Divide into pills. Two* *to be taken each night.*
	℞ Strychniæ gr i Micæ Panis qs ut fiant pilulæ xviii quarum capiatur una ter die	*Take 1 grain Strychnine,* *a sufficient quantity bread crumbs* *to make 18 pills,* *of which let one be taken three times a day.*
16	℞ Mist Acaciæ ʒſs Decoct Hordie ʒi M ft haust tertiis horis sᵈ	*Apr 16. Take ½ ounce Acacia Mixture,* *1 ounce Decoction of Barley.*[44] *Mix.* *Make a draught. To be taken every three hours.*
25	Perstet	*Apr 25. Continue.*
	Cured	*Cured.*

[p.31, *blank*]

[p.32]

Maria Cousins [*age*] 16

[*This is another case of chorea, but the only drug this patient received in common with the previous one was aloes. Galbanum and asafoetida were both used in hysteria, but it seems that Stutter changed his mind about prescribing asafoetida. Maria was also given iron, possibly because she had symptoms of anaemia. For a reason that is not clear, eight leeches were applied behind her ear.*]

1839 Chorea		*1839 Chorea.*
Aprilis 10	℞ Pil Galbani C gr v Ferri sulphatis gr i Aloes gr iv M ft pilulae ii ter die sᵈ. Mitte [*illeg.*] viii [*in margin*]	*Apr 10. Take 5 grains Compound Galbanum Pill,* *1 grain Iron Sulphate,* *4 grains Aloes. Mix.* *Make pills. Two to be taken three times a day.* *Send 8.*
	Applicentur Hirudines viii pone auris	*Apply 8 leeches* *behind the ear.*
April 16	℞ Tinct Sp Ammonii Fetid ʒſs Sodie Sesquicarb gr xv Mist Assafetid ʒi M ft haust bis die	*Apr 16. Take* *½ drachm Tincture Spirit of Foetid Ammonia,* *15 grains Sodium Bicarbonate,* *1 ounce Asafoetida Mixture. Mix;* *Make a draught. [To be taken] twice a day.*

---

44   This decoction was made by boiling barley grains with water, and given as a demulcent or possibly for its nutritive value.

℞ ~~Tinct Valerian ʒxxx~~	~~Take 30 drachms Tincture of Valerian,~~
~~Sodie Sesquicarb ʒſs~~	~~½ ounce Sodium Bicarbonate.~~
~~Aquæ Menth Pip ʒxx~~	~~20 ounces Peppermint Water~~
~~ft mist coch larg ii ter die sd~~	~~Make a mixture. Two tablespoonfuls to be taken~~
	~~three times a day.~~

June 11   ℞ Pil Ferri C ʒii   *June 11. Take ~~2 drachms~~ Compound Iron Pill.*
~~in pil x~~   *~~In ten pills.~~*
no xlviii   *by number 48*
sumᵗ ii ter die   *Let two be taken three times a day.*

       ℞ Pil Aloe c Myrrh   *Take Aloes and Myrrh Pills.*
no xxiv   *by number 24.*
sumᵗ ii o n h s   *Let her take two at night at bedtime.*

       To be out patient[45]   *To be outpatient.*

[p.33]

Mary Emily Bullass [*age*] 19

[*There is little in the prescription record to suggest a diagnosis, but iron was prescribed, so perhaps she was thought to be anaemic. She was also given mixtures containing morphine, to be taken both at night and during the day. This probably indicates that she was in pain.*]

1839   *1839.*

June 4   ℞ Ol Terebinth   *June 4. Take Turpentine Oil.[46]*

       ℞ Liq A A ʒſs   *Take ½ ounce Ammonium Acetate Solution,*
Solut Morph ʒſs   *½ drachm Morphine Solution,*
Mist Camphor ʒi   *1 drachm Camphor Mixture.*
mf haust h s s   *Mix. Make a draught. To be taken at bedtime.*

June 5   ℞ Sodæ Carb ʒiii   *June 5. Take 3 drachms Sodium Carbonate,*
Tinct Valerian ʒi   *1 ounce Tincture of Valerian,*
Solut Morphiæ ʒi   *1 drachm Morphine Solution,*
~~Inf Gentian C //i~~   *~~Compound Infusion of Gentian,~~*
Aquæ puræ //i   *1 pound[47] Pure Water.*
mf mistur sum   *Mix. Make a mixture.*
coch larg iii ter die   *Three tablespoonfuls to be taken three times a day.*

June 11   ℞ Mist Ferri C //i   *June 11. Take 1 pound Compound Iron Mixture.*
sumᵗ coch larg ii   *Let her take two tablespoonfuls*
ter die   *three times a day.*

       To be out patient   *To be outpatient.*

---

45   There are extensive crossings-out on this page, probably done as each item was checked off.
46   No quantity of the oil to be dispensed was given.
47   Equivalent to 12 fluid ounces.

[p.34]

Mary Motte [*age*] 15

[*This patient most likely had an infected eye surrounded by infected eczema. It was treated successfully with local iodine to the eczematous skin (initially applied with a brush) plus eye drops of silver nitrate.*]

1839	Ophthalmia scrofulosa	*1839. Scrofulous ophthalmia [See Appendix II.]*
	℞ Tinct Iodinii C ℥ii applica per penicillum [*illeg.*] et tumori	*Take 2 ounces Tincture of Iodine. Apply by brush to the [illeg.] and swelling.*
	℞ Solution Iodinii ℈ Oi 1/6 ter die	*Take 1 pint Compound Solution of Iodine. One sixth part three times a day.*
29	℞ Argent Nitrat gr x Aq Distill ℥i ft guttæ	*Apr 29. Take 10 grains Silver Nitrate, 1 ounce Distilled Water. Make drops.*[48]
	Cured	*Cured.*

[p.35]

Samuel Chinery [*age not recorded*]

[*This is a very difficult record to interpret. From the use of cantharides and antimony plasters, potassium iodide and quinine, a very tentative diagnosis of rheumatism might be made.*]

1839		*1839.*
June 5	Cucurbitula cruenta ?Ferri[49] sanguin ad ℥x	*June 5. Apply wet cupping glasses and take up to ten ounces of blood.*
	Emp Lyttæ lumbis	*[Apply a] Cantharides Plaster to the loins.*
	℞ Hyd Chlorid gr vi Pulv Opii gr ii mf pil ℈-vi sum^t omne nocte et mane	*Take 6 grains Mercurous Chloride, 2 grains Opium Powder. Mix. Make ℈ 6 pills. Let him take one each night and morning.*
	℞ Potass Iodid ℈ ii Mist Camphor ℔i Tinct Capsici ℨi mf mist sum^t coch larg iii ter die	*Take 2 scruples Potassium Iodide, 1 pound Camphor Mixture, 1 drachm Tincture of Capsicum. Mix. Make a mixture. Let him take three tablespoonfuls three times a day.*
Junii 8	℞ Liq Ammon Acet ℥ii	*June 8. Take 2 ounces Ammonium Acetate Solution,*
	Aquæ ℥iv M cochlear ii 4^tis horis s^d	*4 ounces Water. Mix. Two spoonfuls to be taken every 4 hours.*

---

48 The drops would have been intended for the eyes.
49 The significance of ?*ferri* (iron) in this instruction is not understood.

12	℞ Emp Lyttæ lumbos	*June 12. Take a Cantharides Plaster.* [*Apply*] *to the loins.*
June 22	℞` Hyd c Creta gr xxiv Pulv Ipecac C gr xxiv conf qs ft pil xii sum^t ii o n h s	*June 22. Take 24 grains Mercury with Chalk,* *24 grains Compound Ipecacuanha Powder,* *a sufficient quantity of Confection.*[50] *Make12 pills. Let him take two* *at night, at bedtime.*
Junii 25	℞ Sodæ Carbon ʒſs Aqua ʒxiv	*June 25. Take ½ ounce Sodium Carbonate,* *14 ounces Water.*
	℞ Acid Tartaricis gr xv ft pulv Mitte xii capiatur pulv i cum mistur ʒi in impetu effevescentiæ 4^{tis} horis	*Take 15 grains Tartaric Acid.* *Make a powder. Send 12.* *Let him take a powder with one ounce of the* *mixture*[51] *during effervescence* *every 4 hours.*
	℞ Pil Galbani Comp xxiv sumat duas ter die	*Take 24 Compound Galbanum Pills.* *Let him take two three times a day.*
July 3	℞ Infus Calumb ℔ i sum^t coch larg ii ter die	*July 2. Take 1 pound Infusion of Calumba.* *Let him take two tablespoonfuls* *three times a day.*
9	℞ Tinct Auran ʒvi Tinct Calumb ʒiii Sesquicarb Sodae ʒii Aquæ ℔ i mf mist sum^t coch larg iii ter die	*July 9. Take 6 drachms Tincture of Orange,* *3 drachms Tincture of Calumba,* *2 drachms Sodium Bicarbonate,* *1 pound Water.* *Mix. Make a mixture. Let him take three* *tablespoonfuls three times a day.*

[p.36]

	Samuel Chinery	*Samuel Chinery* [*continued*].
July 18	℞ Quinæ Disulph gr xxiv Pulv Capsici gr xii Confect Rosæ q s ut ft pilulae xxiv quarum capiatur una ter in die	*July 18. Take 24 grains Quinine Disulphate,* *12 grains Capsicum Powder,* *sufficient quantity Confection of Rose* *to make 24 pills.* *Of which let him take one* *three times a day.*
26	℞ Conf Rutae gr x ft conf om mane sm	*July 26. Take 10 grains Confection of Rue.* *Make a confection. To be taken each morning.*
31	℞ Ext Nucis Vomicæ gr xxiv Ext Gentian Ɔii Pulv Glycyrrhis [*sic*] ʒi	*July 31. Take 24 grains Extract of Nux Vomica,*[52] *2 scruples Extract of Gentian,* *1 drachm Liquorice Powder,*

---

50 A simple thick confection would have been used to bind the powders together into a mass suitable for rolling into pills.

51 That is, the mixture of sodium carbonate.

52 This quantity of extract would contain approximately one grain of strychnine.

	vel q s ut fiant pilulæ xxiv quarum capiantur una bis die	*or a sufficient quantity to make 24 pills. Of which let him take one twice a day.*
Aug^{ti} 7	Ommitte pilulas	*Aug 7. Leave off the pills.*
	℞ Quinæ Disulph gr x~~v~~iv Acid Sulph Dil ♏xx Tinct Zingib ʒii Infus Rosæ ℥xiv cochlear iii ampla bis in die	*Take 14 grains Quinine Disulphate, 20 minims Dilute Sulphuric Acid, 2 drachms Tincture of Ginger, 14 ounces Infusion of Rose. Three tablespoonfuls* [*to be taken*] *twice a day.*
	To have a pork chop	*To have a pork chop.*
15	*Aug 15.* ℞ Emp Ant Tart c Ant Tart gr v lumbos	*Take Antimony Tartrate Plaster with 5 grains of Antimony Tartrate.*[53] [*Apply*] *to the loins.*

[p.37]

Isaac Nunn [*age not recorded*]

[*Just two prescriptions seem to have cured this patient, but there is no clue as to a possible diagnosis. He was first given purgative pills of mercury and squill followed by a mildly laxative mixture.*]

1839	*1839.*	
June 5	℞ Pil Hydrarg ʒſs Pulv Ipecac gr vi Pulv Scillæ gr xii Mf pil xii sum^{t} ii o n h s.	*June 5. Take ½ drachm Mercury Pill, 6 grains Ipecacuanha Powder, 12 grains Squill Powder. Mix. Make 12 pills. Let him take two at night, at bedtime.*
	℞ Sp Æther Nit ℥ſs Magnes Sulph ℥i Infus Calumb ℔i mf mist sum^{t} coch larg iii ter die	*Take ½ ounce Spirit of Nitrous Ether, 1 ounce Magnesium Sulphate, 1 pound Infusion of Calumba. Mix. Make a mixture. Let him take three tablespoonfuls three times a day.*
11	Cured	*June 11. Cured.*

[p.38]

John Chinery [*age*] 45

[*This is the second patient mentioned in the casebook who suffered from an enlarged heart. Most probably he had heart failure too. He received digitalis, mercury (considered to aid the diuretic action of digitalis) and potassium iodide. Blood letting, or venesection, would have been* de rigueur *for this condition in 1839 (see Appendix III).*]

---

53 Stutter obviously decided to increase the counter-irritant action of the plaster by the addition of more antimony tartrate.

1839		*1839*
	Hypertrophy of Heart	*Enlarged heart.*

June 19 V S ℥x — *June 19. Venesection. [Up to] 10 ounces [of blood taken].*

℞ Pil Hydrarg gr xxiv
Pulv Digital gr vi
Ext Rhei gr xxiv
mf pil xii sum^t
i ter die

*Take 24 grains Mercury Pill,
6 grains Digitalis Powder,
24 grains Rhubarb Extract.
Mix. Make 12 pills. Let him take
one three times a day.*

25 ℞ Tinct Digitalis ℨiſs
Potass Iodid gr xvi
Mist Camphor ℥xii
m ft mist cujus capiatur
cochlear i magna ter die

*June 25. Take 1½ drachms Tincture of Digitalis,
16 grains Potassium Iodide,
12 ounces Camphor Mixture.
Mix. Make a mixture of which let him take
one tablespoonful three times a day.*

July 3 Perstat mist — *July 3. Continue mixture.*

℞ Pil Galban C
no xxiv sum^t
ii bis die

*Take Compound Galbanum Pills,
24 in number. Let him take
two twice a day.*

4 ℞ Tinct Digital ℨii
Tinct Calumb ℥iſs
Mist Camphor ℔i
mf mist sum^t coch
larg iii bis die

*July 4. Take 2 drachms Tincture of Digitalis,
1½ ounces Tincture of Calumba,
1 pound Camphor Mixture.
Mix. Make a mixture. Let him take three
tablespoonfuls twice a day.*

{Bottle}[54]

{Bottle}

℞ Mist Ferri C ℔i
sum^t coch larg ii
ter die

*Take 1 pound Compound Iron Mixture.
Let him take two tablespoonfuls
three times a day.*

℞ Potass Iodin ℨii
Tinct Capsici ℨi
Mist Camphor ℔i
mf mist sum^t
coch larg iii ter die

*Take 2 drachms Potassium Iodide,
1 drachm Tincture of Capsicum,
1 pound Camphor Mixture.
Mix. Make a mixture. Let him take three
tablespoonfuls three times a day.*

℞ Emp Picis C
c Ant Tart ℨii
ft emp

*Take Compound Plaster of Pitch
with 2 drachms of Antimony Tartrate.
Make a plaster.*

[p.39, *blank*]

---

[54] The significance of this entry is not clear.

[p.40]

George Talbot [*age*] (58)

[*This patient was almost certainly another heart case. He received digitalis and was bled twice, a total of eighteen ounces of blood being taken. The second digitalis mixture was made into an effervescent drink by adding a powder of tartaric acid to each dose (the bicarbonate of potassium in the mixture reacting with the tartaric acid, releasing carbon dioxide). George was also given pills of wild cucumber, which were strongly purgative; this medication was followed by the almost inevitable mercury and colocynth laxative pills.*]

	(Hypertrophy of right side)	*Enlarged right side* [*of heart*].
June 19	℞ Ext Elaterii gr ſs	*June 19. Take ½ grain Extract of Wild Cucumber,*
	Conf q s	*A sufficient quantity Confection*
	ft pil ℏ s s	*[to] make a pill, to be taken immediately.*
	℞ Infus Digital ℥iv	*Take 4 ounces Infusion of Digitalis,*
	Potass Nitrat ℨii	*2 drachms Potassium Nitrate,*
	Mist Camph ℥viii	*8 ounces Camphor Mixture.*
	mf mist sum^t	*Mix. Make a mixture. Let him take*
	coch larg iii ter die	*three tablespoonfuls three times a day.*
20	Rep pil	*June 20. Repeat pill.*
22	Emp Lyttæ laterii	*June 22. [Apply a] Cantharides Plaster to the side.*
July 3	℞ Acid Hydrocyan gtt xxxx	*July 3. Take 40 drops [Dilute] Hydrocyanic Acid,*[55]
	– Nitric D ℥ſs	*½ ounce Dilute Nitric Acid,*
	Tinct Scillæ ℥ſs	*½ ounce Tincture of Squills,*
	Aq Puræ ♯i	*1 pound Pure Water.*
	mf mist sum^t	*Mix. Make a mixture. Let him take*
	cochr larg iii ter die	*three tablespoonfuls three times a day.*
8	[*faint pencilled entry*]	*July 8.*
	℞ Hyd Submur gr vi	*Take 6 grains Mercurous Chloride,*[56]
	Ext Hyosiam [*sic*] gr xii	*12 grains Extract of Henbane,*
	– Coloc C ℨſs	*½ drachm Compound Extract of Colocynth.*
	m pil xii sum^t	*Mix [Make] 12 pills. Let him take*
	ii 2da nocte	*two every second night.*
13	℞ Potass Bicarb ℥ſs	*July 13. Take ½ ounce Potassium Bicarbonate,*
	Sp Æther Nit ℨiii	*3 drachms Spirit of Nitrous Ether,*
	Tinct Digit ℨii	*2 drachms Tincture of Digitalis,*
	Aquae ℥xii M	*12 ounces Water. Mix.*
	adde Tinct Colch ℨiſs [*in margin*]	*Add 1½ drachms Tincture of Colchicum.*

---

[55] The *London Pharmacopœia* of 1836 warned that great caution should be used in the use of this acid, and the initial dose should not exceed five or six minims; Stutter kept within this dose range, the patient taking five minims. See Appendix V.

[56] The common name for this mercury compound was Calomel.

	cochlear ii magna 4^{tis}	Two tablespoonfuls [to be taken] every
	horis cum pulveri seq^n	four hours with the following powder.
	R̵ Acid Tart gr xv	Take 15 grains Tartaric Acid.
	ft pulv mitte xii	Make a powder. Send 12.
	V S ad viii	Venesection. Up to 8 ounces [of blood taken].
14	Repetatur venesectio	July 14. Repeat the Venesection
	ad ʒx	[taking] up to 10 ounces [of blood].
	urine albuminous gravity not known	Albumen in urine. [Specific] gravity not known.
17	urine sp gr 16–17 less albumen	July 17. Urine specific gravity 16–17. Less albumen.
29	To have beer	July 29. To have beer.
Aug^{ti} 7	½ pint of porter twice a day	Aug 7. To have ½ pint of porter twice a day.
Aug 14	Discharged somewhat relieved	Aug 14. Discharged somewhat relieved.

[p.41]

Leah Cross [age] 22

[Leah was purged by taking mercury and colocynth pills. Three days later she had canthar-ides applied to her abdomen, possibly intended to relieve the griping pains that the pills were apt to cause. She was then given an enema, the purging effect increased by the addition of turpentine. Previously a turpentine mixture had been prescribed for her; sometimes this was used internally as a purgative but also as a diuretic for rheumatism and in urinary and kidney disorders. Apart from turpentine Leah had a dozen other drugs administered, but without a diagnosis it is only possible to guess why they were prescribed. The specific gravity of the urine was high (1030), which might suggest dehydration due to fever. There was, however, no albuminuria,[57] which would suggest that the problem did not lie in her kidneys. This theory is also supported by the high specific gravity of the urine. In renal failure the specific gravity is usually low (1010). [See Appendix III under Urine testing.] On 7 August 1839 dyspnoea or breathlessness is mentioned; thus Leah may have had a problem in her heart or lungs.]

1839

July 10	R̵ Mist Assafœtid ℔ i	July 10. Take 1 pound Asafoetida Mixture.
	mf mist sum^t coch	Mix. Make a mixture. Let her take three
	larg iii ter die	tablespoonfuls three times a day.
	R̵ Ferri Sulph gr xxiv	Take 24 grains Iron Sulphate,
	Pil Galban C ʒiſs	1½ drachms Compound Galbanum Pill.
	mf pil xxiv sum^t ii	Mix. Make 24 pills. Let her take two
	c sing dosis mist	with each dose of mixture.
	ommitantur pilulæ	The pills to be left off.

---

57 Albuminuria or albumen in the urine, often a sign of disease in the kidneys. See Appendix III.

July	Ṛ Ferri Potassio Tart gr x	*July 17. Take 10 grains Iron and Potassium Tartrate,*
	Pulv Digitalis gr ½ i	*½ 1 grain Digitalis Powder,*
	Pulv Cinnam C gr iii	*3 grains Compound Cinnamon Powder.*
	ft pulv ter die sumnd	*Make a powder. [One] to be taken three times a*
	mitte xii	*day. Send 12.*
19	Urine sp gr 30 and no precipⁿ by heat or Nit acid	*July 19. Urine specific gravity 30, no precipitation by heat or nitric acid.*
24	Repʳ Linement [sic] Terebinth	*July 24. Repeat Turpentine Liniment.*
Augᵗⁱ 7	Ṛ Sp Æther Sulph C ℨii	*Aug 7. Take 2 drachms Compound Spirit of Sulphuric Ether,*
	Magnesiæ Ɔiv	*4 scruples Magnesia,*
	Aquæ Menth P ℥ vi	*6 ounces Peppermint Water.*
	M ¼ urgente Dyspnoea	*Mix. A fourth part [to be taken] if the difficult breathing is troublesome.*
14	To have new milk for breakfast	*Aug 14. To have new milk for breakfast.*
21	Ṛ Sp Terebinth ℨvi	*Aug 21. Take 6 drachms Turpentine,*
	Mellis Desp ℥i	*1 ounce Clarified Honey,*
	Aq Menth P ℔i	*1 pound Peppermint Water.*
	mf mist sumᵗ coch	*Mix. Make a mixture. Let her take three*
	larg iii ter die	*tablespoonfuls three times a day.*
23	Omitte Mist Terebinth	*Aug 23. Leave off Turpentine mixture.*
	Ṛ Sp Æther Nit ℥i	*Take 1 ounce Spirit of Nitrous Ether,*
	Potass Nit ℨii	*2 drachms Potassium Nitrate,*
	Tinct Hyos ℨvi	*6 drachms Tincture of Henbane,*
	Aquæ ℥xvi	*16 ounces Water.*
	cochlear iii magna 4ᵗⁱˢ	*Three tablespoonfuls*
	horis sumenda	*to be taken every 4 hours.*
25	Ṛ Ext Coloc C gr iv	*25. Take 4 grains Compound Extract of Colocynth,*
	– Hyoscyan [sic] gr ii	*2 grains Extract of Henbane,*
	Hyd Chlorid gr i	*1 grain Mercurous Chloride.*
	mf pil ii sumᵗ ii	*Mix. Make 2 pills. Let her take two*
	4ᵗⁱˢ horis	*every four hours.*[58]

[p.42]

Aug 28	Ṛ	*Aug 28. Take*
	Acet Cantharid ℥iſs	*1½ ounces Vinegar of Cantharides.*
	abdomini applicetur ?pauxill	*Apply a little to the abdomen.*
~~30~~	Ṛ enema communis	~~30~~ *Take Common Enema*[59]
	c Sp Terebinth ℥i	*with 1 ounce Turpentine.*

---

[58] The directions are inexplicable; only two pills were to be made yet two were to be taken every four hours. It is unlikely that such strong laxative pills would be taken so frequently.

[59] One or two tablespoonfuls of common salt dissolved in a pint of warm water.

30	Rep Emenca [*sic*]	*Aug 30. Repeat the enema.*
Sept^i 1	℞ Acid Hydrocyan Dil ℞ xviii Mist Acaciæ ʒ ʃs Aquæ ʒ vʃs M cochlear ii magna 4^tis horis	*Sept 1. Take 18 minims Dilute Hydrocyanic Acid,* *½ ounce Acacia mixture,* *5½ ounces Water. Mix.* *Two tablespoonfuls [to be taken] every 4 hours.*
	omitte altera	*Leave off the other.*
Sept 1	Perstet	*Sept 11. Continue.*

[p.43]

Mary Wade [*age*] (63)

[*The age of the patient combined with administration of sarsaparilla and iodides suggest that rheumatism could be a possible diagnosis.*]

1839

July 31	℞ Potass Iodin 囧ii – Bicarb ʒ iii Ess Sarsae C ʒ ii Decoct Sarsae C ℔ i mf mist sum^t coch larg iii ter die	*July 31. Take 2 scruples Potassium Iodide,* *3 drachms Potassium Bicarbonate,* *2 ounces Compound Essence of Sarsaparilla,* *1 pound Compound Decoction of Sarsaparilla.* *Mix. Make a mixture. Let her take* *three tablespoonfuls three times a day.*
Aug 6	℞ Ung Hydrarg Iodin ʒ i utend nocte et mane	*Aug 6. Take 1 ounce Mercuric Iodide ointment.* *To be used night and morning.*
7	℞ Ext Humuli Pil Saponis C aa ʒ i m ℔ divide in pil xviii ii omni nocte sd	*Aug 7. Take 1 drachms each Extract of Hops,* *Compound Soap[60] Pill.* *Mix. ~~Make~~ Divide into 18 pills.* *Two to be taken each night.*
16	Perstet better	*Aug 16. Continue. Better.*
Augt 19	℞ Ferri Iodid gr xxiv ~~Aquæ~~ Decoct Sarzae ʒ xii m Cochlear iii ter in die	*Aug 19. Take 24 grains Iron iodide,* *12 ounces ~~Water~~ Decoction of Sarsaparilla.* *Mix. Three tablespoonfuls [to be taken]* *three times a day.*
	Omitte misturam Potass Iod	*Leave off the Potassium Iodide mixture.*

[p.44, *blank*]

[p.45]

Robert Gladwell [*age not recorded*]

[*The diagnosis was almost certainly Trigeminal neuralgia or Tic douloureux (see Appendix II for a fuller discussion of this painful condition). A blistering plaster was applied behind the ear and a powder of morphine given to relieve the pain. Leeches were also used, together with powders of iron and a mixture of quinine, nitric acid and hops.*]

---

60 Soap was sometimes used in pill-making to give greater adhesiveness to the mass.

Neuralgic affection, of some portion of the 5th pair		*Neuralgic affection of some part of the fifth cranial nerves.*

1839		
July 31	℞ Quin Sulp gr xxx Acid Nitric D ʒii Tinct Lupuli ʒiii m̶f̶ Aq Puræ ℥ ʃs mf mist sum^t coch larg iii ter die	*July 31. Take 30 grains Quinine Sulphate,* *2 drachms Dilute Nitric Acid,* *3 drachms Tincture of Hops,* *½ pound Pure Water,*[61] *Mix. Make a mixture. Let him take three* *tablespoonfuls three times a day.*
Aug^{ti} 4to	℞ Ferri Sesquioxyd Ɔiii ft pulv bis in die sumend mitte xii	*Aug 4. Take 3 scruples Ferric Oxide.* *Make a powder. [One] to be taken twice a day.* *Send 12.*
7	To have beer	*Aug 7. To have beer.*
12	To have porter and full diet	*Aug 12. To have porter and full diet.*
	perstet in usu Ferri	*Continue to use iron.*
16	Perstet	*Aug 16. Continue.*
19	Perstet	*Aug 19. Continue.*
Oct 22	Rep Mist ℥ ʃs ut Julii 31	*Oct 22. Repeat ½ pound of the mixture of July 31.*
	Rep pulv xii ut Aug 4	*Repeat 12 powders of August 4.*
Oct 28	Hirudines x ?humeri	*Oct 28. [Apply] ten leeches to the ?shoulder.*
	Continue medicament	*Continue medicine.*
Nov 1	Perstet	*Nov 1. Continue.*
4	To have meat every day	*Nov 4. To have meat every day.*
6	Applicetur Emplast Lyttæ post aurem	*Nov 6. Let a Cantharides Plaster be applied* *behind the ear.*
	℞ Morphiæ Chlorid gr ¼ ft pulv cum quo curitur vesicatio	*Take ¼ grain Morphine Chloride.* *Make a powder with which treat* *the blister.*
20^t	Better Perstet	*Nov 20. Better. Continue.*
Nov 22	Perstet	*Nov 22. Continue.*
25	Perstet	*Nov 25. Continue.*
Dec 10	Discharged cured	*Dec 10. Discharged cured.*

[p.46, *blank*]

---

61 Six fluid ounces.

[p.47]

Susan Warren [*age*] (15)

[*Susan was an inpatient from 31 July to 9 October 1839; she then became an outpatient until 18 February 1840 when she was readmitted. During her stay in hospital some forty-four pints of fluid were withdrawn from her abdomen by paracentesis;[62] drugs were also prescribed in an attempt to remove excess fluid. These included elaterium, broom tops, squill, mercury and potassium acetate. Jalap and gamboge were given as purgatives and ten ounces of blood were removed by venesection. This patient almost certainly had cancer of the ovary and one suspects that she died on her second admission to hospital. Towards the end she was given tincture of opium.*]

1839	Disease of ?Ovarium	1839 Disease of Ovary.
Julii 31	℞ ??Sol Iodinii (No 1) Oi 1/6 ter in die	July 31. Take 1 pint Solution of Iodine (No 1).[63] A sixth part three times a day.
Aug^ti ii	Potass bitart ʒi ft pulv ter die sumend	Aug 2. 1 drachm Potassium Bitartrate. Make a powder. To be taken three times a day.
4	urine sp grav 31	Aug 4. urine, specific gravity 31.
14	sp gravity 27 No precipitate	Aug 14. Specific gravity 27. No precipitate.
	perstet in usu medicamentorum	Continue in use of medicines.
16	Complains of intermitting pain in the back and abdomen	Aug 16. Complains of intermitting pain in the back and abdomen.
20	Circumference 2 inches above umbilicus 38$^{7/8}$ in	Aug 20. Circumference 2 inches above umbilicus 38 and seven eighth inches.
21	℞ Ext Elaterii gr i Ex Gentiæ C gr v ft pil s s	Aug 21. Take 1 grain Extract of Elaterium,[64] 5 grains Compound Extract of Gentian. Make a pill. To be taken immediately.
	℞ Decoct Scoparii ℔i Sp Æther Nit ʒvi Tinct Scillæ ʒiv mf mist sum^t coch larg iii 4^tis horis	Take 1 pound Decoction of Broom Tops, 6 drachms Spirit of Nitrous Ether, 4 drachms Tincture of Squill. Mix. Make a mixture. Let her take three tablespoonfuls every 4 hours.
23	℞ Pulv Jalap C ʒſs	Aug 23. Take ½ drachm Compound Jalap Powder.
	ft pulv cras mane sumend	Make a powder. To be taken tomorrow morning.

---

[62] Paracentesis is the removal of fluid from some part of the body. In this case a spiked metal trocar with surrounding metal tube would be inserted into the abdomen. The spiked element of the instrument would be withdrawn and the fluid allowed to drain through the retained tube, which would itself be removed when drainage was complete. This would have been a painful procedure without local anæsthesia.

[63] The hospital presumably had standard formulæ for differing strengths of iodine solutions.

[64] Also known as wild cucumber.

25	Rep^r Pulv Jalap C ℨſs cras mane	*Aug 25. Repeat ½ drachm Jalap Powder tomorrow morning.*
26	Circumference 40½ inches rep pulv J	*Aug 26. Circumference 40½ inches. Repeat Jalap Powder.*
28	Rep Pulv hodie et cras in dosi ʒi	*Aug 28. Repeat the powder in dose of 1 drachm today and tomorrow.*
30	℞ Pil Cambog C no ii nocte	*Aug 30. [Take] 2 Compound Pills of Gamboge at night.*
	℞ Potass Bitart oz ſs cras mane	*Take ½ ounce of Potassium Bitartrate tomorrow morning.*
Sept^i 1	Perstet	*September 1. Continue.*
4	℞ ~~Infus Digital ʒ ivſs~~	*Sept 14. Take ~~Infusion of Digitalis 4½ ounces~~*
	℞ ~~Liq Potass ʒiſs~~ Decot Scoparii ℔i Tinct Scillæ ʒiv mf mist sum^t ut antea	*~~Take 1½ ounces Solution of Potassium~~ 1 pound Decoction of Broom Tops, 4 drachms Tincture of Squill. Mix. Make a mixture. Let it be taken as before.*
	℞ Potass Supertart ℥ii	*Take 2 ounces of Potassium Supertartrate.*
	℞ Pil Hyd Ɵi Pil Scillæ C ʒſs Ɵii mf pil xii sum^t ii o n h s s	*Take 1 scruple Mercury Pill, ~~½ drachm~~ 2 scruples Compound Squill Pill. Mix. Make 12 pills. Let two be taken at bedtime.*

[p.48]

Sep 16	V S ad ℥ x	*Sept 16. Venesection up to 12 ounces of blood withdrawn.*
18	Circumference 41 inches	*Sept 18. Circumference 41 inches.*
20	℞ [sic]	*Sept 20. Take.*
Oct 4	Circumference 42 36 Paracentisis [sic] abdominis evacuatio liquidi Oxix	*Oct 4. Circumference 42, 36 [inches][65] Paracentesis of the abdomen, removal of 19 pints of fluid.*
	℞ [sic] Perstet in usu misturæ cujus singulis ℥xvi adde Potass Bitart ʒiii	*Continue in use of mixture of which to each 16 ounces add 3 drachms of Potassium Bitartrate.*
Oct 9	Circumference 32 inches To be an out patient Circumference 37 [inches]	*Oct 9. Circumference 32 inches. To be an outpatient. Circumference 37 [inches].*
1840 Feb 18	Readmitted	*1840 Feb 18. Readmitted.*

---

65 The two figures represent the measurements before and after the fluid was withdrawn.

22	℞ Mist Acaciæ ʒiʃs	*Feb 22. Take 1½ ounces Acacia mixture,*
	Oxymel Scillæ ʒiii	*3 drachms Oxymel of Squill,*
	Tinct Opii ʒi	*1 drachm Tincture of Opium,*
	Mist Camph ʒviʃs	*6½ ounces Camphor Mixture.*
	m cochlear i magn 4ᵗⁱˢ	*Mix. One tablespoonful [to be taken] every 4*
	horis	*hours.*
26	Circumference 45½ inches	*Feb 26. Circumference 45½ inches*
	after paracentisis	*after paracentisis.*
	twenty four pints	*Twenty four pints of*
	of fluid drawn off	*fluid drawn off.*
	℞ Pil Hydrarg ʒii	*Take 2 drachms Mercury Pill,*
	Pilulæ Scillæ ʒi	*1 drachm Squill pill,*
	Digitalis contrit gr xii M	*12 grains pounded Digitalis. Mix.*
	divide in pil xxiv	*Divide into 24 pills.*
	sumantur ii i 4ᵗⁱˢ horis	*Let ~~two~~ one to be taken every 4 hours.*
	℞ Potass Acetatis ʒi	*Take 1 ounce Potassium acetate,*
	Decoct Scoparii ʒviii	*8 ounces Decoction of Broom Tops.*
	cochlear iii magna	*Three tablespoonfuls [to be taken] every 4*
	horis	*hours.*
27	Comfortable, pulse 100	*Feb 2. Comfortable, pulse 100.*
March 2	P 100 Kidneys act well [*illeg.*]	*Mar 2. Pulse 100. Kidneys act well [illeg.].*
	Perstet.	*Continue.*
4	tumour (ovarian?) again	*Mar 4. (ovarian?) tumour again*
	distinctly felt. Perstet	*distinctly felt. Continue.*

[p.49]

Eliz Mathews [*age not recorded*]

[*Stutter did not write down any diagnosis, and little indication of it can be gained from the drugs given during her stay. On admission, asafoetida mixture and iron pills were prescribed, followed ten days later by a pain relieving liniment of soap, opium and colchicum. Her treatment was completed with laxatives, namely mercury compound pills and decoction of aloes.*]

1839

History [*blank*]

July 31	Mist Assafoetid ℔i	*July 31. 1 pound Asafoetida Mixture.*
	sumᵗ coch larg iii	*Let her take three tablespoonfuls*
	ter die	*three times a day.*
	℞ Pil Ferr C no xxiv	*Take Compound Iron Pills 24 in number.*
	sumt ii c sing	*Let her take two with each*
	dosis mist	*dose of mixture.*
Aug 10	Tinct Colchici ʒii	*Aug 10. 2 ounces Tincture of Colchicum,*
	– Opii ʒi	*1 ounce Tincture of Opium,*
	Lin Saponi C ʒiii	*3 ounces Compound Soap Liniment.*
	mf liniment utend	*Mix. Make a liniment, to be used*
	ter die	*three times a day.*

25	Ŗ Ext Col C gr v	*Aug 25. Take 5 grains Compound Extract of Colocynth,*
	Ext Hyos gr iv	*4 grains Extract of Henbane,*
	Hyd Chlorid gr iii M	*3 grains Mercurous chloride. Mix.*
	divide in pil ii cras mane	*Divide into pills. Two to be taken tomorrow*
	s^d	*morning.*
26	Ŗ Decoct Aloe C ʒiſs	*Aug 26. Take Compound Decoction of Aloes 1½ ounces.*
	omne mane sumnd	*To be taken each morning.*
Sep^ti 1	Perstet	*Sept 1. Continue.*
11	Perstet	*Sept 11. Continue.*
	To be out	*To be out [patient].*

[p.50]

Elizabeth Pawsey [*age*] (22)

[*Again there is no diagnosis for this patient. She received just three prescriptions during her stay in hospital; the mixture of morphine taken three times a day indicates that her condition was causing some pain. In common with the previous patient (Elizabeth Matthews) Elizabeth Pawsey was given iron pills and aloes decoction, a combination of drugs that Stutter seemed to use for young ladies with a diagnosis of anaemia.*]

[p.51][66]

History [*blank*]

Aug 20	Tinct Valerian ʒi	*Aug 20. 1 ounce Tincture of Valerian,*
	Solutio Morphiæ ʒiii	*3 drachms Morphine solution,*
	Mist Camphor ℔ ſs	*½ pound Camphor Mixture.*
	mf mist sum^t	*Mix. Make a mixture. To be taken in three large*
	larg [*sic*] iii ter die	*[spoonfuls] taken three times a day.*
	Common diet with ~~beer~~ porter[67]	*Common diet with ~~beer~~ porter.*
	Ŗ Pil Ferri C no	*Take Compound Iron Pills,*
	xxiv sum^t ii	*24 in number. Let two be taken*
	c sing dosis mist	*with each dose of mixture.*
25	Ŗ Decoct Aloes C	*Aug 25. Take Compound Decoction of Aloes.*
	ʒiſs singulis auroris	*1½ ounces each morning.*
Sep^ti 1	Continua	*Sept 1. Continue.*
11	Perstet	*Sept 11. Continue.*

---

66 A new layout appears on this page, with columns headed 'Treatment' and 'Diet'.
67 A heavy dark-brown beer brewed from browned or charred malt.

[p.52]

Minter Ling [*age*] (45)

[*The drugs prescribed appear to be directed to the relief of the stomach. Bismuth, hops and hydrocyanic acid were believed to reduce nausea caused by stomach problems. Nitric acid was frequently combined with hydrocyanic acid as in the prescription of 3 September. The pitch plaster with antimony would act as a counter-irritant, possibly to relieve severe dyspepsia or heartburn. All in all it sounds as if Minter had a peptic ulcer.*]

1839

1839

History

Aug 21 Has been complaining for 7 months of a fullness and uneasiness in the region of the stomach after foods with nausea, also of pain and numbness of legs and arms and says he has wasted much in his limbs; his appetite is bad and feels faint after eating. Tongue white and a little coated. P weak B regular

Aug 2. For the past seven months he has been complaining of nausea and a fullness and uneasiness in the region of the stomach after foods. He has also complained of pain and numbness of his legs and arms. He says he has become much wasted in his limbs. His appetite is bad and he feels faint after eating. The tongue is white and a little coated. Pulse weak. Bowels regular.

Aug 28   feels better

Aug 28. Feels better.

Sept 10   Made an out patient

Sept 10. Made an outpatient.

[p.53]

Aug 21   ℞ Oxyd Bismuth
Ext Humuli a a ℥i
mf pil xxiv
sumt ii ter die

Aug 21. Take 1 drachm each Bismuth oxide and Extract of Hops.
Mix. Make 24 pills.
Let him take two three times a day.

Common diet.

℞ Emp Picis C
Ant Tart gr iii
ft emp scorb cord[68]
To have porter
a pint and
meat daily

Take Compound Pitch Plaster,
3 grains Antimony Tartrate.
Make a plaster [for] the pit of the stomach.
To have porter
a pint and
meat daily.

Sep 3   ℞ Acid Hydrocyan gtt xxx
Acid Nitric D ℥ſs
Tinct Lupuli ℥i
Aq Puræ ℔i

Sept 3. Take 30 drops[69] Hydrocyanic Acid,[70]
½ ounce Dilute Nitric Acid,
1 ounce Tincture of Hops,
1 pound Pure Water.

---

[68] This is an abbreviation for *scrobiculum cordis*, 'The pit of the stomach called by some the heart pit, the word scrobiculum standing for a little pit or furrow': D. Turner, *The Art of Surgery*, vol. II, 1742.

[69] Drops were usually interpreted to be equivalent to minims and were measured using a small glass 'minim' measure.

[70] This would have been the dilute acid of the *London Pharmacopœia*, 1836.

mf mist sum^t	Mix. Make a mixture. Three tablespoonfuls [to
coch larg iii ter	be taken] three times
die	a day.

[p.54]

Charlotte Smith [age] (25)

[On her first day she was prescribed an ointment of antimony tartrate. This was sometimes used for ulcerated legs or applied to boils. At the same time Charlotte was given an iron mixture and pills of rhubarb, which were mildly laxative. Two months later she was prescribed powders containing mercury with chalk, ipecacuanha with opium (Dover's powder) and potassium nitrate. Dover's powder was much used in fevers and rheumatism.]

History [not written]

[p.55]

Aug 21	℞ Ung Ant Tart ʒi	Aug 21. Take 1 ounce Antimony Tartrate Ointment.
	utend omne nocte	To be used each night
	part affect	[on] the affected part.
	Common	Common [diet].
	℞ Mist Ferri Co	Take Compound Iron Mixture
	℔i	1 pound.
	sum^t coch larg ii	Let her take two tablespoonfuls
	ter die	three times a day.
	℞ Pil Rhei C	Take Compound Rhubarb Pills,[71]
	no xii	12 in number.
	sum^t ii o n	Let her take two every night.
Oct 26	℞	Oct 26. Take
	Hyd c Creta Ӡii	2 scruples Mercury with Chalk,
	Pulv Ipecac C ʒi	1 drachm Compound Ipecacuanha Powder,
	Potass Nitrat ʒiſs	1½ drachms Potassium Nitrate.
	mf pulv xii	Mix. Make 12 powders.
	sum^t i ter die	Let her take one three times a day.

[p.56]

Susan Welch [age] (18)

[This patient may have had fluid in the peritoneal cavity. Leeches, mercury liniment and a counter-irritant ointment of antimony were applied to the abdomen and its circumference was measured on two occasions. In addition she was prescribed squill, mercury and digitalis, presumably for their diuretic effect, plus two powerful purgatives (wild cucumber and croton oil) which would have caused copious liquid evacuations.]

History [not entered]

---

[71] Contained aloes and myrrh in addition to rhubarb; used as a laxative and for dyspepsia.

Circumference 2 inches about the umbilicus
34½ in [*this is opposite entry for 23 August
on facing right-hand page – p.57*]

[p.57]   [*Susan Welch, continued*]

		Common	*Common [diet]*
Aug 21	℞ Ext. Elaterii gr ſs		*Aug 21. Take ½ grain Extract of Wild Cucumber,*
	Ext. Gentian gr v		*5 grains Extract of Gentian.*
	ft pil cras mane		*Make a pill. [To be taken] tomorrow morning.*

℞ Ferri Potassio Tart gr xv — *Take 15 grains Iron and Potassium Tartrate,*
Potass Bitrat [*sic*] ʒſs — *½ drachm Potassium Bitartrate,[72]*
Pulv Zing gr v — *5 grains Ginger Powder.*
ft pulv sum^t — *Make powders. Let her take*
i ter die Mitte xii — *one three times a day. Send 12.*

℞ Liniment Hydrarg — *Take Compound Liniment of Mercury*
C ʒi — *1 ounce.*
utend abdomi — *To be used on the abdomen*
bis die — *twice a day.*

23   ℞ P̶i̶l̶ Ext Col C — *Aug 23. Take P̶i̶l̶l̶ Extract of Colocynth*
gr v Ol Croton ℥ i — *5 grains, 1 minim Croton Oil.*
ft pilula cras — *Make a pill. To be taken*
mane sumenda — *tomorrow morning.*

continuentur pulveres — *Continue [to take] powders.*

25   Pulv Jalap C — *Aug 25. Take Compound Jalap Powder*
ʒi — *1 drachm.*
s s — *To be taken immediately.*

26   ℞ Pulv Jalap — *Aug 26. Take Jalap Powder,*
Potass Bitart — *Potassium Bitartrate,*
Sodie Sesquicarb sing ʒi — *Sodium Bicarbonate each 1 drachm.*
Ipecac contrit gr i M — *1 grain Ipecacuanha, pounded. Mix.*
ft pulv st. s — *Make powders. To be taken immediately*
et rep^t 4^tis horis — *and repeat four hourly*
si opus sit — *if necessary.*
Mitte viii — *Send 8 [powders].*

30   Applicentur Hirud — *Aug 3. Let 12 leeches be applied*
xii abdomini — *to the abdomen.*

℞ Pil Cambog C gr x — *Take 10 grains Compound Gamboge Pill,*
Hyd Chlorid gr iii M — *3 grains Mercurous chloride. Mix.*
divide in pil — *Divide into pills.*
ii n s. — *Two to be taken at night.*

℞ Potass bitart — *Take ½ ounce Potassium Bitartrate,*
ʒſs cras mane — *to be taken tomorrow morning*
sumend in elect — *in an electuary.*

---

[72] Commonly known as cream of tartar.

| Sep^{ti} 1 | Perstet | *Sept 1. Continue.* |

| 4 | Rep pil ii h s s | *Sept 4. Repeat pills take 2 at night.* |

| 6 | Rep pulv cras m | *Sept 6. Repeat powder tomorrow morning.* |

[p.58]   [*Susan Welch, continued*]

| Sept 9 | Circumference 34 ¼ inches | *Sept 9. Circumference 34¼ inches* |

[p.59]

Sept 6	R℥	*Sept 6. Take*
	Pil Hydrarg Əi	*1 scruple Mercury Pill,*
	Pulv Digit gr vi	*6 grains Digitalis Powder,*
	Pil Scillæ C gr ʒ ʃs⁷³	*½ drachm Compound Squill Pill.*
	mf pil xii sum^t	*Mix. Make 12 pills. Let her take*
	~~ii~~ i ter die	*~~two~~ one three times a day.*
	rep pil aper	*Repeat aperient pills.*
	rep pulv c m	*Repeat powder with m[ixture].*
	rep liniment	*Repeat liniment.*

9	R℥ Ung Ant Pot	*Sept 9. Take 1 ounce Antimony and Potassium*
	Tart ʒi Ol Crot	*Tartrate Ointment,*
	onis ʒi ~~M~~ ft	*1 drachm Croton Oil. ~~Mix.~~ Make*
	Ung abdomini	*an ointment*
	applicand omni nocte	*to be applied to the abdomen each night.*

| 11 | Perstet | *Sept 11. Continue.* |

27	R℥ Sp. Æther Nit ʒiʃs	*Sept 27. Take 1½ drachms Nitrous Ether Spirit,*
	Potass Nit Əii	*2 scruples Potassium Nitrate,*
	Tinct Hyos ʒiʃs	*1½ drachms Tincture of Henbane,*
	Aquæ ʒviiʃs	*7½ ounces Water.*
	cochlear ii magn	*Two tablespoonfuls to be taken*
	4^{tis} horis sd	*every four hours.*

30	Perstet in usu unguenti	*Sept 30. Continue in use of the ointment*
	R℥ Hyd Chlorid gr ~~iii~~ vi	*Take ~~3~~ 6 grains Mercurous Chloride,*
	Ant Potass Tart gr i	*1 grain Antimony and Potassium Tartrate,*
	Pulv Opii gr iʃs M	*1½ grains Opium Powder. Mix.*
	divide in pulveris xii	*Divide into 12 powders.*
	i 4^{tis} horis sd	*One to be taken every 4 hours.*

Oct 4	R℥ Misturæ Efer	*Oct 4. Take 16 ounces*
	vescentis a a ʒxvi	*Effervescent Mixtures,*⁷⁴
	4^{tis} horis sumend	*[A dose] to be taken every four hours.*

---

73   Stutter appears to have changed the dosage of this powder inserting ʒʃs (half a drachm) over the number of grains originally entered and forgetting to delete the 'gr'.

74   Consisted of two mixtures, one containing an alkali, usually sodium bicarbonate, and the other an acid such as tartaric or citric. The patient mixed a dose of each in a suitable glass and drank the resulting effervescent liquid. The popular Seidlitz powders had the same dry ingredients wrapped individually in

| 14 | Perstet | *Oct 14. Continue.* |
| 23 | Perstet | *Oct 23. Continue* |

[p.60]

Esther Isaacson [*age*] (19)

[*This patient was discharged cured after treatment by venesection,*[75] *wet cupping,*[76] *purging, and the prescription of a mixture of nitric ether spirit with nitrate of potassium. The latter combination was often used in fevers (as was bloodletting in all its forms) but the only recorded evidence that the patient might have been feverish is a rather rapid pulse rate of 100 per minute. Purging was achieved with a domestic purge (probably containing senna), and pills of jalap and calomel. It was obviously successful. On 11 October 1839, Stutter reported that her bowels had been opened and that she felt better, so Esther was allowed to get up. It is difficult to make a modern diagnosis, but because the patient seemed to recover quite quickly it may be that her main problem was back pain and sciatica, in which case the rest from work would probably have done more good than anything else.*]

Oct 2

History

Was taken six months ago with pain and numbness of left foot ~~extending gradually to the hip & across the loins~~ which, after a time was transferred to the right hip and across the lower part of the loins. Great tenderness about the 3rd and 4th dorsal vertebrae and also when the Head of the Femur is pressed against the acetabulum or when the joint is jarred in any way, is not regular being so every fortnight or three weeks but not so much as ought to be. She suffer [*sic*] great pain at that time, ~~has~~ complains of constant pain and giddiness in the head, is a very robust florid girl, P 100 small ~~but~~ tongue coated and red at tip. Bowels costive. Has been able to remain in service till within a week, has been subject to repeated and copious attacks of epistaxis. Her menstrual periods do not occur at times for six weeks – has not had any Epistaxis for the last 12 months during which time the menstrual discharge has diminished in quantity. Complains of tenderness on percussion over the left subclavicular region.

Six months ago she was taken with pain and numbness of the left foot, which after a time was transferred to the right hip and across the lower part of the loins. Great tenderness about the 3rd and 4th dorsal vertebrae and also when the head of the femur is pressed against the acetabulum, or when the joint is jarred in any way. Is not regular, being so every fortnight or three weeks, but not so much as ought to be. She suffers great pain at that time. [The patient] complains of constant pain and giddiness in the head. [She is] a very robust, florid girl. Pulse [rate] 100 [per minute] – small. The tongue is coated and red at the tip. Her bowels are costive. [She] has been able to remain in service up until a week ago. [She] has been subject to repeated and copious attacks of epistaxis.[77] *Her menstrual periods do not occur at times for six weeks. [She] has not had any epistaxes for the last 12 months, during which time the menstrual discharge has diminished in quantity. [She] complains of tenderness on percussion over the left subclavicular region.*[78]

---

white and blue papers. When required, the patient stirred one of each powder into a tumbler of water. See Appendix V.

[75] Venesection is the opening of a vein to release blood. See Appendix IV.

[76] For wet cupping, see Appendix IV.

[77] Epistaxis means nose bleeding.

[78] The region of the chest just below the left collar-bone.

Oct 4 Feels much the same
9 P....taken unwell today
11 P 80 bowels opened. Says she feels
better, allowed to get up this afternoon

22 Discharged cured

[p.61]

1839
Date

Oct 2

V S ad ℥ xv
hodie applicentur
curcurbitulæ cruentae cras
et distrahantur sanguinis ℥xii
e lumbis loco dolenti

Common

℞ Ext Jalapæ gr vii
Hyd Chloridi gr v
ft pilulæ duæ
st sumenda

℞ mist purgantis
domestice ℥iʃs horis
4 post pilulas sdæ
si opus

℞ Sp Æther Nit ʒiʃs
Potass Nit ℈ii
Aque ℥viii M
cochlear ii magna
4ᵗⁱˢ horis

4   Perstet in usu misturæ

        Rep pilulæ
        nocti sumend

9   Perstet

11   Perstet

14   Perstet in usu
        misturæ

        Dismissed cured

Oct 4. Feels much the same.
Oct 9. P[ulse] [not given]. Taken unwell today.
Oct 11. P[ulse rate] 80 [per minute]. Bowels
opened. Says she feels better, [so] allowed to get
up this afternoon.
Oct 22. Discharged cured.

Oct 2.
Venesection, 15 ounces [of blood] withdrawn
today.
Let cupping glasses be applied tomorrow
and withdraw 12 ounces of blood
from the painful area of the back.

Common [diet].

Take 7 grains Extract of Jalap,,
5 grains Mercurous Chloride.
Make two pills.
To be taken immediately.

Take 1½ ounces domestic purging mixture.
To be taken 4 hours
after the pills
if required.

Take 1½ drachms Spirit of Nitrous Ether,
2 scruples Potassium Nitrate,
8 ounces Water. Mix.
Two tablespoonfuls [to be taken]
every 4 hours.

Oct 4. Continue in use of the mixtures.

Repeat the pills,
to be taken at night.

Oct 9. Continue.

Oct 11. Continue.

Oct 14. Continue in use
of the mixture.

Dismissed cured.

[p.62]

Ann Copping [*age*] 30

[*Ann is one of the few patients who were not given any laxative medicine. On admission Stutter noted that her bowels were open. Later during her stay in hospital he gave her a mixture of chalk and opium, which suggests that she might have had diarrhoea. An analgesic liniment containing opium was used each evening, presumably being applied for the abdominal pain that was troubling her. The history tells us that she had had no menstrual discharge. This might be because she was anaemic and thus the administration of iron would be logical, but it seems strange that both powders and pills containing iron were considered necessary. The vomiting of blood and the tenderness over the stomach suggests a possible gastric ulcer. The dark stools may also have been due to bleeding into the gut from such an ulcer. Whatever the diagnosis, the treatment seems to have been successful because the patient was discharged 'cured'.*]

1837 [*sic*] Nov[r] 13 Has enjoyed good health till her present illness which commenced about three months ago by a pain in the abdomen. Has been married 12 years, has had five children all of which died within four months. The last born 12 months ago, died at the end of a fortnight. Her menses were regular from the period of her last confinement till her present illness since when she has had no menstrual discharge. Has no suspicion of being enceinte.[79] Comitenamo pale with a tinge of yellow tongue coated slightly. P. 72 without much volume. Bowels open, motions dark coloured, some tenseness and fullness of the abdomen. Has had ascites and anasarca. Makes a great deal of water, has had hemitemisis [*sic*] at the same time as great tenderness in the epigastrium.

1839 Nov 13. [She] has enjoyed good health till the present illness, which commenced about three months ago with a pain in the abdomen. [She] has been married [for] 12 years [and] has had five children, all of [whom] died within four months [of birth]. The last, born 12 months ago, died at the end of a fortnight.[80] Her menses were regular from the time of her last confinement till her present illness [started], since when she has had no menstrual discharge. [She] has no suspicion of being [pregnant]. Countenance pale with a tinge of yellow. Tongue coated slightly. Pulse [rate] 72 [per minute] without much volume. Bowels open. Motions dark coloured. Some tenseness and fullness of the abdomen. Has had ascites[81] and anasarca.[82] She makes a great deal of water. [She] has had haematemesis[83] at the same time as great tenderness in the epigastrium.[84]

[p.63]

Married

Married

Nov[r] 13.   ℞ Ferri Tart gr viii
        Pulv Cinnam C gr ii
        ft pulv ter in die
        sumend Mitte xii

To have meat daily

Nov 13. Take 8 grains Iron Tartrate,
2 grains Compound Cinnamon Powder.
Make powders. [One] to be taken three times a day. Send 12.

To have meat daily.

---

[79] Pregnant (French).
[80] A disastrous obstetric history.
[81] Ascites is a collection of fluid in the abdominal cavity.
[82] Dropsy is a collection of fluid in the tissues of the lower limbs.
[83] Haematemesis means the vomiting of blood.
[84] Epigastrium is that part of the abdomen immediately over the stomach.

	℞ misturæ et pulveram effervesc entium dos vi capiatur dos i ter in die	*Take 6 doses of* *effervescent mixture and powders.* *One dose to be taken* *three times a day.*
Novr 15	Omitte pulveres	*Nov 15. Leave off the powders.*
	℞ Pil Ferri C ʒi divide in pil xii quarum sumantur duæ ter in die	*Take 1 drachm Compound Iron Pill.* *Divide into 12 pills.* *Of which two to be taken three times a day.*
20	Perstet	*Nov 20. Continue.*
	℞ Liniment Sapon ʒii Tinct Opii ʒii ft liniment omni vespere applicand	*Take 2 ounces Soap Liniment,* *2 drachms Tincture of Opium.* *Make a liniment.* *To be applied every evening.*
22	Perstet	*Nov 22. Continue.*
24	℞ Mist Cretæ ʒviii Tinct Opii ʒſs	*Nov 24. Take 8 ounces Chalk Mixture,* *½ drachm Tincture of Opium.*[85]
25	Perstet	*Nov 25. Continue.*
Decr 17	Discharged cured	*Dec 17. Discharged cured.*

[p.64]

Susan Sharpe [*age*] (18)

[*The only medication Susan received was a mixture containing iron. This was probably very appropriate since her pale colour, absent periods and carotid murmurs certainly suggest a diagnosis of anaemia. The iron, coupled with a full diet, porter to drink and a few weeks off work seem to have effected a cure. The symptom of early morning sickness would suggest the possibility of pregnancy to most people, but Stutter does not seem to have entertained this thought.*]

1839
History

Has been out of health a year and a half and has been a servant to a washerwoman, having a hard place. Never been regular, but complains of pain in head and loins at stated periods feels very weak, and pain in side; her ancles swell towards night. B. regular. T. pale and clean. P. 80, weak. Generally feels sick in the morning, no appetite, looks very pale and lips whitish. Her catameniae have never appeared. Bellows

History

Has been out of Health a year and a half. [She] has been a servant to a washerwoman, having a hard place [of work]. [Her periods] have never been regular but [she] complains of pain in head and loins at [the] stated periods. [She] feels very weak, and [has this] pain in [her] side. Her ankles swell towards night. Bowels regular. Tongue pale and clean. Pulse [rate] 80 [per minute]. [It is] weak. [She] generally feels sick in the morning [and has] no appetite. Looks very pale [with] whitish lips. Her

---

85 No dose was indicated for this mixture.

sound in the carotids, on both sides very marked. Slightly so in the heart. Complains of appetite being capricious.

catameniae[86] have never appeared. [There is a] bellows sound in the carotids on both sides [which is] very marked. Slightly so in the heart.[87] [She] complains of [her] appetite being capricious.

Oct 11 Feels better, colour rather improved

Oct 11. Feels better. Colour rather improved.

Oct 14 P.96 complains of headache

Oct 14. P [pulse rate] 96 [per minute]. Complains of a headache.

[p. 65]

Oct 2

Full diet with beer

Oct 2.

Full diet with beer

R̷
Misturæ Ferri C
℥viii ℥xvi
cochlear iii ii magna
capiantur ter in die

Take
8 ounces 16 ounces
Compound Iron Mixture.
Let three two tablespoonfuls.
be taken three times a day.

Common [diet] with meat daily and beer

Common [diet] with meat daily and beer.

5   Perstet

Oct 5. Continue.

11   Perstet 1 pint of Porter

Oct 11. Continue. 1 pint of Porter

14   Perstet omit the porter

Oct 14. Continue, leave off the porter.

21   Perstet

Oct 21. Continue.

23   Perstet

Oct 23. Continue.

28   Perstet

Oct 28. Continue.

Nov 1   Perstet To have a pint of porter

Nov 1. Continue. To have a pint of porter.

25   Discharged cured

Nov 25. Discharged cured.

[p.66]

Kezia Atkins [age] 20

[In the nineteenth century it was considered that galbanum was useful in the treatment of hysteria,[88] particularly when the mental problems were accompanied by amenorrhoea.[89] The first prescription the patient received was for pills containing galbanum and iron, the latter substance frequently being used when young ladies had deficient or absent menstrual periods. Spirits of sulphuric ether and of ammonia with asafoetida were also commonly recommended for hysteria, and Kezia was given mixtures containing both these substances. Mixtures of the bitter tonics, gentian and chiretta were prescribed, presumably in an attempt to improve Kezia's appetite. Pains in her side and elsewhere were treated by the application of

---

86   Catamenia is menstrual discharge.
87   The patient could have had rheumatic heart disease or severe anaemia.
88   For a discussion of hysteria see Appendix II.
89   Amenorrhoea – the absence of menstrual periods.

leeches, plasters of galbanum and of cantharides as well as liniments of camphor or of ammonia and opium. Although the notes indicate that this patient was not constipated, she was given several doses of castor oil as well as aperient pills and an electuary of senna. The combination of acacia, ipecacuanha, camphor and poppy syrup was a traditional formula used in the making of cough mixtures.]

Nov 15 Has enjoyed good health till about twelve months ago when in consequence of a fright she had an attack of hysteria, to which she has been occasionally subject since that time. Her menses have been very irregular in frequency and quantity, began to appear a little after she was thirteen – subject at times to fainting fits. For the last three months she has had pain in the side and elsewhere with swelling of the legs towards night – has not had any menstrual discharge for the last four months. No emaciation, colour not leucophegmatic, bowels are open – pulse 88, ?small. No anormal [*sic*] sound at the heart or in the carotids, tongue clean and moist. Appetite bad, digestion not good.

Nov 15. Enjoyed good health till about twelve months ago when in consequence of a fright she had an attack of hysteria, to which she has been occasionally subject since that time. Her menses have been very irregular in frequency and quantity. [They] began to appear a little after she was thirteen. [She is] subject at times to fainting fits. For the last three months she has had pain in the side and elsewhere with swelling of the legs towards night. [She] has not had any menstrual discharge for the last four months. No emaciation. Colour not leucophegmatic.[90] [Her] bowels are open. Pulse [rate] 88 [per minute], [and of] small [volume]. No abnormal sound at the heart or in the carotids. Tongue clean and moist. Appetite bad. Digestion [poor].

[p.67]

Nov ʳ 15	℞ Pil Ferri C Pil Galbani C a a ℈i M divide in pil xxiv quarum sumantur duæ ter in die	*Nov 15. Take Compound Iron and Compound Galbanum Pills,* *1 drachm of each. Mix.* *Divide into 24 pills,* *of which let two be taken* *three times a day.*
	To have meat every day with beer.	*To have meat every day with beer.*
	℞ Mist Gentian C ℥viii sumantur cochlear iii magna omni mane	*Take 8 ounces Compound Gentian Mixture.* *Let three tablespoonfuls be taken* *each morning.*
20	Repʳ mistura adde Ammon sesquicarb gr xxiv	*Nov 20. Repeat the mixture.* *Add 24 grains of Ammonium Bicarbonate.*
	Repʳ pilulæ	*Repeat the pills.*
22	Applica Emplast Galbani C lateri	*Nov 22. Apply a Compound Galbanum* *Plaster to the side.*
24	℞ Mist Aper ℥iſs	*Nov 24. Take 1½ ounces Aperient Mixture.*
25	Perstet	*Nov 25. Continue.*
27	Perstet	*Nov 27. Continue.*

---

90 Leucophlegmatic means 'having a dropsical tendency' – *OED*.

5. Typical pages from the casebook (pp. 66 and 67) showing Kezia Atkins' medical history on the left and the medicines prescribed for her on the right.

	R̵ Decoct Aloes ʒvi	*Take 6 ounces Decoction of Aloes.*
	cochlear iii magna	*Three tablespoonfuls [to be taken]*
	alternis auroris	*every other morning.*
28	R̵ Sp Æther S C ℈xl	*Nov 28. Take 40 minims Compound Spirit of Sulphuric Ether,*
	Tinct Opii ℈x	*10 minims Tincture of Opium,*
	Mist Camphor ʒifs	*1½ ounces Camphor Mixture.[91]*
29	R̵ Pil Aper C ii	*Nov 29. Take two Compound Aperient Pills.*
	R̵ Olii Ricini ʒifs	*Take 1½ ounces Castor Oil.*

[91] Presumably this was a single-dose draught.

	℞ Sp Ammon Fetid ʒii Sp Æther S C ʒiʃs Mist Camphor ʒviii cochlea ii magna ter in die	*Take 2 drachms of Foetid Spirit of Ammonia,*[92] *1½ drachms Compound Spirit of Sulphuric Ether,* *8 ounces Camphor Mixture.* *Two tablespoonfuls [to be taken] three times* *a day.*
Decr 2	℞ Ol Ricini ʒi	*Dec 2. Take 1 ounce Castor Oil.*
	℞ Liniment Camphor C ʒiʃs abdomini infricand	*Take Compound Camphor Liniment* *1½ ounces.* *Rub on the abdomen.*
	Rep^r mistura	*Repeat the mixture.*
Dec 8	Applica Hirudines viii abdomini	*Dec 8. Apply 8 leeches* *to the abdomen.*
	℞ Ol Ricini ʒʃs 4^{tis} horis donec alvus responderit	*Take ½ ounce Castor Oil.* *[Give] every 4 hours until* *the bowels respond.*
11	Omitte Decoct Aloes	*Dec 11. Leave off the Decoction of Aloes.*
	Rep^r Ol Ricini omni mane	*Repeat the Castor Oil each morning.*
16	℞ Liq Potass ♏ xl Infus Chirettæ ʒiv Aqua Menth ʒiv M cochlear ii magna ter in die	*Take 40 minims Solution of Potassium,* *4 ounces Infusion of Chiretta,* *4 ounces Peppermint Water. Mix.* *Two tablespoonfuls [to be taken] three times a* *day.*
Dec 16	℞ Pil Aper C ii o n	*Dec 16. Take two Compound Aperient Pills at* *night.*
21	℞ Liq Amm ʒiii Tinct Opii ʒʃs Lin Sapon ʒvi Mf Lin utend freq ?fauci	*Dec 21. Take 3 drachms Solution of Ammonia,* *½ ounce Tincture of Opium,* *6 ounces Soap Liniment. Mix. Make* *a liniment [to be applied] frequently to the* *?throat.*[93]

[*The above two prescriptions were written at the bottom of the previous page, i.e. page 66.*]

[*Prescriptions for this patient continue on page 91 but for clarity are entered below.*]

[p. 91]

	Kesia [sic] Atkins from page 66	*Kesia [sic] Atkins from page 66.*
Dec ^r 23	℞ Ferri Sesquioxyd ʒi Confect Sennæ ʒiʃs M	*Dec 23. Take 1 ounce Iron Oxide,* *1½ ounces Confection of Senna. Mix.*

---

92 This contained asafoetida in addition to the ammonia.
93 The liniment was applied externally to the throat (the anterior surface of the neck).

	ft elect cujus capiatur cochlear i parv ter in die	*Make an Electuary, of which let one teaspoonful be taken three times a day.*
27	Perstet	*Dec 27. Continue.*
30	Rep^r Empl Galban C	*Dec 30. Repeat the Compound Galbanum Plaster.*
Jan 12	℞ Mist Acaciæ ʒii Vin Ipecac ʒii Syr Papaver ʒſs Mist Camphor ʒiv cochlear i magnum M 3^{tiis} horis	*Jan 12. Take 2 ounces Acacia Mixture, 2 drachms Ipecacuanha Wine, ½ ounce Syrup of Poppies, 4 ounces Camphor Mixture. One tablespoonful [to be taken] every 3 hours.*
15	Omitte elect	*Jan 15. Leave off the Electuary.*
17	Applica Empl Lyttæ	*Jan 17. Apply a Plaster of Cantharides.*
	℞ Pil Aper fort ii nocte s^d	*Take two Strong Aperient Pills at night.*

[p.68]

Susan Plumbe [*age*] (19)

[*This patient almost certainly had rheumatic heart disease (see Appendix II) with what sounds like a leaky mitral[94] valve. She had a long stay in hospital. While she was an inpatient her drug regime included mixtures containing digitalis. This medicine, derived from the leaves of the humble foxglove, had been recognised for its beneficial effects in cardiac conditions since the eighteenth century. Susan suffered from palpitations, and it is probably for that reason that she was given hydrocyanic acid. Her periods seem to have been irregular, and so, knowing some of Stutter's prescribing habits, it is no surprise to see that iron, in the form of mixtures, powders and pills, appeared on her drug list. In order to keep the patient's bowels open, the following medicines were given – aperient powders and mixture, calomel and rhubarb powders, calomel and scammony powders, calomel and opium powders, mercury and jalap pills. When these failed a domestic enema was given. Mixtures containing potassium nitrate and spirit of nitric ether were often prescribed to reduce fever, whilst medicines containing ipecacuanha, opium and camphor were usually given to patients when they were suffering from a cough. Leeches may have been applied to the upper abdomen with the intention of relieving discomfort due to an engorged liver secondary to heart failure. More leeches were later placed on the lower abdomen. A blistering plaster and some antimony ointment (which were both counter-irritants), as well as a large poultice and mercury liniment were also used on the upper abdomen. Later in her stay she was given opium powders, presumably to reduce any pain she may have had and perhaps to ease her state of mind too. The general conclusion must be that this patient was very ill, and it is extremely unlikely that she would have lived very long.*]

---

[94] The mitral valve is situated on the left side of the heart. It is frequently affected in rheumatic heart disease. See Appendix II.

Octr 2 History
Nearly two years ago was taken with cold chills followed by fever and palpitation of the heart with pain. Was ~~not~~ never ~~regular~~ unwell until she has been ill half a year ago she was so but only two or three times since, feels pain in the head & side, feels pain and sickness after eating and feels relief immediately she vomits. P.130 weak. Tongue coated in centre & red at edges, tenderness of Epigastrium, B. open, has wasted very much the last three months. During her illness 2 years ago she was confined to bed for six months. Still subject to palpitations accompanied with pain in the region of the heart at intervals, which are always bro^t [sic] on by walking quickly. Dullness on percussion on the precordium extending from ½ an inch to the right of the miscal line of the sternum as far as the left nipple, very distinct and intense bellows sound in the region of the cartilage of the sixth rib which disappears towards the centre and apex of the heart, heart beats visibly to the eyes over the whole front of the chest.

Nearly two years ago [she] was taken with cold chills followed by fever and palpitation of the heart, with pain. [Her periods were regular until about half a year ago. She has only had them two or three times since.] [She] feels pain in the head and side, and has pain and sickness after eating. [She] feels relief immediately she vomits. P[ulse rate]130 [per minute] – weak. Tongue coated in centre and red at edges. Tenderness of epigastrium.[95] B[owels] open. Has wasted very much in the last three months. During her illness two years ago she was confined to bed for six months. Still subject to palpitations, accompanied [by] pain in the region of the heart at intervals, which are always brought on by walking quickly. Dullness on percussion [over] the precordium[96] extending from ½ an inch to the right of the miscal[97] line of the sternum as far as the left nipple, very distinct and intense bellows sound in the region of the cartilage of the sixth rib which disappears towards the centre and apex of the heart. [The] heart beats visibly to the eyes over the whole front of the chest.

Oct 4 Hearts action quieter, pulse 90. Had to take a dose of domestic aperient, after which bowels were twice relieved. Tongue cleaner.

Oct 4. Heart's action quieter, pulse [rate] 90 [per minute]. Had to take a dose of domestic aperient, after which bowels were twice relieved. Tongue cleaner.

11 P.80. Heart action quiet. No abnormal sound, impulse confined to its natural limits, bowels relieved after two doses of the aperient powder ordered on the 9th. 14 pulse 72, better.

Oct 11. Pulse [rate] 80 [per minute]. Heart is quiet. No abnormal sound, impulse confined to its natural limits, bowels relieved after two doses of aperient powder ordered on the 9th. Oct 14. Pulse [rate] 72 [per minute]. Better.

16 P. 64

Oct 16. [Pulse rate] 64 [per minute].

[p.69]

Oct 2   ℞ Mist Ferri C ℥viii
           Tinct Digitalis ʒiiʃs
           Mist Camph ℥viiʃs
           Tinct Hyos ʒiii M
           cochlear ii magna
           ter in die

Oct 2. Take 8 ounces Compound Iron Mixture, 2½ drachms Tincture of Digitalis, 7½ ounces Camphor Mixture, 3 drachms Tincture of Henbane. Mix. Two tablespoonfuls [to be taken] three times a day.

       [Diet] ~~Common~~ Full without beer

~~Common~~ Full diet without beer.

---

95   The epigastrium is that part of the abdomen immediately over the stomach.
96   The area in front of the heart.
97   The middle line of the sternum.

	℞ Hyd Chlorid gr iv Pulv Rhei gr x ft pulvis nocte sd M	*Take 4 grains Mercurous Chloride,* *10 grains Rhubarb Powder. Mix.* *Make a powder. To be taken at night.*
4	Perstet in usu misturæ	*Oct 4. Continue in use* *of the mixture.*
	℞ Ext Col C gr v Hyd Chlorid gr v M ft pil ii nocte s^d	*Take 5 grains Compound Extract of Colocynth,* *5 grains Mercurous Chloride,* *Mix. Make pills. Two to be taken at night.*
5	Omitte misturam interim ℞ Sp Æther Nit ℥ſs Tinct Digitalis ℥ii Tinct Hyoscam ℥ſs Misturæ Camph ℥viii xvi cochlear ii 4^tis horis	*Oct 5. Leave off the mixture.* *In the meantime,* *take ½ ounce Nitrous Ether Spirit,* *2 drachms Tincture of Digitalis, ½ ounce* *Tincture of Henbane.* *8 16 ounces Camphor mixture.* *Two spoonfuls[98] [to be taken] every four hours.*
Oct 9	℞ Hyd Chlorid gr ii Pulv Scam C gr x ft pulv s s	*Oct 9. Take 2 grains Mercurous Chloride,* *10 grains Compound Powder of Scammony.* *Make a powder. To be taken at once.*
11	℞ Tinct Digit ℥ii Tinct Hyoscyam ℥ſs Sodæ Carb ℥iſs Aq Puræ ℔i mf mist sum^t coch larg ii 4^tis hori^s c sequentis pulv	*Oct 11. Take 2 drachms Tincture of Digitalis,* *½ ounce Tincture of Henbane,* *1½ drachms Sodium Carbonate,* *1 pound Pure Water.* *Mix. Make a mixture. Let her take two* *tablespoonfuls every 4 hours* *with the following powder.*
	℞ Acid Tartar ℥iſs in pulv xxi	*Take 1½ drachms Tartaric Acid.* *[Divide into] 21 powders.[99]*
14	Perstet in usu potus effervescentis	*Oct 14. Continue in use* *of the effervescent drink.*
16	℞ Acid Hydrocyan gtt xxiv Mucilag Acac ℥i Aq Puræ ℔ſs mf mist sum^t coch larg iii 4^tis horis	*Oct 16. Take 24 drops Hydrocyanic Acid* *[Dilute],* *1 ounce Mucilage of Acacia,* *½ pound Pure Water.* *Mix. Make a mixture. Let her take* *three tablespoonfuls every 4 hours.*
	Omittat mist et pulv ut 9	*Leave off the mixture and powder of the 9th.*
18	℞ Hyd Chlorid gr vi Ant Tart gr i Pulv Opii gr iſs mf pulv vi sum^t i nocte et mane	*Oct 18. Take 6 grains Mercurous Chloride,* *1 grain Antimony Tartrate,* *1½ grains Opium Powder.* *Mix. Make 6 powders. Let her take one [each]* *night and morning.*

---

[98] The size of the spoonful was not recorded; it is probable that two tablespoonfuls were intended.
[99] The addition of the acid powder to the alkaline mixture would produce effervescence, and help to mask the unpleasant taste of the tinctures.

[p.71] [*This page was written before page 70. To maintain chronological sequence it has been printed before p.70.*]

Oct 21	Rep mist	*Oct 21. Repeat mixture.*
	rep pulv	*Repeat powder.*
	Hirudines vi epigast	*[Apply] 6 leeches to the epigastrium.*
23	Rep^r pulveres	*Oct 23. Repeat powders.*
	Rep^r mistura	*Repeat Mixture.*
	℞ Ung Ant Potass Tart ℨi	*Take 1 ounce Antimony and Potassium Tartrate ointment.*
	applicetur abdomini nocte maneque	*Let it be applied to the abdomen night and morning.*
Octr 31	Habeat Emplast Lyttæ regione epigastrico	*Oct 31. Let her have a Cantharides Plaster on the epigastric area.*
Novr 1	Perstet	*Nov 1. Continue.*
4	Perstet	*Nov 4. Continue.*
6	Sumatur pulv i o n	*Nov 6. Let her take one powder at night.*[100]
8	℞ Liniment Hydr ℨii utatur nocte maneque	*Nov 8. Take 2 ounces Mercury Liniment. Let it be used night and morning.*
	℞ Solutionis Morphii Chlor ʒii Mist camphor ℨviii sumantur cochlear ii magna ter in die	*Take 2 drachms Solution of Morphine Chloride, 8 ounces Camphor Mixture. Let her take two tablespoonfuls three times a day.*
	Omitte pulveres	*Leave off the powders.*
	℞ Ext Jalapæ Əii Pil Hyd Əi M divide in pil xii quarum sumantur duæ singulis noctibus	*Take 2 scruples Extract of Jalap, 1 scruple Mercury Pill. Mix. Divide into 12 pill, of which let her take two each night.*
15	Perstet	*Nov 15. Continue.*
20	Applica Hirudines vi epigastrio	*Nov 20. Apply 6 leeches to the epigastrium.*
	℞ Potass Nitratis Əii Tinct Hyocyam ʒii Sp Æther Nitrici ʒiiſs ~~Mist~~ Aquæ ℨviii M cochlear ii ter in die	*Take 2 scruples Potassium Nitrate, 2 drachms Tincture of Henbane, 2½ drachms Spirit of Nitrous Ether, 8 ounces ~~Mixture~~ Water. Mix. Two spoonfuls [to be taken] three times a day.*

[100] The powder originally prescribed on 18 October, the dose being reduced from night and morning to just one at night.

47

	Omitte Mist Morphii	*Leave off the morphine mixture.*
22	Perstet	*Nov 22. Continue.*
25	Applica Hirudines x hypogast habeat enema domesticam	*Nov 25. Apply 10 leeches to the hypogastrium.* *To have a domestic enema.*[101]
26	Cataplasma ?largina abdom	*Nov 26. [apply] a large poultice to the* *abdomen.*
27	Perstet	*Nov 27. Continue.*
29	Applica Hirudines x hodie et repetantur cras mane	*Nov 29. Apply 10 leeches* *today and repeat* *tomorrow morning.*
Decr 1	Rep^r Hirudines x	*Dec 1. Repeat 10 leeches.*
2	R Hydr Chlorid gr xxiv Pulv Opii gr ii M divide in pulv vi i 4^{tis} horis	*Take 24 grains Mercurous Chloride,* *2 grains Opium Powder. Mix.* *Divide into 6 powders.* *One [to be taken] every 4 hours.*
	R Haust aper cras mane	*Take Aperient Draught* *tomorrow morning.*

[*back to p.70*]

[p.70]

~~Oct 21~~	~~p96 sharpe tenderness in~~ ~~epigastrium~~ ~~a~~	*~~Oct 21. p[ulse] 96. Sharp tenderness in~~* *~~epigastric region.~~*
~~Nov~~		*~~Nov~~*
Decr 9	R Mist Alkal ℥xii Tinc Cinchon ʒi Pulv Acid[103] q s capiatur dosis in effevescentiæ 4^{tis} horis	*Dec 9. Take 12 ounces Alkaline Mixture,*[102] *1 drachm Tincture of Cinchona,* *A sufficient quantity of [?]Tartaric Acid.* *Let her take a dose whilst effervescing every 4* *hours.*
13	Omitte pulveres	*Dec 13. Leave off the powders.*
	R Liq Sodæ Chlor ʒii Aquæ ℥viii M ft gargarum sæpe utend	*Take 2 drachms Sodium Chloride Solution,* *8 ounces Water, Mix.* *Make a gargle, to be used frequently*
28	R Ferri Ammon Tart	*Dec 29. Take Iron and Ammonium Tartrate.*

---

[101] One or two tablespoonfuls of common salt dissolved in a pint of warm water.

[102] Probably a mixture containing sodium or potassium bicarbonate, which when the acid powder was added would have produced effervescence.

[103] The name of the acid is partially obliterated but is probably tartaric acid.

	ft pulv ter in die gr vi	*Make [into] powders of 6 grains. [One to be taken] three times a day.*
Jan 3	Omitte Pulv Ferri	*Jan 3. Leave off the Iron powders.*
16	℞ Sp Æther Nit ʒiii Vin Ipecac ʒi Tinct Opii ʒi Mist Camphor ℥viii cochlear ii magna 4ᵗⁱˢ horis	*Take 3 drachms Spirit of Nitrous Ether, 1 drachm Ipecacuanha Wine, 1 drachm Tincture of Opium, 8 ounces Camphor Mixture. Two tablespoonfuls [to be taken] every four hours.*
	Omitte alia	*Leave off the rest.*
23	Omitte misturam	*Jan 23. Leave off the mixture.*
	Repʳ Pulv Ferri	*Repeat the Iron Powders.*
~~Nov 11......P 88~~		~~*Nov 11. P[ulse] 88.*~~
Feb 7	℞ Pil Ferri C ʒiʃs Ext Colocynth C ʒʃs M	*Feb 7. Take 1½ drachms Iron Pill, ½ drachm Compound Extract of Colocynth, Mix.*
	ft [illeg.] in pil xxiv ii ter in die	*Make [illeg.] into 24 pills. Two [to be taken] three times a day.*

[p.72]

George Channell [age] (16)

[This patient had rheumatic pains in his hips, shoulders and knees. He was given one prescription only. This was a mixture of quinine (sometimes prescribed for rheumatism, but also used as a tonic) plus the laxative magnesium sulphate (Epsom salts) flavoured with infusion of rose petals. He was discharged cured after a relatively short stay in the ward. It sounds as if he had rheumatic fever (see Appendix II) and was in fact recovering when he was admitted to hospital.]

Has been a baker's boy for 2 years at Mildenhall, has been ill for six weeks, had good health previously at which period he was confined to bed for a week, with pain in the hips, knees and shoulders of rheumatic character. Was under medical treatment during that week, since which time he has been unable to work, has lost flesh considerably, his countenance is expressive of illness being pale, pain at present confined to left shoulder with pain occasionally in the left knee. T. slightly coated, large, & thick. Appetite good. B. regular. P. 72. Respiration normal.

He has been a baker's boy at Mildenhall for two years. He has been ill for six weeks [but] had good health previously. [Six weeks ago] he was confined to bed for a week with pain in the hips, knees and shoulders of rheumatic character. He was under medical treatment during that week. Since [then] he has been unable to work and has lost flesh considerably. His countenance is expressive of illness being pale. [The] pain [is] at present confined to [the] left shoulder with pain occasionally in the left knee. T[ongue] slightly coated, large and thick. Appetite good. B[owels] regular. P[ulse rate] 72 [per minute]. Respiration normal.

49

[p.73]

Oct 2	R̸ Quin Disulph gr viii Infusion Rosæ ℥ ʃs Magnes Sulp ʒi mf mist sum^t coch larg ii ter die	*Oct 2. Take 8 grains Quinine Disulphate,* *½ pound Infusion of Rose,* *1 ounce Magnesium Sulphate.*[104] *Mix. Make a mixture. Two tablespoonfuls to be* *taken three times a day·*
	Common diet with beer	*Common diet with beer.*
	Full diet	*Full diet.*
5	Perstet	*Oct 5. Continue.*
14	Perstet	*Oct 14. Continue.*
	Cured	*Cured.*

[p.74]

John Scott (Carpenter)
Ætatis 25 (Purpura urticans)

Age 25 with a diagnosis of purpura and urticaria.

[*John Scott was one of two patients for whom Stutter prescribed ergot. The treatment of purpura was not one of the main uses of ergot, but it was nevertheless sometimes employed as a remedy for that condition during the nineteenth century. The patient's other medications were quinine mixture, iron pills and laxatives in the form of calomel and colocynth pills, as well as draughts of senna. The modern diagnosis may have been simple urticaria (nettle rash) or more likely erythema multiforme (see Appendix II) which could well have followed the herpes infection.*]

Oct. 23 Fair complexion with ~~chestnut~~ auburn hair. Thin whiskers – has enjoyed good health until five weeks ago when he perceived that in the afternoons his legs ached, which encreased so much that he was obliged to take to his bed. At the same time he was affected with an eruption he described as resembling nettle rash followed by spots of purpura. Last Tuesday (9 days ago) week he describes that he had a dryness of the nostrils and cold in the head followed in two days by a copious efflorescence of the vesicles of herpes labialis round the lips and left nostril, at which time he felt feverish. On examination there is a copious efflorescence of spots of purpura on the legs and arms, from which the trunk is free, and on some portions of the

Oct. 23 [The patient has] a fair complexion with auburn hair and thin whiskers. [He] enjoyed good health until five weeks ago when he perceived that in the afternoons his legs ached. [This] increased so much that he was obliged to take to his bed. At the same time he was affected with an eruption he describes as resembling nettle rash followed by spots of purpura.[105] Last Tuesday week (nine days ago) he describes that he felt feverish, had a dryness of the nostrils and cold in the head followed two days [later] by a copious efflorescence of the vesicles of herpes labialis[106] round the lips and left nostril. On examination there is a copious efflorescence of spots of purpura on the legs and arms from which the trunk is free. On some portions of the back part of the leg the eruption has the appearance of urticaria with itching. The patient has observed that the eruption has

---

104 Epsom salts.
105 See Appendix II.
106 Herpes of the lip or cold sore.

back part of the leg and. The eruption has the appearance of urticaria with itching. The patient has observed that the eruption has generally been in its most intense stage in one leg and the opposite arm at the same time. No headache – crusts of herpes round the mouth and nose, tongue brown and coated, not dry – bowels regular, urine natural in quantity. Pulse 56, small in the recumbent posture, increased to 76 by sitting in bed.

28 Eruption almost gone.

Pulse 62

[p.75]

| Oct 23 | ℞ Infus Rosæ ℥xvi Quinie disulph ʒſs M cochlear ii magna 4ᵗⁱˢ horis sd |
| Full diet A pint of porter |
| ℞ Ext Colocynth C gr iv Hyd Chlorid gr v ft pil ii st s |
| Oct 28 | Rep pil hac nocte et repet omne 2ᵈᵃ nocte |
| ℞ Haust Sennæ ℥iſs sequente mane |
| Nov 1 | Perstet |
| Nov 4 | Perstet |
| ℞ Ergotæ Ɲi ft pulv omne meridie sumend cum mistura |
| 8 | Perstet |
| To have two pints of Porter |
| Nov 20 | ℞ Pil Ferri C ʒii ft pilulæ xxiv quaram sumat ii ter in die |

generally been in its most intense stage in one leg and the opposite arm at the same time. He has no headache. [There are] crusts of herpes round the mouth and nose. Tongue brown, coated and not dry. Bowels regular. Urine natural in quantity. Pulse [rate] 56 [per minute]. Small in the recumbent posture, increased to 76 [per minute] by sitting [up] in bed.

Oct 28. Eruption almost gone.

Pulse 62.

Oct 23. Take 16 ounces Infusion of Rose, Quinine Disulphate ½ drachm. Mix. Two tablespoonfuls to be taken every 4 hours.

Full diet. A pint of porter.

Take 4 grains Extract of Colocynth, 5 grains Mercurous Chloride. Make 2 pills. To be taken at once.

Oct 28. Repeat the pills to-night and [then] repeat every second night.

Take 1½ ounces Senna Draught the following morning.

Nov 1. Continue.

Nov 4. Continue.

Take 1 scruple Ergot,[107] Make a powder. To be taken every mid-day with the mixture.

Nov 8. Continue.

To have two pints of porter.

Nov 20. Take 2 drachms Compound Iron Pill. Make 24 pills, of which let him take two three times a day.

---

[107] Ergot is a fungus that occurs in the ovary of rye. See Appendix V.

	Omitte misturam	*Leave off the mixture.*
25	Exeat	*Nov 25. He may leave.*

[p.76]

Samuel Burman æt 20

age 20

[*There seems little doubt that this patient had tuberculosis of the lung with a cavity in the right upper lobe. The first mixture prescribed for him contained hydrocyanic acid, which was often used in pulmonary conditions. It had a transient sedative action, and it was useful for reducing the frequency of coughing fits. Hemlock pills, which were narcotic, were administered twice; on the second occasion, lead acetate was added. This substance was often prescribed when internal bleeding was suspected, and so it was frequently employed in tuberculosis of the lung when blood appeared in the sputum. Samuel was given a quarter of a grain of morphine at night. The morphine would have helped to ease his cough and control any pain, but if he had a demonstrable cavity in the right lung and was coughing up blood, death would probably soon intervene.*]

Phthisis Pulmonaris. Cavity under right clavicle	*Tuberculosis with cavities [in the] right [upper lung].*

[*no other history recorded*]

[p.77]

Oct 23	℞ Acid Hydrocyan ʒi	*Oct 23. Take 1 drachm [Dilute] Hydrocyanic Acid,*
	Acid Nitric D ʒſs	*½ ounce Dilute Nitric Acid,*
	Aquæ puræ ℔i	*1 pound Pure Water.*
	mf mist sum^t	*Mix. Make a mixture. Three tablespoonfuls to be*
	coch larg iii ter die	*taken three times a day.*
28	℞ Ung Ant Tart ʒi	*Oct 28. Take 1 ounce Antimony Tartrate Ointment.*
	utend nocte et mane	*To be used night and morning.*
	℞ Pil Conii C gr x	*Take 10 grains Compound Pill of Hemlock.*
	omne nocte sumend	*To be taken each night.*
	℞ Morphii Ch gr ii	*Take 2 grains Morphine Ch[loride],*
	Mist Camphor ʒ viii	*8 ounces Camphor Mixture.*
	M cochlear ii magna	*Mix. Two tablespoonfuls [to be taken]*
	omni nocte	*each night.*
	Omitte pilulas	*Leave off the pills.*
Novr 1	Perstet	*Nov 1. Continue.*
Nov 20		*Nov 20.*
	℞ Pil Conii C Ͻii	*Take 2 scruples Compound Pill of Hemlock,*
	Plumbi Acet gr xv	*15 grains Lead Acetate.*
	ft pil ~~xxii~~ xii M	*Mix. Make ~~22~~ 12 pills.*
	sumatur pil i on	*Let one pill be taken at night.*
Nov 25	Exeat	*Nov 25. He may leave.*

[p.78]

Sarah Ford [age] 18

[*A blistering plaster of cantharides was applied to her right hypochondrium (right upper abdomen), presumably in an attempt to relieve a pain in that region. Stutter's notes lead us to suspect that Susan may have had a fever (flushed appearance and raised pulse rate), in which case the prescription of potassium nitrate was in accordance with contemporary practice. As usual, the symptom of amenorrhoea[108] seems to have been treated with galbanum, iron and aloes. It is difficult to make a modern diagnosis, but recurrent pains in the right hypochondrium might suggest a diagnosis of gall stones and/or inflammation of the gall bladder.*]

Nov 15 Has enjoyed good health untill three months ago when she was seized with pain in the side encreases on taking a full inspiration, this pain has been relieved on two occasions by the application of a blister. Has never had the least appearance of menstrual secretion – bowels are generally open. No cough. Face rather flushed. Tongue a little coated and pointed, with red spots. Pulse 96. Chest clear on percussion. Respiration easy.

Nov 15 [She] enjoyed good health until three months ago when she was seized with pain in the side. [This] increases on taking a full breath. [The] pain has been relieved on two occasions by the application of a blister. Has never had the least appearance of menstrual secretion. [Her] bowels are generally open. No cough. Face rather flushed. Tongue a little coated and pointed, with red spots. Pulse [rate] 96 [per minute]. Chest clear on percussion.[109] Respiration easy.

[p.79]

Nov 15	℞ Pil Ferri C Ɔii Pil Galbani C Ɔii Aloes Ʒſs M divide in pil xxiv quaram sumantur duæ ter in die	*Nov 15. Take 2 scruples Compound Iron Pill, 2 scruples Compound Galbanum Pill, ½ drachm Aloes. Mix. Divide into 24 pills. Of which two to be taken three times a day.*
	Common diet	*Common diet.*
	℞ Misturæ Camphor Ʒviii Potass Nit Ʒi solve sumantur cochlear ii magna ter in die	*Take 8 ounces Camphor Mixture, 1 drachm Potassium Nitrate, dissolve [in the Camphor Mixture]. Let her take two tablespoonfuls three times a day.*
20	Omitte misturam	*Nov 20. Leave off the mixture.*
22	Perstet	*Nov 22. Continue.*
25	Perstet	*Nov 25. Continue.*
27	 Applica emplast Lyttæ ~~parv~~ modiiæ amplitudinis hypochond dextro	*Nov 27. Apply a ~~small~~ moderate sized Cantharides Plaster to the right hypochondrium.*

---

108 Absence of menstrual periods.
109 See Appendix III for explanation of percussion.

[p.80]

James Carter [*age not recorded*]

[*remainder of page blank*]

[*Sulphur was used extensively for skin conditions, especially 'the itch' (scabies);*[110] *it may be that this is why James was given a sulphur vapour bath twice a week. Ammonia liniment was a stimulant and rubefacient.*[111] *Colocynth had a violent purging action, as did colchicum, which was often prescribed in cases of gout, rheumatism and water retention.*]

[p.81]

Oct 25[r]	Habeat balneum Vaporis Sulphuris bis in hebdomada	*Oct 25. Let him have a Sulphur Vapour Bath twice a week.*
Nov[r] 6	℞ Liniment Ammon Fort ℥ii bis die applicand	*Nov 6. Take 2 ounces Strong Ammonia Liniment. To be applied twice a day.*
20	℞ Ext Col C gr iv Ext Colchici Acet gr ii M ft pil ii alternis noctibus s[d]	*Nov 20. Take 4 grains Compound Extract of Colocynth, 2 grains Acetic Extract of Colchicum. Mix. Make 2 pills. To be taken every other night.*
	Dismissed relieved	*Dismissed relieved.*

[p.82]

John Cocksedge [*age*] 39

[*John Cocksedge's abdominal pain and vomiting after meals was treated with a mixture of henbane and hydrocyanic acid, supplemented by the application of ten leeches to the upper abdomen. He was given repeated doses of castor oil for his habitual constipation. Unfortunately, it sounds very much as though this patient had cancer of the stomach or head of the pancreas.*]

1839

Nov 29 Has for seven years been subject to pain in the epigastric region with pyrosis and vomiting after meals. For the last five months has been unable to work: bowels habitually constipated. Features sharp – general emaciation. Occasional headaches – tongue dry and coated – bowels relieved yesterday. Colour yellowish. Tenderness in the epigastric

Nov 29. Has for seven years been subject to pain in the epigastric[112] *region, with pyrosis*[113] *and vomiting after meals. For the last five months has been unable to work. [His] bowels [are] habitually constipated. Features sharp. General emaciation. Occasional headaches. Tongue dry and coated. Bowels relieved yesterday. Colour yellowish. Tenderness in the epigastric region on pressure – also in the right*

---

110 See Appendix II.
111 A rubefacient is an application producing a redness or slight inflammation of the skin.
112 Epigastrium: the upper part of the abdomen, immediately over the stomach.
113 Pyrosis: a burning sensation in the stomach and oesophagus with the eructation of watery fluid (water brash).

region on pressure – also in the right hypochondriac region where there is felt a tumour whose surface is unequal – Stomach and bowels much distended with wind – abdominal muscles very rigid – skin cool, Pulse 88.

hypochondriac[114] *region a tumour can be felt whose surface is unequal. Stomach and bowels much distended with wind. [His] abdominal muscles [are] very rigid. Skin cool. Pulse [rate] 88 [per minute]*

℞ Tinct Hyos ʒii
Acid Hydrocyan Dil ♏xx
Mist Acaciæ ʒii
Aquæ ʒvi M
cochlear ii magna ter in die

Take 2 drachms Tincture of Henbane, 20 minims Dilute Hydrocyanic Acid, 2 ounces Acacia Mixture, 6 ounces Water. Mix. Two tablespoonfuls [to be taken] three times a day.

Applica Hirudin x epigastrio

Apply ten leeches to the epigastric region.

Decr 8

Dec 8.

℞ Ol Ricini ʒʃs st s

Take ½ ounce Castor Oil. To be taken immediately.

Rep^r mistura

Repeat mixture.

27   Perstet

Dec 27. Continue.

Jan 10   Rep^r Ol Ricini

Jan 10. Repeat Castor Oil.

Jan 13   Rep^r Oli Ricini

Jan 13. Repeat Castor Oil.

Rep^r mistura

Repeat mixture.

[p.83, *blank*]

[p.84]

George Brame [*age not recorded*]

[*During George Brame's stay he was bled twice by venesection*[115] *and had more blood withdrawn by 'cupping'.*[116] *He also had blistering plasters applied to his side and back. On admission he was given aperient pills and an ounce of castor oil, repeated after two hours. Two days later this drug regime was used again. In addition, mercury and rhubarb pills were prescribed. These were to be taken each night. This combination of drugs must surely have resulted in considerable purging, but nevertheless a week later George was given a mixture of Epsom salts (magnesium sulphate) and magnesia each morning with mercury pills at night. The use of mixtures containing first dandelion extract and then serega, as well as the administration of fever-reducing drugs such as ammonium acetate and potassium nitrate, suggest that the patient may have been suffering from rheumatic fever. The last medicine prescribed contained morphine and camphor, but there are no clear instructions as to the dosage or time of administration.*]

---

114   The right hypochondrium is that part of the abdomen lying just under the ribs on the right side.
115   See Appendix IV.
116   See Appendix IV.

Jan 6		*Jan 6.*
	℞ Ext Taraxici ʒi	*Take 1 drachm Extract of Dandelion,*
	Plumbi Diacetat Ɔi	*1 scruple Lead Acetate.*
	M ft pilulæ xii quarum	*Mix. Make 12 pills, of which let him take two*
	sumantur duæ ter in die	*three times a day.*

[p.85]

Dec 4	℞ Pil Aper ii s s	*Dec 4. Take 2 Aperient Pills.*
		To be taken immediately.
	℞ Ol Ricini ʒ i	*Take 1 ounce Castor Oil*
	post duas horas	*after two hours.*[117]
6	Rep pil ii	*Dec 6. Repeat pills 2.*
	Rep Ol Ricini	*Repeat Castor Oil.*
	℞ Hyd c Creta Ɔi	*Take 1 scruple Mercury with Chalk Powder,*
	Ext Rhei ʒſs	*½ drachm Extract of Rhubarb,*
	Sapon Hisp gr x	*10 grains Spanish Soap.*
	Mf pil 12 sum^t	*Mix. Make 12 pills.*
	ii o n h s	*Two to be taken at night at bedtime.*
	℞ Sodæ Sesquicarb ʒſs	*Take ½ ounce Sodium Bicarbonate,*
	Ext Taraxaci ʒſs	*½ ounce Extract of Dandelion,*
	Inf Gent C. ℔i	*1 pound Compound Infusion of Gentian.*
	Mf mist sum^t coch	*Mix. Make a mixture. Three tablespoonfuls to be*
	larg iii ter die	*taken three times a day.*
9	V S ad ʒx	*Dec 9. Venesection withdrawing 10 ounces of*
		blood.
	℞ Liq Ammon Acet ʒi	*Take 1 ounce Solution of Ammonium Acetate,*
	Potass Nit ʒſs	*½ drachm Potassium Nitrate,*
	Vin Ipecac ʒi	*1 drachm Ipecacuanha Wine,*
	Mist Camphor ʒviii M	*8 ounces Camphor Mixture. Mix.*
	cochlear ii magna 4^tis horis	*Two tablespoonfuls [to be taken] every 4 hours.*
	Omitte cætera	*Leave off the others.*
11	V S ad ʒxii	*Dec 11. Venesection withdrawing 12 ounces of*
		blood.
Dec 13	Applicantur cucurbitulæ	*Dec 13. Wet cupping glasses to be applied*
	cruentæ hypochond dextro	*to the right hypochondrium.*
	℞ Pil Hyd gr v o n s	*Take 5 grains Mercury Pill. To be taken at*
		night.
	℞ Magnesiæ Sulph ʒiii	*Take 3 drachms Magnesium Sulphate,*
	Magnesiæ Ɔi	*1 scruple Magnesia,*
	Aquæ Menth Pip ʒiſs	*1½ ounces Peppermint Water.*
	omni mane	*[To be taken] each morning.*

---

[117] That is, two hours after taking the aperient pills.

16	Applican^d Emplast Lyttæ lateri 6 inches by 4	*Dec 16. Apply a Cantharides Plaster 6 inches by 4 [inches] to the side.*
20	ꝶ Decoct Senegæ ℥ vi Ammon Sesquicarb ʒi Liq Ammon Aceta ℥ii M cochlear ii magna 4^{tis} horis	*Dec 20. Take 6 ounces Decoction of Senega, 1 drachm Ammonium Bicarbonate, 2 ounces Solution of Ammonium Acetate. Mix. Two tablespoonfuls [to be taken] every 4 hours*
	Omitte pilulas	*Leave off the pills.*
Dec 23	ꝶ Morphiæ Solution ʒii Mist Camphor ℥viii M cochlear [illeg.]	*Dec 23. Take 2 drachms Morphine Solution, 8 ounces Camphor Mixture. Mix. Spoonful [illeg.].*
28	Emplast Lyttæ dorso	*Dec 28. [Apply a] Cantharides Plaster to back*
29	Perstet	*Dec 29. Continue.*

[p.86]

James Clark [*age*] (36)

[*This patient was admitted with pneumonia (see Appendix II) on 8 December 1839. He was seriously ill and died on the same day. All that Stutter could do was to try and ease his symptoms with pills containing opium and an infusion of senega.*]

Decr 8	Pneumonia with tendency to Delirium Tremens	*Dec 8. Pneumonia with tendency to Delirium Tremens.*[118]

[p.87]

		Dec 8.
Decr 8	ꝶ Ant Potassio Tart gr iv ~~Tinct~~ Pulv Opii gr v ~~Mistura Camphor~~ Pil Saponis C ꝙs ʒſs	*Take 4 grains Antimony and Potassium Tartrate, 5 grains ~~Tincture~~ Opium Powder, ~~Camphor Mixture~~ ~~A sufficient quantity~~ ½ drachm Compound Soap Pill.*
	M divide in pil ꭓ vi pil i 4^{tis} horis	*Mix. Divide into ~~10~~ 6 pills. One [to be taken] every four hours.*
	ꝶ Infus Senegæ ℥viii cochlear ii magna 4^{tis} horis	*Take 8 ounces Infusion of Senega. Two tablespoonfuls [to be taken] every 4 hours.*
	Mortuus est	*He died.*

[p.88]

Thomas Ruddock [*age*] 41

[*The only information given in the casebook is that Thomas had a coated tongue and a pulse rate of 60 per minute. Chiretta, present in two of the mixtures he was given, was a bitter tonic used in dyspepsia and to improve appetite. Both ipecacuanha and poppy syrup were prescribed for the relief of coughs.*]

---

[118] This patient was admitted and died on the same day. His delirium may simply have been a toxic confusional state due to pneumonia.

1839
Decr 16th Tongue coated, white.
Pulse 60

Dec 16. Tongue coated white.
Pulse 60.

[p.89]

Decr 13 ℞ Pil Aper xii
ii alternis noctibus

Take 12 Aperient Pills.
Two [to be taken] every other night.

~~℞ Infus Chirettæ ℥viii~~
~~cochlear ii magna~~
~~ter in die~~

~~Take 8 ounces Infusion of Chirretta~~
~~Two tablespoonfuls~~
~~three times a day~~

℞ Infus Chirettæ ℥vi
Sp Ammon Ar ʒ ſs
Mist Camphor ℥iſs M
cochlear ii magna
ter in die

Take 6 ounces Infusion of Chiretta,[119]
½ ounce Aromatic Spirit of Ammonia,
1½ ounces Camphor Mixture. Mix.
Two tablespoonfuls
[to be taken] three times a day.

℞ Vin Ipecac ʒi
Syr Papav ℥i
Mist Camphor ℥viii M
cochlear i magna
4^{tis} horis

Take 1 drachm Ipecacuanha Wine,
1 ounce Syrup of Poppies,
8 ounces Camphor Mixture. Mix.
One tablespoonful [to be taken]
every 4 hours.

Omitte Mist Chirettæ

Leave off the Chiretta mixture.

Omitte Mist ~~Camph~~
cum Vino Ipecac

Leave off the ~~Camphor~~ mixture
with Ipecacuanha Wine.

Rep^r Mist Chirrettæ
et Ammon

Repeat the Chiretta
and Ammonia mixture.

[p.90] [*90 crossed out and 91 inserted*]

Kesia [*sic*] Atkins

[*On this page prescriptions etc. were written for Kezia Atkins, which follow on from those appearing on pages 66–7 and for the sake of clarity have been recorded on that page.*]

[p.92, *blank*]

[p.93]

William Shepherd [*age not recorded*]

[*William had a blistering plaster applied to the chest wall over the heart on no less than three occasions. This, together with the prescription of digitalis, may be an indication that he was thought to have a cardiac condition. He may also have had a fever, because he was given powders that were normally given to reduce body temperature. On one occasion these were made up of ipecacuanha with antimony, whilst on another potassium nitrate and tartrate were the active ingredients.*]

---

[119]   Used as a bitter tonic. See Appendix V.

Dec 25	℞ Tinct Digitalis ʒii Tinct Hyoscyam ʒiii Mist Camphor ℥viiſs cochlear ii magna ter in die	*Dec 25. Take 2 drachms Tincture of Digitalis,* *3 drachms Tincture of Henbane,* *7½ ounces Camphor Mixture.* *Two tablespoonfuls [to be taken]* *three times a day.*
28	Applica Emplast Lyttae ovale pollices 5 longum regioni cordis	*Dec 28. Apply an oval Cantharides Plaster* *5 inches long* *to the region of the heart.*
30	℞ Pulv Ipecac gr xv Ant Potass Tart gr i ft pulv st sd	*Dec 30. Take 15 grains Ipecacuanha Powder,* *1 grain Antimony and Potassium Tartrate.* *Make a powder. To be taken at once.*
Jan 6	Emplast Lyttæ ejusdem magnitudinis	*Jan 6. [Apply] Cantharides Plaster* *of the same size.*[120]
10	℞ Potass Nit gr L Ant Potass Tart gr iſs Pulv Ipecac C gr x M divide in pulv vi quarum capiatur i ter in die	*Jan 10. Take 50 grains Take Potassium Nitrate,* *1½ grains Antimony and Potassium Tartrate,* *10 grains Compound Ipecacuanha Powder.* *Mix. Divide into 6 powders, of which* *let him take one three times a day.*
15	Omitte mistura et pulveres	*Jan 15. Leave off the mixture and powders.*
	℞ Sp Ammon Ar ʒſs Sodæ Sesquicarb ʒii Infus Chirettæ ℥viiſs cochlear ii magna ter in die	*Take ½ ounce Aromatic Spirit of Ammonia,* *2 drachms Sodium Bicarbonate,* *7½ ounces Infusion of Chiretta.* *Two tablespoonfuls [to be taken] three times a* *day.*
	℞ Morphiæ Chlorid gr ~~iii~~ ii Mist Camphor ℥viii cochlear ii magna omni nocte	*Take ~~3~~ 2 grains Morphine Chloride,* *8 ounces Camphor Mixture.* *Two tablespoonfuls [to be taken]* *each night.*
17	℞ Ol Ricini ℥i	*Jan 17. Take 1 ounce Castor Oil.*
23	℞ Magnes Sulphat ℥iſs Quinæ Disulph gr xii Infus Rosæ ℥vii M cochlear iii magna ter in die	*Jan 23. Take 1½ ounces Magnesium Sulphate,* *12 grains Quinine Disulphate,* *7 ounces Infusion of Rose.* *Mix. Three tablespoonfuls [to be taken]* *three times a day.*
	Omitte Mist Chirettæ	*Leave off Chiretta mixture.*
Feb 10	Applicaʳ Emp Lytt parv ovale 4 pollices longum	*Feb 10. Apply a small oval Cantharides Plaster* *4 inches long.*
18	Applica Emplast Galban C ~~dorso~~ lumbis	*Feb 18. Apply a Compound Galbanum Plaster* *to the ~~back~~ loins.*

[p.94, *blank*]

---

[120] That is, the same size as the plaster applied on 28 December.

[p.95 *does not exist*]

[p.96]

Sarah Bryant [*age*] 25

[*This patient almost certainly suffered from tuberculosis. She had a cavity in the right upper lung and was eventually discharged incurable. The first prescription she was given was for a confection of senna because she was constipated. Hydrocyanic acid (prescribed in a mixture on the same day as the senna), was considered to be of value in easing difficult breathing and reducing coughing. Anaemia may have been suspected because of the patient's delicate appearance and irregular periods; no doubt this is why iron was given, both in pills and in a mixture. Iron oxide was also added to the senna confection. The mixture of squills, ammonium acetate and spirit of nitric acid would have been given in the hope of reducing fever and control the patient's cough. Morphine was administered at night. This would have acted both as a sedative and a further cough suppressant.*]

1840

Jan 15 Has been delicate ever since she remembers, subject to headache, pain in side and constipated bowels. Menstruated at 14, after which her health improved a little. Menses have continued regular until 2 months ago. About 4 months ago she was seized with what was called inflammation on the chest (for which she was blistered and had nauseating medicine) with cough and difficulty of breathing, which two symptoms have continued until this moment. Present appearance delicate with hectic flushing of the cheeks and emaciation, has had nightly perspirations within some weeks, which have now disappeared. Expectoration frothy, tongue coated, lips dry. Pulse 109, exceedingly small. Clear sound on percussion over the whole chest. Respiration puerile – tenderness in the epigastrium and in a slight degree over the whole abdomen.

25 Looks better P 100

31 Much worse. Expectoration altered in character from being clear and frothy it has become purulent with one or two granular particles.
Feb 3 Gurgling and pectoriloquy at the summit of right lung-cavity.

Jan 15. Has been delicate ever since she [can] remember. Subject to headache, pain in the side and constipated bowels. [She] menstruated at 14 after which her health improved a little. [Her] menses have continued regular until two months ago. About four months ago she was seized with what was called inflammation on the chest [for which she was blistered and had nauseating medicine]. [She had a] cough and difficulty in breathing. These two symptoms have continued until this moment. Her present appearance is delicate with hectic flushing of the cheek and emaciation. [She] has had nightly perspirations for some weeks.[121] [These have] now disappeared. Expectoration frothy. Tongue coated. Lips dry. Pulse [rate] 109 [per minute]. [Volume] exceedingly small. Clear sound on percussion over the whole chest. Respiration puerile.[122] Tenderness in the epigastrium, and in a slight degree over the whole abdomen.

Jan 25. Looks better. P[ulse rate] 100 [per minute].
Jan 31. Much worse. Expectoration altered in character. From being clear and frothy it has become purulent with one or two granular particles.
Feb 3. Gurgling and pectoriloquy[123] at the summit of right lung-cavity.

---

121   Night sweats are a classic sign of pulmonary tuberculosis.
122   In this context 'puerile' must mean 'childlike'.
123   The transmission of the sound of the voice through the wall of the chest to the ear on auscultation. This is usually the sign of a cavity in the lung.

[p.97]

Jan 15	℞ Confection Sennæ ʒi Ferri Sesquioxyd gr lxxx cochlear i parv ter in die	*Jan 15. Take 1 ounce Confection of Senna,* *80 grains Iron Oxide,* *1 teaspoonful [to be taken] three times a day.*
	℞ Tinct Hyos ℩ lxxx Acid Hydrocyan Dil ʒſs Mist Acaciæ ʒi Aquæ ʒviii M cochlear ii magna bis in die	*Take 80 minims Tincture of Henbane,* *½ drachm Dilute Hydrocyanic Acid,* *1 ounce Acacia Mixture,* *8 ounces Water. Mix.* *Two tablespoonfuls [to be taken]* *twice a day.*
17	℞ Pil Ferri C ʒi ft pil xii ii ter in die	*Jan 17. Take 1 drachm Compound Iron Pill.* *Make 12 pills.* *Two [to be taken] three times a day.*
22	Omitte pilulas	*Jan 22. Stop taking the pills.*
	℞ Mist Ferri ʒviii cochlear i magna ter in die	*Take 8 ounces Iron Mixture.* *One tablespoonful [to be taken]* *three times a day.*
23	Perstet	*Jan 23. Continue.*
25	Perstet	*Jan 25. Continue.*
27	Omitte misturam	*Jan 27. Leave off the mixture.*
	℞ Oxymel Scillæ ʒiii Liq Ammon Acet ʒi ~~Tinct Opii ʒi~~ Sp Æther Nit ʒſs Mist Camphor ʒviſs M cochlear ii magna 4^tis horis	*Take 3 drachms Oxymel of Squills,* *1 ounce Solution of Ammonium Acetate,* *~~1 drachm Tincture of Opium~~* *½ ounce Spirit of Nitrous Ether,* *6½ ounces Camphor Mixture.* *Mix. Two tablespoonfuls [to be taken]* *every four hours.*
29	℞ Oli Ricini ʒſs	*29. Take ½ ounce Castor Oil.*
31	℞ Morphii Chlorid Sol ʒii Mist Camphor ʒviii M cochlear iii magna hora somni	*31. Take 2 drachms Solution of Morphine* *Chloride,* *8 ounces Camphor Mixture.* *Mix. Three tablespoonfuls to be taken at* *bedtime.*[124]
Feb 3	Perstet Discharged incurable	*Feb 3. Continue.* *Discharged incurable.*

---

[124] Literally 'at the hour of sleep'.

[p.98]

Phoebe Horrex [*age*] 28

[*The diagnosis is shrouded in mystery. The patient may just have had lumbar back strain but kidney stones and/or a urinary tract infection are other more serious possibilities. Stutter recorded that Phoebe was habitually constipated; he treated her with aperient pills and mixture as well as a confection of senna with added sulphur and Epsom salts. Two large blistering plasters were applied to her painful loins and a plaster of galbanum to her back. The latter treatment was sometimes used when patients were suffering from rickets, but there is nothing in the history to suggest that Phoebe definitely had that condition. A bitter tonic mixture of chiretta and another containing gentian completed her medication.*]

1840

Jan 15 Enjoyed perfectly good health till the age of 19. Menstruated at 14 since which she has been quite regular. Married about 20, has never been pregnant, has an impediment in her speech which has been the same since a child, which however is confined to the first syllable, after pronouncing which she talks fluently. Her health has not been as good since she married, since when she has been generally ailing in the autumn. Has had Leucorrhoa which ceased after a year ~~not~~ spontaneously – has habitually pain in the loins and always feels most comfortable in bed. Feels a sinking when she gets up. Her complexion is generally [*illeg.*]. Yesterday and today her countenance is much flushed – bowels habitually constipated. Appetite almost voracious and never satisfied; tongue brown, moist skin bedewed with perspiration. Pulse 74, soft. A good deal of tenderness in the region of the liver. Bowels have been only slightly relieved on Sunday (13) and yesterday morning.

Jan 15. Enjoyed perfectly good health till the age of 19. [She] menstruated at 14 since when she has been quite regular. Married about 20, [but] has never been pregnant. She has an impediment in her speech, which has been the same since [she was] a child. [It is], however, confined to the first syllable, after pronouncing which she talks fluently. Her health has not been as good since she married, since when she has been generally ailed in the autumn. Has had leucorrhoea[125] which ceased after a year spontaneously. [She] has habitually [had] pain in the loins and always feels most comfortable in bed. [Has] a sinking feeling when she gets up. Her complexion is generally [?fair]. Yesterday and today her countenance is much flushed. Bowel habitually constipated. Appetite almost voracious and never satisfied. Tongue brown and moist. [Her] skin [is] bedewed with perspiration. Pulse [rate] 74 [per minute] – soft. A good deal of tenderness in the region of the liver. Bowels have been only slightly relieved on Sunday [13th] and yesterday morning.

Feb 3 Her menses began yesterday – the period at which they were expected

Feb 3. Her menses began yesterday – the period at which they were expected.

Feels better

Feels better.

[p.99]

Jan 15 ℞ Pil Aper fortiori ii
       st sd

Feb 15. Take 2 Strong Aperient Pills. To be taken at once.

℞ Misturæ Aper ʒiſs

Take 1½ ounces[126] Aperient Mixture.

---

[125] Leucorrhoea is a white vaginal discharge. See Appendix II.
[126] Approximately equivalent to three tablespoonfuls.

	post horas quatuor et repetatur omni bihora donec alvus responderit	*[To be taken] after four hours*[127] *and repeated every two hours until the bowels respond.*
17	℞ Sp Ammon Ar ℨiii	*Feb 17. Take 3 drachms Aromatic Spirit of Ammonia,*
	Infus Chirettæ Mist Camphor a a ℥ii cochlear ii magna ter in die	*2 ounces each Infusion of Chiretta [and] Camphor Mixture. Two tablespoonfuls [to be taken] three times a day.*
	℞ Applica Emplast Galban C magnum lumbis	~~*Take*~~ *Apply a large Compound Plaster of Galbanum to the loins.*
29		*Jan 29.*
	Applia Emplast Lyttæ magnum lumbis	*Apply a large Cantharides Plaster to the loins.*
Jan 31	℞ Confect Sennæ ℨi Sulphur Sublim ℨii M ft elect cujus capiantur cochlear i parv alvo astrict[128]	*Jan 31. Take 1 ounce Confection of Senna, 2 drachms Sublimed Sulphur.*[129] *Mix. Make an Electuary, of which let one teaspoonful be taken for constipation.*
	Omitte Misturam Chiretæ	*Leave off the Chiretta mixture.*
Feb 7	Applica Emplast Galban C magnum lumbis	*Feb 7. Apply a large Compound Galbanum plaster to the loins.*
	℞ Infus Gentian ℥vii Tinct Aurantii ℥i Tinct Cinchon ℥ſs ~~Liq Potass ℨſs~~ M cochlear ii magna ter in die	*Take 7 ounces Infusion of Gentian, 1 ounce Tincture of Orange, ½ ounce Tincture of Cinchona, ~~½ drachm Solution of Potassium.~~ Two tablespoonfuls [to be taken] three times a day.*
March 4	Adde Magnes Sulph ℨiii misturam	*Mar 4. Add 3 drachms Magnesium Sulphate to the mixture.*[130]

[p.100]

Frances Baker [age] 34

*[This may have been yet another case of pulmonary tuberculosis. The productive cough and
dullness on the left side of the chest are very suggestive of that malady, although there are
several other possibilities. Leeches were applied to left side of the chest twice. The patient was
bled once, and up to 15 ounces of blood taken. A blistering plaster of cantharides was also
applied (presumably to the chest). A plaster of antimony tartrate was later applied to the right
upper abdomen. She was given mercury pills or powder twice, but they affected her mouth*

---

127 Stutter intended that this mixture should be taken four hours after the aperient pills.
128 *Alvo astricto*, the bowels being confined.
129 Commonly known as Flowers of Sulphur.
130 That is, to the mixture of Gentian etc. dispensed on 7 February.

and were replaced with castor oil and a mixture of Epsom salts and antimony tartrate. Potassium acetate dissolved in a decoction of broom tops was also administered. Both these drugs were diuretics. The final mixture prescribed was for dilute sulphuric acid, made more pleasant by dilution with infusion of roses. In the nineteenth century sulphuric acid was used for dyspepsia, diabetes, menorrhagia[131] and some skin conditions.]

Jan 15 Never has enjoyed very good health since the age of 16. Menstruated at 17, married at 24, has never been pregnant but has menstruated regularly till within 8 months from which period she dates her present illness. Since then the menses have appeared once, two months ago. The illness began by violent pain in the back part of the head succeeded by inflammation in the chest (as she describes) for which she was twice bled with but little relief. Subject to hysterical affections. Complains at present of pain in the precordial region – countenance flushed. Pulse 100. Skin dry – cough with slight fluid ~~evacuation~~ expectoration, pain in the left side of the chest in the region of the false ribs – dull sound on that side over the whole chest, measurement of this side under the mamma 15 inches, the other side under 14, on which side the sound is clear and respiration distinct. While on the left side respiration is inaudible excepting at the summit. With distinct egophony in the region of the angle of the left scapula. 21 Left of thorax 14½ inches. Pulse 100

Jan 25 Pulse 92. Mouth affected by the Calomel
Jan 31 Much better. P.76
Feb 7 P 80 tongue clearer. Egophony disappeared, respiration distinct

Jan 15. Never has enjoyed very good health since the age of 16. She menstruated at 17 and married at 24. She has never been pregnant but has menstruated regularly. [She] has been ill for the past eight months, and during that time she has menstruated only once – two months ago. The illness began [with] violent pain in the back part of the head [and was] succeeded by inflammation in the chest [as she describes it], for which she was twice bled with but little relief. Subject to hysterical affections, at present she complains of pain in the precodial[132] region. Countenance flushed. Pulse [rate] 100 [per minute]. Skin dry. Cough with slight fluid expectoration. Pain in the left side of the chest in the region of the false ribs – dull sounds on that side over the whole chest. Measurement of this side under the mamma – 15 inches, the other side under 14 inches, on which side the sound is clear and respiration distinct. On the left side respiration is inaudible excepting at the summit, with distinct egophony[133] in the region of the angle of the left scapula. Jan 21. Left [side] of thorax 14½ inches. Pulse [rate] 100 [per minute].
Jan 25. Pulse [rate] 92 [per minute]. Mouth affected by the Calomel.
Jan 31. Much better. Pulse rate [6 per minute].
Feb 7. P[ulse rate] 80 [per minute]. Tongue clearer. Egophony disappeared. Respiration distinct.

[p.101]

Jan 15 Applica Hirudines xx to the left side of the chest

R̶ Hydrarg Chlorid gr v
Pulv Ant Comp gr vi
Ext Col C gr v M
ft pilulæ ii st sd

Jan 15. Apply 20 leeches to the left side of the chest.

Take 5 grains Mercurous Chloride, 6 grains Compound Antimony Powder, 5 grains Compound Extract of Colocynth. Mix. Make 2 pills. To be taken immediately.

---

131 Excessive flow of the menses.
132 The precordial region is the front part of the chest.
133 Aegophony or egophony is a noise like the bleating of a kid which may be heard in pleurisy.

	℞ Magnes Sulphat ℨi	*Take 1 ounce Magnesium Sulphate,*
	Sp Æther Nit ℨii	*2 drachms Spirit of Nitrous Ether,*
	Tincti Juniper C ℨii	*2 drachms Compound Tincture of Juniper,*
	Aqua ℥viii M	*8 ounces Water. Mix.*
	cochlear iii magna	*Three tablespoonfuls [to be taken]*
	4tis horis	*every 4 hours.*
17	V S ad ℥ xv	*Jan 17. Venesection. 15 ounces of blood withdrawn.*
	[*Pencilled entry*]	
	Hyd Chlorid gr xii	*12 grains Mercurous Chloride,*
	P Opii gr [*illeg.*][134]	*[illeg.] grains Opium Powder.*
	divide in pulveres sex	*Divide into six powders, of*
	quorum sumatur i 4tis	*which let her take one every 4*
	horis	*hours.*
	Repr misturam	*Repeat mixture.*
18		*Jan 18.*
	℞ mist et pulveres	*Take Effervescent Mixture and Powders.*
	effervescentes capiatur	*Take*
	dosis 4tis horis	*a dose every 4 hours.*
19	Perstet	*Jan 19. Continue.*
21	Perstet	*Jan 21. Continue.*
23	Perstet	*Jan 23. Continue.*
25	Omitte Pulveres Hydrarg	*Jan 25. Leave off Mercury powders.*[135]
27	℞ Decoct Scoparii ℥viii	*Jan 27. Take 8 ounces Decoction of Broom Tops,*
	Potass Acetat ℥iſs M	*1½ ounces Potassium Acetate. Mix*
	cochlear iii magna	*Three tablespoonfuls [to be taken]*
	ter in die	*three times a day.*
29	Omitte haust eferves	*Jan 29. Leave off the effervescent draught.*
31	℞ Ol Ricin ℥ſs	*Jan 31. Take ½ ounce Castor Oil.*
Feb 3	℞ Magnes Sulphatis ℥ſs	*Feb 3. Take ½ ounce Magnesium Sulphate,*
	Antimonii Pot Tart gr i	*1 grain Antimony and Potassium Tartrate,*
	Sp Æther Nitrici ℨiii	*3 drachms Nitrous Ether Spirit,*
	Aquæ ℥viii M	*8 ounces Water. Mix.*
	cochlear ii magna 4tis	*Two tablespoonfuls [to be taken] every 4*
	horis	*hours.*
	Omitte alia	*Leave off the rest.*

---

[134] The number of grains intended is illegible.

[135] The patient history notes that the mercury powders were affecting the patient's mouth. As she had been taking these every four hours, possibly with a high mercury content, for a week, it is not surprising that adverse effects occurred.

Feb 13	Emplast Lyttæ 4/5 inches	*Feb 17. [Apply] a Cantharides Plaster 4/5 inches.*
25	Ry misturæ ℥viii at page 106 Susan Reeve	*Feb 25. Take 8 ounces Mixture at page 106.* *Susan Reeve*

[p.106]

Frances Baker, continued
from p. 100 [*sic*]

Frances Baker [continued]

March 2	Ry Infus Rosæ ℥viii	*March 2. Take 8 ounces Infusion of Rose.*
	Omitte alia	*Leave off the rest.*
4	Emplast Ant Tart hypochondrio dextro	*March 4. [Apply] Antimony Tartrate Plaster to right hypochondrium.*
	Common diet	
10	~~Discharged~~ Out patient	*March 10. ~~Discharged~~.* *Outpatient.*
April 29	Ry Infus Rosæ ℥viii Acid Sulph Dil ʒſs M cochlear i magnum in aquæ cyatho 4tis horis	*Apr 29. Take 8 ounces Infusion of Rose,* *½ drachm Dilute Sulphuric Acid. Mix.* *One tablespoonful [to be taken] in a glass of* *water every* *4 hours.*

[p.102]

Mary Cook [*age*] 44

[*There is no case history for this patient and it is difficult to suggest a diagnosis from the drugs prescribed. In common with the previous patient, Frances Baker, Mary was prescribed antimony plaster and a mixture of sulphuric acid and infusion of rose, but on this occasion quinine was also added. Pills of squill and hemlock were given at night, the hemlock most likely as a narcotic, the squills possibly as an expectorant. Stomach powders of rhubarb, ginger and bicarbonate of soda were given for several days. On the last day on which a prescription was recorded, the quinine mixture was replaced by one containing tincture of ergot.*]

[p.103]

Jan 15	Ry Emp Ant Tart	*Jan 15. Take Antimony Tartrate plaster.*
	Ry Pil Aper ii nocte sd	*Take Aperient Pills. Two to be taken at night.*
	Ry Quinæ Disulphate gr xii Infus Rosæ ℥viii Acid Sulphur Dil ʒſs M cochlear iii magna ter in die	*Take 12 grains Quinine Disulphate,* *8 ounces Infusion of Rose,* *½ drachm Dilute Sulphuric Acid. Mix.* *Three tablespoonfuls [to be taken] three* *a day.*

66

℞ Pil Scillæ C ʒſs	*Take ½ drachm Compound Squill Pill,*
Ext Conii ʒſs	*½ drachm Extract of Hemlock.*
Mf pil xii	*Mix. Make 12 pills.*
sum^t ii o n h s	*Let her take two at night, at bedtime.*
Full diet	*Full diet.*

March 2	Rep^r mistura et pil	*March 2. Repeat mixture and pills.*
9		*March 9.*
	℞ Pulv Rhei gr xl	*Take 40 grains Rhubarb powder,*
	Pulv Zingib ʒſs M	*½ drachm Ginger Powder,*
	Sodæ Sesquicarb ʒi	*Sodium Bicarbonate 1 drachm. Mix.*
	divide in pulv viii	*Divide into 8 powders.*
	i bis in die in aqua	*One [to be taken] twice a day, in water.*
12	Perstet	*March 12. Continue.*
17	Perstet	*March 17. Continue.*
	Rep^r pulveres vi	*Repeat 6 powders.*
24	℞ Infus Rosæ ʒviii	*March 24. Take 8 ounces Infusion of Rose,*
	Tinct Ergot ʒii M	*2 drachms Tincture of Ergot. Mix.*
	cochlear ii magna bis	*Two tablespoonfuls [to be taken] twice*
	in die	*a day.*
	Omitte Mist Quinæ	*Leave off the Quinine mixture.*

[p.104]

Samuel Scott [age] 44

[*A very brief record, the patient being admitted on 15 January and transferred to the surgeon of the week on the 17 January. This was just long enough for him to be prescribed aperient pills and solution of iodine.*]

[p.105]

Jan 15		*Jan 15.*
	℞ L̶i̶q̶ Sol Iodin C ʒ viii	*Take 8 ounces Compound solution of Iodine.*
	cochlear i mag bis	*One tablespoonful [to be taken] twice*
	in die	*a day.*
	℞ Pil Aper ii	*Take Aperient pills. Two*
	nocte s^d	*to be taken at night.*
Jan 17	To be transferred to the surgeon of the week	*Jan 17. To be transferred to the surgeon of the week.*

[p.106]

William Wilkinson [age] 12

[*Presumably this patient had had a fit, because a possible diagnosis of epilepsy was made. The only treatment he received was a few doses of aperient powders. (See Appendix II for a discussion of epilepsy.)*]

1840
Jan 25   No fits since before the 17

1840
Jan 25. No fits since before 17 [January].·

[There follows on this page further prescriptions for Frances Baker which have been included with her records on pp. 101–2.]

[p.107]

Epilepsy ?

A possible diagnosis of epilepsy was made.

Jan 17
℞ Pulv Aper C gr xii
nocte s^d

Jan 17.
Take 12 grains Compound Aperient Powder.
To be taken at night.

Jan 19   Rep^r Pulv Aper bis in
hebdomada

Jan 19. Repeat the Aperient Powders twice a
week.

Continued from P.100[136]

[p.108]

Susan Reeve [age] 23

[The thing to note here is the way in which infectious diseases had affected Susan's life. Both her parents had already died of pulmonary tuberculosis and she herself was blind in the left eye due to childhood measles. Pills of calomel (mercury) with colocynth followed by a dose of castor oil were prescribed as aperients. The patient had had a fractured left ankle and now seemed to have pains in other joints too. Camphorated oil (compound liniment of camphor) was a long-established remedy for the relief of joint pains. Susan had it applied to her knee. Later, lead lotion with colchicum was used twice a day, presumably for the pain and swelling in her right foot. On 25 February she was given a typical cough mixture containing camphor, squills and acacia. Both potassium nitrate and antimony tartrate were used in fevers, and these were present in two of the mixtures prescribed. On 17 March ten ounces of blood were taken by venesection, this being another indication that she may have had a fever.]

1840
Feb 7 Extremely tall, nearly 6 feet, of a florid complexion – loosely made. The whole? family tall. Parents both dead of Phthisis. Enjoyed good health till the ?age of 19 when she began to? feel the bad effects of amenorrhoea, her menses having? never appeared up to that time. From that period she has been laid up by pains in? the limbs and sinking in the precordia [sic], liable to faint? on the slightest emotion – about 21 her menses began to come at irregular intervals and in small quantity – but have gradually been improving. Had measles at 10 or 11,

1840
Feb 7. Extremely tall, nearly 6 feet. [She has] a florid complexion and is loosely made. The whole family are tall. [Her] parents both dead of Phthisis.[137] Enjoyed good health till the age of 19 when she began to feel the bad effects of amenorrhoea,[138] her menses having never appeared [until then]. From that time she has been laid up with pains in the limbs and sinking in the precordia.[139]· [She is] liable to faint on the slightest emotion. [At] about 21 her menses began to come at irregular intervals and in small quantity but [they] have gradually been improving. [She] had measles at 10 or 11.

---

136   This remark refers to p. 106 opposite and the case of Frances Baker.
137   Pulmonary tuberculosis.
138   Lack of periods.
139   The region around the heart.

soon after which she had inflammation of both eyes, apparently of a strumous character, during which she completely lost? the sight of the left eye, the cornea of which is quite opake [*sic*]. 29 weeks ago fractured her left leg in the region of the ankle. About 6 or 8 weeks has been afflicted? with pain and swelling of the right foot, which has incapacitated her from walking. Pulse 116, with occasional irregularity. Strength of pulse at wrist small compared with force of the hearts action. Tongue coated – moist – ?left foot a little swelled, right not so but painful, no heat however appreciable. 14 Menses have appeared

Soon after [this] she had inflammation of both eyes apparently of a strumous[140] *character. She completely lost the sight of the left eye, the cornea of which is quite opaque. 29 weeks ago [she] fractured her left leg in the region of the ankle, [and for] about six or eight weeks [she] has been affected with pain and swelling of the right foot, which has incapacitated her from walking. Pulse [rate] 116 [per minute] with occasional irregularity. The strength of [the] pulse at [the] wrist [is] small compared with the force of the heart's action. Tongue coated and moist. Left foot a little swelled. [The] right not so, but [it is] painful. No appreciable heat, however.* [141]

March 14. Menses have appeared.

March 30 Common diet

March 30. Common diet.

    R̉ Ext Col C gr iv
    Hydrarg Chlorid gr v M
    ft pil n s

Take 4 grains Compound Extract of Colocynth, 5 grains Mercurous Chloride. Mix. Make a pill. [To be taken] at night.

    R̉ Ol Ricini ʒſs mane

Take ½ ounce Castor Oil in the morning.

[p.109]

Feb 5 R̉ Ext Colchici Acet gr iii

Feb 5 Take 3 grains Acetic Extract of Colchicum,

    Ext Colocynth C ϴi
    Hydrag [*sic*] Chlorid gr vi M
    divide in pil vi
    ii omni nocte sᵈ

1 scruple Compound Extract of Colocynth, 6 grains Mercurous Chloride. Mix. Divide into 6 pills. Two to be taken at night.

    R̉ Magnes Sulphat ʒi
    Ant Potass Tart gr i
    Mist Camphor ʒviii
    M cochlear ii magna
    bis in die

Feb 7. Take 1 ounce Magnesium Sulphate, 1 grain Antimony and Potassium Tartrate, 8 ounces Camphor Mixture. Mix. Two tablespoonfuls [to be taken] twice a day.

    Common Diet

Common diet.

7   Perstet

Feb 7. Continue.

16   Perstet

Feb 16. Continue.

20   ~~Applica Emplast Lyttæ parv regioni cordis~~

Feb 20. ~~Apply a small Cantharides Plaster to the region of the heart.~~

---

140 An appearance similar to scrofula. Her eyes obviously became infected and she developed scarring of the cornea as a result. Measles is a serious illness.
141 Stutter must have palpated both joints to check for heat (or calor) which would indicate underlying infection. He was obviously a hands-on doctor.

22	℞ Lin Camphor C ʒii	*Feb 22. Take 2 ounces Compound Liniment of Camphor.*
	genubus applicandum	*To be applied to the knee.*
25	℞ Tinct Camphor C ʒiii	*Take 3 drachms Compound Tincture of Camphor,*[142]
	Oxymel Scillæ ʒii	*2 drachms Oxymel of Squill,*
	Mist Acaciæ ʒiſs	*1½ ounces Acacia Mixture,*
	Mist Camphor ʒvi M	*6 ounces Camphor Mixture. Mix.*
	cochlear i mag	*One tablespoonful [to be taken]*
	urgente tusi	*if the cough is troublesome.*
27	Perstet in usu emulsionis	*Feb 27. Continue to use Emulsion.*[143]
	Omitte alia	*Leave off the rest.*
	℞ Sp Ammon Fœtid ʒiii	*Take 3 drachms Foetid Spirit of Ammonia,*[144]
	Sodæ Sesquicarb ʒiſs	*1½ drachms Sodium Bicarbonate,*
	Mist Camphor ʒviii	*8 ounces Camphor mixture.*
	M cochlear iii magna	*Mix. Three tablespoonfuls [to be taken]*
	ter in die	*three times a day.*
March 2	Perstet – common diet	*March 2. Continue. Common diet.*
9	℞ Tinct Colchici ʒſs	*March 9. Take ½ ounce Tincture of Colchicum,*
	Liq Plumbi Acet Dil ʒviii	*8 ounces Dilute Solution of Lead Acetate.*
	M ft lotio bis in die	*Mix. Make a lotion.*[145] *Apply twice a day.*
	applicand	
	Common diet, ½ a pint	*Common diet with ½ pint*
	of beer	*of beer.*
March 17	VS ad ʒx	*March 17. Venesection 10 ounces of blood taken.*
	Repʳ linimentum	*Repeat the liniment.*
March 24		*March 24.*
	℞ [deletion] Potass Nit ʒiſs	*Take 1½ drachms Potassium Nitrate,*
	Ant Potassio Tart gr ii	*2 grains Antimony & Potassium Tartrate,*
	Aquæ ʒ viii	*8 ounces Water.*
	cochlear ii magna 4ᵗⁱˢ horis	*Two tablespoonfuls [to be taken] every 4 hours.*
	℞ Jalapæ Rhei a a gr viii	*Take 8 grains each Jalap and Rhubarb,*
	Hydrag [sic] Chlorid gr v M	*5 grains Mercurous Chloride.*[146] *Mix.*
	ft pulv st sᵈ	*Make a powder. To be taken immediately.*
	Vide p.112. [marginal note].	*See p.112.*

---

142 This tincture (commonly known as 'paregoric') contained a small dose of opium; its use for allaying coughs continued well into the twentieth century.

143 That is, the cough mixture of 25 February.

144 A combination of aromatic spirit of ammonia with asafœtida.

145 A pain-relieving lotion probably for Susan's swollen right foot.

146 The jalap and rhubarb combined with the mercury would have produced a strong purgative action.

[p.112] **Susan Reeve** [*continued from page 109*]

April 1	
	Complains much of head ache, tongue much coated

Apr 1.
Complains much of headache, tongue much coated

[p.113]

R̃ Quinæ Disulph gr viii
Magnes Sulphatis ʒi
Infus Rosæ ʒvii
Tinct Zingib ʒii M
cochlear ii magna
ter in die

Take 8 grains Quinine Disulphate.
1 ounce Magnesium Sulphate,
7 ounces Infusion of Rose,
2 drachms Tincture of Ginger. Mix.
Two tablespoonfuls [to be taken]
three times a day.

Omitte
½ a pint of beer

Half a pint of beer.

Omitte pilulas

Leave off the pills.

[p.110]

Thomas Scott [*age*] (19)

[*Stutter noted that Thomas's bowels were confined. The House Apothecary prescribed purgative pills of colchicum, colocynth and mercury with a mildly laxative mixture of Epsom Salts (magnesium sulphate), pleasantly flavoured with infusion of rose petals. The use of sixteen leeches on the same day was apparently successful, because Stutter noted that the patient was much relieved by them. Camphorated oil was the only other treatment that the young tailor was given before he was discharged cured. It may be he had had an attack of rheumatic fever.*]

5th Feb By trade a tailor, has worked for nearly six years and enjoyed good health until five weeks ago, when he was seized with pain in the left foot which was much swollen and to which poultices were applied and a stimulating liniment which relieved the foot, but at that time a pain appeared in the left hip at its latero posterior part where it has continued ever since, feels occasionally pain for a short time in the right calf. Skin cool. Pulse 104. Tongue slightly coated moist. Has become emaciated since his illness. Countenance pale, appetite good. No cough. Chest clear on percussion, respiration normal, hearts action intense, sounds loud, impulse considerable, abdomen soft. Bowels confined – generally so.

Feb 7 Much relieved by the leeches.

5th Feb. By trade a tailor, [he] has worked for nearly six years and enjoyed good health until five weeks ago, when he was seized with pain in the left foot, which was much swollen. Poultices were applied and a stimulating liniment which relieved the foot, but at that time a pain appeared in the left hip at its latero posterior[147] part where it has continued ever since. He occasionally feels pain for a short time in the right calf. Skin cool. Pulse [rate] 104 [per minute]. Tongue slightly coated and moist. [He] has become emaciated since his illness. Countenance pale. Appetite good. No cough. Chest clear on percussion. Respiration normal. Heart's action intense. Sounds loud. Impulse considerable. Abdomen soft. Bowels confined – [they are] generally so.

Feb 7. Much relieved by the leeches.

---

147   The upper and outer part of the thigh.

[p.111]

5th Feb	℞		*Feb 5. Take*
	Ext Colchici Acet gr vi		*6 grains Acetic extract of Colchicum,*
	Ext Colocynth C Ɔii		*2 scruples Compound Extract of Colocynth,*
	Pulv Digitalis gr v		*5 grains Digitalis Powder,*
	Hyd Chlorid gr xii		*12 grains Mercurous Chloride.*
	divide in pil vi ii o n		*Divide into 6 pills, [take] two at night.*

℞ Magnes Sulphatis ℥iſs — *Take 1½ ounces Magnesium Sulphate,*
Infus Rosæ — *4 ounces each Infusion of Rose [and]*
Aquæ a a ℥iv M — *Water. Mix.*
cochlear iii magna ter — *Three tablespoonfuls [to be taken] three*
in die — *times a day.*

Applica Hirudines xvi — *Apply 16 leeches.*

Common Diet

Feb 7	Perstet	*Feb 7. Continue.*

28 — *Feb 28.*
℞ Lin Camphor C ℥ii — *Take 2 ounces Compound Liniment of Camphor.*
bis die applicand — *Apply twice a day.*

March 10 Discharged cured — *Mar 10. Discharged, cured.*

[p.112]

Elizabeth Payne [*age*] 12

[*Small doses of strychnine were believed to restore muscle tone. Sufferers from chorea[148] often develop irregular uncontrollable movements, and so the logic of giving Elizabeth pills containing one twentieth of a grain of strychnine can be seen. She was also given aperient powders of calomel, rhubarb and jalap to be taken every other morning, later changed to a teaspoonful of senna confection to be taken each night.*]

1840
March 18th Chorea which has visited six weeks, confined more particularly to the left arm and head.

She has had Chorea for the past six weeks, mainly affecting the left arm and head.

[p.113]

March 18 ℞ Strychiæ [*sic*] gr i — *Mar 18. Take 1 grain Strychnine,*
Micæ Panis ℨi M — *1 drachm Bread crumbs. Mix.*
divide in pilulas xx — *Divide into 20 pills.*
i ter in die — *[Take] one three times a day.*

℞ Hydrarg Chlorid gr iii — *Take 3 grains Mercurous Chloride,*
Pulv Rhei — *5 grains each of Rhubarb Powder and*

---

[148] See Appendix II.

Pulv Jalap a a gr v M
ft pulv alternis ~~noctibus~~
auroris

Jalap Powder. Mix.
Make a powder. [Take] every other ~~night~~
morning.

Common diet

Common diet.

March 20 Omitte ?pulverum aper[*illeg.*]

Mar 20. Leave off the aperient powder.[149]

March 26
    ℞ Confect Sennae Opt
    ʒi nocte s^d

Mar 26.
Take Best Confection of Senna.
1 teaspoonful to be taken at night.

[p.114]

Mary Death [*age*] 41

[*Mercury was considered to be beneficial in chronic hepatitis and rheumatism and so Mary Death was prescribed mercury pills, despite the fact that thirteen years earlier she had lost nearly all her teeth as a result of similar treatment. An aperient mixture of Epsom Salts and magnesia was given each morning. It seems likely that this proved to be too effective, since the mixture was later stopped and replaced by powders of chalk and opium (present in the ipecacuanha compound powder). Both chalk and opium were used in the treatment of diarrhoea. She was relieved of twelve ounces of blood by venesection[150] and a further ten ounces by cupping.[151] A counter-irritant ointment of antimony and potassium tartrate ointment was used each night and morning.*

The patient had pain in the right side of her upper abdomen and her shoulders. She had also been jaundiced for two weeks and had tenderness over the liver. It seems possible that she did not have hepatitis as we understand it at all. Instead, she might have had an obstructive jaundice due to gall stones, which were eventually passed through her common bile duct into the bowel, allowing the jaundice to subside and making her appetite good enough for her to be able to face a normal diet. (See Appendix II under hepatitis for further discussion of this case).]

1840 Has never enjoyed very good health, but for the last five years has been almost constantly ill, suffering from severe pains in the right side shoulders and neck – which were called by her medical attendant rheumatic. For two years she has been unable to walk from pain in the loins. No great emaciation, great yellowness of skin and conjunctivae of 2 weeks standing, during which period she has had more pain in her right side – at times suffers from dyspnoea, has lost all her teeth but one in consequence of excessive salivation 13 years ago. Bowels habitually constipated. Pulse 96, small.

1840 She has never enjoyed very good health, but for the last five years, she has been almost constantly ill, suffering from severe pains in the right side, shoulders and neck. Her medical attendant called these rheumatic. For two years she has been unable to walk because of pain in the loins. There is no great emaciation but there is great yellowness of skin and conjunctivae of two weeks standing. During this period she has had more pain in her right side.[152] At times she suffers from dyspnoea and has lost all her teeth but one in consequence of excessive salivation thirteen years ago.[153] Her bowels are habitually constipated. Pulse 96,

---

149   That is, those containing mercury, rhubarb and jalap.
150   See Appendix IV.
151   See Appendix IV.
152   As mentioned above, the patient's problem may have been gallstones obstructing the biliary duct. But Stutter had no way of investigating the condition and it would be many years before surgeons ventured to operate on such cases.
153   This was undoubtedly iatrogenic, due to the excessive prescription of mercury.

Tongue dryish – thirst, respiration healthy – sounds of the heart not normal. Cannot bear the slightest pressure in the region of the liver.	*small. Tongue dryish [she is thirsty]. Respiration healthy. Sounds of the heart are not normal.*[154] *Cannot bear the slightest pressure in the region of the liver.*

[p.115]

	Chronic Rheumatism. Hepatitis.	*Chronic Rheumatism. Hepatitis.*
	℞ Pil Hydrarg ʒi ~~gr v~~ divide in pil xii i ter in die sumend	*Take ~~5 grains~~ 1 drachm Mercury pill,* *Divide into 12 pills.* *One to be taken three times a day.*
	℞ Magnes Sulphatis ℥iſs Magnes Carbon ℈iv Aquæ bullientis ℥viii sumatur pars quarta omni mane	*Take 1½ ounces Magnesium Sulphate,* *4 scruples Magnesium Carbonate,* *8 ounces Boiling Water.* *Let a fourth part be taken* *each morning.*
	V S ad ℥ xii statim	*Venesection of up to 12 ounces [of blood to be taken] at once.*
	Applica cucurbitulas cruentas cras et ditrahantur sanguinis ℥x si opus e regione hypocondriaco dextro	*Apply wet cupping glasses* *tomorrow and draw* *10 ounces of blood if needed* *from the right hypochondrial region.*
	cataplasma eidem regioni	*[Apply] a poultice*[155] *to the same region.*
	low diet	*To have a low diet.*
20	~~Omn~~ Sumatur pil i o n et cochlear ii magna misturæ omni mane	*Mar 20. ~~Each~~ Let one pill* *be taken at night and two tablespoonfuls* *of the mixture each morning.*
24	℞ Ung Ant Potassio Tart ℥i nocte maneque utend	*Mar 24. Take 1 ounce Antimony and Potassium Tartrate ointment.* *To be used night and morning.*
26	Cataplasma largam lateri sinistro	*Mar 26. [Apply a] large poultice* *to the left side.*
30	Repr pilulæ alternis noctibus	*30. Repeat the pills on alternate nights.*
April 1	Omitte Misturam Magnes Sulphatis	*Apr 1. Leave off the Magnesium Sulphate mixture.*
	℞ Confectionis Arom ℥ſs Pulv Creta C ℈ii Tinct Cinnam ʒii Mist Camphor ℥viii	*Take ½ ounce Aromatic Confection,* *2 scruples Compound Powder of Chalk,* *2 drachms Tincture of Cinnamon,* *8 ounces Camphor mixture.*

---

[154] Stutter is not committing himself here. He thinks the heart sounds are abnormal but cannot quite describe the abnormality. At least he is being intellectually honest.

[155] The type of poultice is not specified.

	cochlear ii magna ter in die	*Two tablespoonfuls [to be taken] three times a day.*
	Common diet	*Common diet*
3	Cataplasma	*Poultice*
April 13	℞ Pulv Creta C gr x	*Apr 13. Take 10 grains Compound Chalk Powder,*
	Pulv Ipecac C gr v M ft pulv 4ᵗⁱˢ horis sumendas Mitte vi	*5 grains Compound Ipecacuanha Powder. Mix. Make a powder. One to be taken every 4 hours. Send 6.*
	Omitte misturam interim Rice and milk	*Leave off the mixture in the meantime. [To have] rice and milk.*
15	℞ Confect Arom Ɔii Tinct Opii ʒi Tinct Cinnam ʒii Sp Ammon Ar ʒiſs Aquæ ℥viii M cochlear ii magna ter in die	*Apr 15. Take 2 scruples Aromatic Confection, 1 drachm Tincture of Opium, 2 drachms Tincture of Cinnamon, 1½ drachms Aromatic Spirit of Ammonia, 8 ounces Water. Mix. Two tablespoonfuls [to be taken] three times a day.*

[p.116]

David Tweed [age] 40

[The pills of colocynth, colchicum and mercury would have had a strong purgative action. Stutter may have been using them solely for this effect or for the supposed pain-relieving properties of colchicum. This drug was (and is) very effective in gout, and because of this its use seems to have been extended to all cases of joint and muscle pain. In addition, contemporary opinion still held that mercury was helpful in rheumatism. Antimony and potassium tartrate and potassium iodide were further drugs which were recommended for the same problem. They were prescribed for this patient as mixtures, the first having the aperient Epsom Salts included in the brew.]

1840
March 18 Has enjoyed good health until the last two months, during which time he has been unable to work from rheumatic pains in the right arm and thigh. P. 82, tongue moist with a brown mark in the centre.

Mar 18. [He] enjoyed good health until two months ago when he became unable to work on account of rheumatic pains in the right arm and thigh. Pulse [rate] 82 [per minute]. Tongue moist with a brown mark in the centre.[156]

[p.117]

March 18	℞ Ext Colchici Acet gr viii Ext Colocynth C ʒi Hyd chlorid gr xvi M divide in pil xii ii omni nocte	*Mar 18. Take 8 grains Acetic Extract of Colchicum, 1 drachm Compound Extract of Colocynth, 16 grains Mercurous chloride. Mix. Divide into 12 pills. Two [to be taken] each night.*

---

156   This is probably insignificant.

	Rᵉ Magnesiæ Sulphatis ʒi	*Take 1 ounce Magnesium Sulphate,*
	Ant Potassio Tart gr i	*1 grain Antimony and Potassium Tartrate,*
	Aquæ ʒviiiM	*8 ounces Water. Mix.*
	¼ omni mane	*A fourth part [to be taken] each morning.*
	Rᵉ Potassii Iodidi Ꙗi	*Take 1 scruple Potassium Iodide,*
	Mist Camphoræ ʒviii	*8 ounces Camphor Mixture,*
	Syrupi Croci ʒi M	*1 drachm Syrup of Saffron.[157] Mix.*
	cochlear ii magna ter	*Two tablespoonfuls [to be taken] three times*
	in die	*a day.*
	Low diet	*Low diet.*
24	Sumatur pil i alternis	*Mar 24. Let him take one pill on alternate*
	noctibus	*nights.*
30	Common diet	*Mar 30. Common diet.*
	Perstet in aliis	*Continue with the others.*
April 7	Perstet	*Apr 7. Continue.*
15	A pint of beer	*Apr 15. [To have] a pint of beer.*

[p.118]

James Fane [*age*] 10

[There is no recorded medical history for this young lad, and on the strength of just two prescriptions it is almost impossible to suggest a diagnosis, although the use of digitalis does raise the possibility of a heart condition. Despite the fact that he was only ten years old, James was prescribed beer and wine. The latter was thought to be very beneficial for almost anybody in a poor state of health.]

1840 from Dr Jackson

	Rᵉ Tinct Digital ʒi	*Take 1 drachm Tincture of Digitalis,*
	Tinct Hyoscyam ʒiſs	*1½ drachms Tincture of Henbane,*
	Aquæ ʒvi	*6 ounces Water.*
	cochlear i magnum ter in die	*One tablespoonful [to be taken] three times a*
		day.
	Rᵉ Pil Ferri C Ꙗii	*Take 2 scruples Compound Iron Pill,*
	Saponis Ꙗi M	*1 scruple Soap. Mix.*
	ft pil xx i ter in die	*Make 20 pills, [take] one three times a day.*
April 7	Omit wine	*Apr 7. Leave off the wine.*
	to have a pint of beer a day	*To have a pint of beer a day.*

[p.119, *blank*]

---

[157] Chiefly used to impart colour to mixtures.

[p.120]

Jonathon Sturgeon [*age not recorded*]

[*This is yet another patient whose medical history was not recorded. He received just two prescriptions before being discharged as cured. Purgatives dominated his drug therapy. He was given pills of mercury, colocynth, scammony and ipecacuanha as well as a mixture that included Epsom Salts as one of the ingredients.*]

1840

℞ Pil Hyd ʒſs	*Take ½ drachm Mercury Pill,*
Ext Colocynth	*10 grains each Extract of Colocynth,*
Scam Resinæ a a gr x	*Scammony Resin,*
Pulv Colchici	*5 grains each Colchicum Powder,*
– Ipecac a a gr v	*Ipecacuanha Powder.*
[*New hand*] divide in pil xii sum^t i	*Divide into 12 pills. Let him take one*
nocte maneque	*night and morning.*
℞ Sulph Magnes ʒiſs	*Take 1½ ounces Magnesium Sulphate,*
Mist Camph ʒv	*5 ounces Camphor Mixture,*
Liq Ammon Acet ʒiv	*4 ounces Solution of Ammonium Acetate,*
Vin Colchici ʒiii	*3 drachms Colchicum Wine,*
Spt Æth Nit ʒv	*5 drachms Spirit of Nitrous Ether.*
mf mist sum^t coch ii larga	*Mix. Make a mixture. Let him take two*
ter die	*tablespoonfuls three times a day.*
[*orginal hand*] Discharged cured	*Discharged, cured.*
Mrs Woodroffe	*Mrs Woodroffe [matron]*

[p.121, *blank*]

[p.122]

Matthew Sindell [*age*] 40

[*This patient may have had a severe attack of chilblains following exposure to cold. The lesions on his buttocks sound remarkably similar to those which were sometimes seen in winter in the nineteen sixties, the sufferers in that era being young women who had been wearing the then fashionable miniskirts. Matthew was given an astringent lotion containing alum and zinc sulphate and a yeast poultice. Yeast poultices, made from yeast and flour, were said to be antiseptic and were usually applied to putrefying areas. As usual, Stutter prescribed aperient draughts as well as laxative pills containing colocynth and mercury. The administration of powders of chalk and opium (in compound ipecacuanha powder) and the iron nitrate suggest that diarrhoea may have been consequent on the purgation. Iron nitrate solution was thought to be a valuable remedy in chronic diarrhoea.*]

1840
April 1 A waterman between Lynn and Bury – strong and muscular, has enjoyed excellent health until about a year ago when he was ill and under medical treatment at Lynn for pain in the neck and shoulders. He had also shortness of breathing which has continued ever since on making any exertion, but has

1840
Apr 1. A waterman between Lynn and Bury. [He is] strong and muscular [and] has enjoyed excellent health until about a year ago when he was ill and under medical treatment at Lynn for pain in the neck and shoulders. He also had shortness of breathing, which has continued ever since on making any exertion. [Nevertheless], he continued with his work

77

continued with his work until a week ago when, after exposure to severe cold he observed that his face was much swollen and blue, his ankles also became swollen and his water became diminished in quantity and has been very turbid even when first voided. He also found that he had tumours on the nates[158] which itched and were tender. Bowels have been regularly relieved once a day till now. His countenance is today natural, tongue white and coated, chest clear on percussion, respiration natural, sounds of heart muffled – hearts action not in accordance with the pulse at the wrist, being much stronger in proportion, no tenderness of abdomen. On the left hip there is a considerable [sic] the skin of which has ulcerated and is replaced by a dry black eschar – the right hip is also the seat of a similar tumour, the skin unbroken, resembling chilblains, veins of legs varicose, slight puffiness of ankles.

until a week ago, when, after exposure to severe cold he observed that his face was much swollen and blue. His ankles also became swollen and his water became diminished in quantity and has [since] been very turbid, even when first voided. He also found that he had tumours on the buttocks, which itched and were tender. [His] bowels have been regularly relieved once a day till now. His countenance is today natural, tongue white and coated, chest clear on percussion. Respiration natural. Sounds of heart muffled. [The] heart's action [is] not in accordance with the pulse at the wrist being much stronger in proportion. [There is] no tenderness [of the] abdomen. On the left hip there is a considerable [tumour], the skin of which has ulcerated and is replaced by a dry black eschar.[159] The right hip is also the seat of a similar tumour, [but] the skin [is] unbroken, resembling chilblains. [He has] varicose veins of [the] legs [and] slight puffiness of [the] ankles.

[p.123]

April 1	℞ Ext Col C gr v	Apr 1. Take 5 grains Compound Extract of Colocynth,
	Pil Hyd gr iv M divide in pil ii ~~nocte s~~d st sd	4 grains Mercury Pill. Mix. Divide into 2 pills to be taken ~~at night~~ immediately.
	℞ Haust Aper post horas sex	Take Aperient Draught after six hours.[160]
	℞ Sp Æther Nit ʒſs Tinct Hyos ʒiii Mist Camphor ʒviii cochlear ii magna ter in die	Take ½ ounce Spirit of Nitrous Ether, 3 drachms Tincture of Henbane. 8 ounces Camphor Mixture. Two tablespoonfuls [to be taken] three times a day.
	℞ Liq Alumin C O i ft Lotio tumoribus assidue applicand	Take 1 pint Compound Solution of Aluminium.[161] Make a lotion for the swelling To be applied frequently.
	Cataplasmata	[Apply a] Poultice.
	Common diet	Common diet.

[158] 'Nates' means 'buttocks'.
[159] 'Eschar' means 'a dry slough'.
[160] That is, six hours after the pills.
[161] Contained alum and zinc sulphate.

3	Rep^r pilulæ ii hac nocte	*3 Repeat the pills. Two [to be be taken] tonight.*
	Rep^r Haust. Aper cras mane	*Repeat the Aperient Draught tomorrow morning.*
	Cataplasma fermenti	*[Apply a] Yeast Poultice.*[162]
Ap^r 7	R̸ Quinæ Disuphat ʒſs Tinct Zinzib ʒiii Infus Rosæ ℥viii M cochlear ii magna 4^tis horis	*Apr 7. Take ½ drachm Quinine Disulphate, 3 drachms Tincture of Ginger, 8 ounces Infusion of Rose, Mix. Two tablespoonfuls [to be taken] every 4 hours.*
	1 pint of beer	*[To have] one pint of beer.*
11	To have two pints of beer Perstet	*To have 2 pints of beer. Continue.*
	R̸ Pulv Cretæ C gr x	*Apr 18. Take 10 grains Compound Chalk Powder.*
	Pulv Ipecac C gr iii M ft pulv ter in die sum Mitte iv	*3 grains Compound Ipecacuanha Powder. Mix. Make 4 powders. One to be taken three times a day. Send 4.*
Maii 1	Omitte pulveres	*May 1. Leave off the powders.*
	R̸ Ferri Persesquinitratis ʒii Aquæ ℥viii M Cochlear iii magna bis in die	*Take 2 drachms [Solution of] Iron Nitrate,*[163] *8 ounces Water. Mix. Three tablespoonfuls [to be taken] twice a day.*
May 19	Cured	*May 19. Cured.*

[p.124]

Frances Steggles [age] (25)

[*In the first half of the nineteenth century symptoms were treated as though they were illnesses in themselves. Iron and decoctions of aloes were recognised as being useful for amenorrhoea, and this is no doubt why Frances received them. Calomel and colocynth pills were given to relieve constipation. To combat the patient's stomach pains Stutter prescribed a mixture of hydrocyanic acid by mouth and an application of antimony ointment to the skin of the upper abdomen. The latter would have acted as a counter-irritant.*]

1840
April 15 Enjoyed good health until 4 months ago though she did not menstruate regularly and not at all till	*Apr 15. She enjoyed good health until four months ago, though she did not menstruate regularly and not at all till she was 20.*[164]

---

162   This poultice was described as 'antiseptic' in 1820, fifty years before the Listerian concept of sepsis, being defined in Webster's *Dictionary* of 1828 as 'a medicine which resists or corrects putrefaction'. The modern definition is a substance that destroys micro-organisms which carry disease without harming body tissues.
163   Prepared by dissolving iron wire in nitric acid.
164   Later onset of menstruation was commoner in those who were malnourished.

she was 20. Suffers from pains in the head and stomach. Menses have not at all shown themselves for the last three months. P. 70, languid. Bowels have not been relieved for three days.

Suffers from pains in the head and stomach. Menses have not at all shown themselves for the last three months. Pulse [rate] 70 [per minute and] languid. Bowels have not been relieved for three days.

[p.125]

℞ Pil Ferri C ʒi
divide in pilulas xii
capiantur duæ ter
in die

Take 1 drachm Compound Iron Pill. Divide into 12 pills. Let two be taken three times a day.

℞ Decoct Aloes C ʒiv
Sol Magnes Bicarb ʒi
Infus Aurantii ʒiii
M.cochlear ii magna
4ᵗⁱˢ horis

Take 4 ounces Compound Decoction of Aloes, 1 ounce Solution of Magnesium Bicarbonate, 3 ounces Infusion of Orange. Mix. Two tablespoonfuls [to be taken] every 4 hours.

℞ Ext Colocynth C gr vi
Hyd Chlorid gr iiii
Ext Hyos gr iii M
divide in pil duas
hac nocte sumend

Take 6 grains Compound Extract of Colocynth, 4 grains Mercurous Chloride, 3 grains Extract of Henbane. Mix. Divide into 2 pills to be taken tonight.

Common diet

Common diet

18 ℞ Decoct Aloes C ʒvi

Apr 18. Take 6 ounces Compound Decoction of Aloes,

Infus ~~Aurantii~~ Gentian ʒii
M cochlear ii magna
ter in die

2 ounces Infusion of ~~Orange~~ Gentian. Mix. Two tablespoonfuls [to be taken] three times a day.

Omitte Misturam Magnes

Leave off the Magnesium mixture.

26 ℞ Ferri Potassio Tart gr viii

Apr 26. Take 8 grains Iron & Potassium Tartrate,

Potass Bitart ʒſs
Zingiberis gr iii M
ft pulv ter in die
sumend Mitte viii

½ drachm Potassium Bitartrate, 3 grains Ginger [powder]. Mix. Make a powder, to be taken three times a day. Send 8.

Omitte pilulas Ferri

Leave off the Iron Pills.

Maii 1 Omitte pulveres

May 1. Leave off the powders.

℞ Potass Nitrat gr xlviii
Tinct Hyos ʒiii
Mist Camphor ʒviii
Acid Hydrocyan Dil ʒſs
cochlear ii magna
ter in die

Take 48 grains Potassium nitrate, 3 drachms Tincture of Henbane, 8 ounces Camphor Mixture, ½ drachm Dilute Hydrocyanic Acid. Two tablespoonfuls [to be taken] three times a day.

℞ Ung Ant Potass Tart ʒi

Take 1 ounce Antimony and Potassium Tartrate Ointment

	epigastrio applicand	To be applied to the epigastrium.
May 25		*May 25.*
	℞ Mistura Ferri ℥vii	*Take 7 ounces Iron Mixture.*
	cochlear ii magna	*Two tablespoonfuls [to be taken]*
	ter in die	*three times a day.*
	Omitte alia	*Leave off the others.*

[p.126]

Hannah Pratt [*age*] (58)

[It sounds very much as though this patient had rheumatoid arthritis. Guaiacum and colchicum were both recognised treatments for 'rheumatism' in the early nineteenth century whilst the practice of applying soap liniment to painful rheumatic areas of the body had a long tradition behind it. Although Hannah's bowels were regular she still was given laxative pills containing calomel and colocynth.]

1840

April 15th Enjoyed tolerable health till the age of 48, at which time her menses stopped. Since then she has suffered from Rheumatic pains which have frequently confined her to bed for as long as 3 months. She is at present suffering from Rheumatism in all the smaller joints of her hands and feet with enlargement of them. Bowels regular, tongue coated. Pulse 72. Countenance florid.	*Apr 15. Enjoyed tolerable health till the age of 48, when her menses stopped. Since then she has suffered from rheumatic pains which have frequently confined her to bed for as long as three months. She is at present suffering from rheumatism in all the smaller joints of her hands and feet, with enlargement of them.*[165] *Bowels regular. Tongue coated. Pulse 72 [per minute]. Countenance florid.*

[p.127]

15	℞ Tinct Colchici ℨii	*Apr 15. Take 2 drachms Tincture of Colchicum,*
	Sol Magnes Bicarb ℥i	*1 ounce Solution of Magnesium Bicarbonate,*
	Aquæ ℥vii	*7 ounces Water.*
	cochlear ii magna 4tis horis	*Two tablespoonfuls [to be taken] every 4 hours.*
	℞ Ext Colchici Acet gr i	*Take 1 grain Acetic Extract of Colchicum,*
	Ext Col C gr vi	*6 grains Compound Extract of Colocynth,*
	Hyd Chlorid gr v M	*5 grains Mercurous Chloride. Mix.*
	ft pilulæ duæ nocte sd	*Make 2 pills. To be taken at night.*
	Low diet	*Low diet.*
18	Repr pilulæ alternis noctibus	*Apr 18. Repeat the pills on alternate nights.*
Maii 4	Perstet	*May 4. Continue.*
6	℞ Tinct Guaiaci C ℥ſs	*May 6. Take ½ ounce Compound Tincture of Guaiacum,*
	Mist Acaciæ ℥i	*1 ounce Acacia Mixture,*
	Mist Camphor ℥viſs	*6½ ounces Camphor Mixture.*

---

165   These are classical symptoms of rheumatoid arthritis. See Appendix II.

M cochlear magna ii ter in die	*Mix. Two tablespoonfuls [to be taken]* *three times a day.*
Omitte Misturam Colchici	*Leave off the Colchicum mixture.*

May 20

R̥ Liniment Saponis ʒii bis die applicand	*May 20.* *Take 2 ounces Soap Liniment.* *To be applied twice a day.*

25 A pint of beer daily — *[To have] a pint of beer daily.*

Common diet — *Common diet.*

[p.128]

Harriet Scarf [age] (24)

[*This patient was prescribed iron and aloes, which were the usual contemporary drugs for sufferers from anaemia and amenorrhoea.*]

1840
April 15 Enjoyed good health till the age of 20 when she began to suffer from amenorrhea. Up to this time she had menstruated regularly from the age of 14. Her menses have been scanty for the last 12 months. Suffer [*sic*] from pains in the back and loins, bowels much confined, ankles swell at times. P. 96, tongue clear. Bruit detectable, very marked in the right carotid, less so in the left.

Apr 15. Enjoyed good health till the age of 20 when she began to suffer from amenorrhoea. Up to this time she had menstruated regularly from the age of 14. Her menses have been scanty for the last twelve months.[166] [She suffers] from pains in the back and loins, bowels much confined, ankles swell at times. Pulse 96 [per minute], tongue clear. Bruit[167] detectable, very marked in the right carotid, less so in the left.

May 1 Menses appeared

[p.129] Anæmia — *[Anaemia]*

R̥ Mist Ferri C ʒvi Tinct Aurantii ʒii Mist Camphor ʒii M. cochlear duo magna ter in die	*Take 6 ounces Compound Iron Mixture,* *2 drachms Tincture of Orange,* *2 ounces Camphor Mixture. Mix.* *Two tablespoonfuls [to be taken]* *three times a day.*
R̥ Decoct aloes C ʒvi cochlear iii magna bis in die	*Take 6 ounces Compound Decoction of Aloes.* *Three tablespoonfuls [to be taken]* *twice a day.*

Common diet — *Common diet.*

---

[166] This fits with a diagnosis of anaemia. In females with severe anaemia the periods may well shut down to conserve blood.
[167] A bruit is a noise heard on auscultation (usually) with a stethoscope. A bruit over the carotids may be heard in carotid artery stenosis, which is a narrowing of the arteries caused by atheroma. But bruits can also occur in anaemia.

21	℞ Pil Ferri C xii sumatur 2 c mistura ter in die	*May 21. Take 12 Compound Iron Pills.* *Let her take two with the mixture* *three times a day.*
25	½ a pint of beer	*[To have] half a pint of beer.*
May 19	Made out-patient	*May 19. Made an outpatient.*

[p.130, *blank*]

Robert Nelson [*age*] (60)

[*This patient was thought to have bronchitis (see Appendix II) and the medicines he was given are very much in accordance with that diagnosis. Presumably he had a fever, because he was treated with a fever mixture and with cascarilla, which had weak fever-reducing properties. The combination of ipecacuanha, camphor and opium (the latter was an ingredient of the compound camphor tincture) constituted a typical cough mixture. It was reinforced with a counter-irritant plaster applied to the back, between the shoulder blades. Tincture of Henbane (present in the cough mixture) was frequently used as a substitute for opium, its aim being to induce mild sedation.*]

[p.131]	Bronchitis	*Bronchitis*
1840 April 15	Low diet	*Apr 15. Low diet*
	℞ Vin Ipecac ʒiſs Tinct Hyoscyam ʒii Mist Febris ℔ſs Tinct Camph C ʒii Mf mist sum^t coch larg iii 4^tis horis	*Take 1½ drachms Ipecacuanha Wine,* *2 drachms Tincture of Henbane,* *½ lb Fever mixture,*[168] *2 drachms Compound Tincture of Camphor.* *Mix. Make a mixture. Let him take three* *tablespoonfuls every four hours.*
	℞ Applica Emplast Lyttæ dorso inter scapulas	*Apply a Cantharides Plaster* *to the back, between the shoulder blades.*
21	~~Perstet~~ ℞ Infusi Cascarillæ Mist Camphor a a ʒiii M cochlear iii magna ter in die	*Apr 21. ~~Continue~~ Take Infusion* *of Cascarilla [and]* *Camphor Mixture, of each* *3 ounces. Mix.* *Three tablespoonfuls [to be taken]* *three times a day.*
24	Common diet Perstet in aliis	*Apr 24. Common diet* *Continue with the others.*
May 2	A pint of beer	*May 2. [To have] a pint of beer.*
19	Cured	*May 19. Cured.*

---

168   Intended to reduce the patient's temperature.

[p.132]

Mary Willingham [age] (35)

[*This patient was dying from tuberculosis, which had invaded both her chest and abdomen. Her abdominal pains were partly relieved by the application of six leeches, and a week later turpentine liniment was applied twice a day in a further attempt to relieve her discomfort. Mary was given a dose of castor oil for constipation. This appears to have resulted in diarrhoea, because three days later she was prescribed a medicine containing chalk and opium, a formula much used to control loose motions. The mixture of ammonium acetate and spirit of nitric ether prescribed on 7 May was a recognised medicine for reducing body heat when the sufferer had a fever. It was all to no avail. The patient died on 17 May 1840.*]

1840 (April 30)

Is married. Never enjoyed very good health. First menstruated about 17. Married at 20, had one child born alive – lived one day. The 2nd was still-born rather before the full period. Has had not been since pregnant for 13 years. Has been subject to constipation and felt her health gradually deteriorating till 3 months ago when she began to suffer from pains in the abdomen accompanied with anorexia and sickness. Cessation of menses during same period. Has been confined to bed for six weeks – under medical treatment – gradually getting worse, 6 leeches applied last week to abdomen afforded some relief. Considerable emaciation, yellowish tinge, dryness of skin. Tongue clear and moist, thirst. P.112, exceedingly small. Has expectorated some viscid mucus with one or two pellets of purulent matter, which she says is unusual with her. Respiration normal excepting in the left supra scapular region where there is mucous râles. Bowels relieved yesterday and today once, motions watery – which has been the case for ten days. Great tenderness with considerable fullness over whole abdomen. Water scanty.

1840 (April 30)

[*She*] *is married.* [*She has*] *never enjoyed very good health. The patient first menstruated at about* [*the age of*] *17.* [*She*] *married at 20 and had one child born alive.* [*It*] *lived one day. The second was stillborn.* [*It was born*] *rather before the full period.* [*She*] *has not been pregnant since* [*that time, which was thirteen years ago*]. [*She*] *has been subject to constipation and has felt her health gradually deteriorating. Three months ago she began to suffer from pains in the abdomen with anorexia, sickness and the cessation of menses. She has been confined to bed for six weeks – under medical treatment.* [*Despite this she has been*] *gradually getting worse. Six leeches were applied to the abdomen last week.* [*This*] *afforded some relief.* [*There is*] *considerable emaciation. The skin is dry,* [*with a*] *yellowish tinge. The tongue is clear and moist.* [*She is*] *thirsty. Pulse rate 112* [*per minute*][169] *and exceedingly small in volume. She has expectorated some viscid mucus with one or two pellets of purulent matter, which she says is unusual. Her respiration is normal except in the left supra scapular region*[170] *where there* [*are*] *mucous râles.*[171] [*Her*] *bowels were relieved yesterday and once again today.* [*Her*] *motions are watery.* [*They*] *have been like this for ten days.* [*There is*] *great tenderness with considerable fullness over the whole abdomen.* [*Her*] *water* [*is*] *scanty.*

---

169 Pulse rate of 112 per minute. This is high, suggesting that the patient was very ill, as indeed she was.
170 The region above the shoulder blade.
171 A râle is a crackling sound (French). The stethoscope had been invented in 1816 by the Frenchman René Théophile Hyacinthe Laennec (1781–1826), and so naturally a lot of the terminology associated with its use came from France. Early stethoscopes were one-ear wooden tubes about nine inches long. They were usually made in two pieces which screwed together, and in addition they had detachable ear and chest pieces. Laennec-type stethoscopes were available in England from about 1825. See Appendix III.

May 2 Mucous râles and pectoriloquy under the right clavicle.

May 2. Mucous râles and pectoriloquy[172] under the right clavicle

[p.133] Chronic Peritonitis. Pulmonary tubercles.

Aprilis 30 ℞ Hydrarg c Creta gr ʃs
    Pulv Ipecac C gr v M
    ft pulv 4^tis horis sumend
    Mitte vi

Apr 30. Take ½ grain Mercury with Chalk,[173] 5 grains Compound Ipecacuanha Powder. Mix. Make a powder, to be taken every 4 hours. Send 6.

    ℞ Ol Ricini ʒii
    cras mane sumendi

Take 2 drachms Castor Oil. To be taken tomorrow morning.

    ℞ Liniment Terebinth
    abdomini applicandum
    bis in die

Take Turpentine Liniment. To be applied to the abdomen twice a day.

    Rice and milk
    ℞ To have ʒii of
    wine in a pint of
    water daily

[To have] Rice and Milk. ~~Take~~ To have 2 ounces of wine in a pint of water daily.

Maii 4   Omitte pulveres

May 4. Leave off the powders.

    ℞ Mist Cretæ ʒvi
    Confectionis Arom Эii
    Mist Camphor ʒii
    Tinct Opii ~~ʒiiʃs~~ ʒii M
    cochlear ii magna
    4^tis horis

Take 6 ounces Chalk Mixture, 2 scruples Aromatic Confection, 2 ounces Camphor Mixture, 2½ 2 drachms Tincture of Opium. Mix. Two tablespoonfuls [to be taken] every 4 hours.

5`   ~~℞ Sp Æther Nit ʒiii~~
    ~~Liq Ammon Acet ʒiv~~
    ~~Aquæ Cinnam ʒ viiʃ~~ M
    cochlear ii magna
    ter in die

May 5. ~~Take 3 drachms Spirit of Nitrous Ether, 4 ounces Solution of Ammonium acetate, 7½ ounces Cinnamon Water~~. Mix. Two tablespoonfuls [to be taken] three times a day.

7   ℞ Sp Æther Nit ʒiii
    Liq Ammon Acet ʒi
    Aquæ ʒvii M
    cochlear ii mag
    ter in die

May 7. Take 3 drachms Spirit of Nitrous Ether, 1 ounce Solution of Ammonium Acetate, 7 ounces Water. Mix. Two tablespoonfuls [to be taken] three times a day.

    Omitte Misturam Cretæ

Leave off the Chalk mixture.

10   Rep^r Mistura Cretæ
    c Tinct Opii ʒii

May 10. Repeat the Chalk mixture. with 2 drachms Tincture of Opium [added].

---

[172] Pectoriloquy is a term used to describe the transmission of the sound of the voice through the wall of the chest to the ear in auscultation (usually with a stethoscope). It is frequently the sign of a cavity in the lung, such as might well be present in tuberculosis.

[173] A popular preparation for administering mercury, commonly known as 'Grey Powder'.

11	¼ of a pint of beer daily	*May 11. [To have] ¼ of a pint of beer daily.*
17	Died	*May 17. Died.*

[p.134]

James Sharp [*age*] 42

[*No history is recorded and there are only a few clues in the list of prescriptions which help us to make any sort of retrospective comment. Treatment started with the usual purgative of calomel and colocynth (with henbane added to prevent griping). A mixture of potassium nitrate and nitric ether followed the purgatives. Both these substances were used in cases of fever. Lastly, an ointment of antimony tartrate was applied to the stomach area. This was typically employed as a counter-irritant and its use implies that the patient might have been suffering from abdominal pain.*]

[p.135]

1840

April 29	℞ Ext Col C gr v	*Apr 29. Take 5 grains Compound Extract of Colocynth,*
	Ext Hyos gr ii	*2 grains Extract of Henbane,*
	Hyd Chlorid gr iii M	*3 grains Mercurous Chloride. Mix.*
	ft pilulæ ii	*Make pills two*[174]
	alternis noctibus sumendæ	*to be taken on alternate nights.*
	℞ Potass Nitrat ʒi	*Take 1 drachm Potassium Nitrate,*
	Sp Æther Nit ʒii	*2 drachms Spirit of Nitrous Ether,*
	Tinct Hyos ʒii	*2 drachms Tincture of Henbane,*
	Aquæ ℥viiʃs M	*7½ ounces Water. Mix*
	cochlear ii magna	*Two tablespoonfuls [to be taken]*
	ter in die	*three times a day.*
	Low diet	*Low diet.*
3		*May 3.*
	℞ Ung Ant Pot tart ℥i	*Take 1 ounce Antimony & Potassium Tartrate Ointment.*
	bis in die appicand epigast	*To be applied to the epigastrium twice a day.*
May 9	Common diet	*May 9. Common diet.*
16	1 pint of beer daily	*May 16. [To] have one pint of beer daily.*
19	Cured	*May 19. Cured.*

---

[174] It is not clear whether two pills were to be made and one to be taken on alternate nights, or an unspecified number of pills made of which two were be taken every other night.

[p.136]

Caroline Wayfield [*age*] (19)

[*Castor and asafoetida (present in the foetid spirit of ammonia) were both commonly prescribed for hysteria.*[175] *Hydrocyanic acid (given in the same mixture) was sometimes used for treating palpitations; Caroline may well have been experiencing this symptom due to anxiety. On 21 May she was given a mixture containing morphine, which, following the fashion of the time, could have been prescribed just as a sedative. Naturally, she did not escape without being given laxatives. They were as follows – a confection of senna, some castor oil, colocynth pills and aloes and myrrh pills. Included in the colocynth pills was a small dose (1/10th grain) of strychnine, which was sometimes prescribed in cases of nervous exhaustion. This may be why Stutter used it on this occasion. A liniment of strong ammonia solution and camphor was applied to the patient's back. Using strong ammonia in this way could cause blistering. Iron pills were also given, suggesting that she might have been anaemic.*]

[p.137]

Hysteria 1840		Hysteria
May 20	℞ Tinct Castorie ʒiii Sp Ammon Fœtid ʒiii Acid Hydrocyan ʒſs Mist Camphor ʒvii M cochlear ii magna ter in die	May 20. Take 3 drachms Tincture of Castor,[176] 3 drachms Foetid Spirit of Ammonia, ½ drachm [Dilute] Hydrocyanic Acid, 7 ounces Camphor Mixture. Mix. Two tablespoonfuls [to be taken] three times a day.
	℞ Confection Sennæ ʒiſs nocte sumend	Take 1½ drachms Confection of Senna. To be taken at night.
	Low diet	Low diet.
21	Rep^r Confection Sennæ ʒii 4^{tis} horis donec alvus responderit.	May 21. Repeat the Confection of Senna. Two drachms [to be taken] every 4 hours until the bowels respond.
	℞ Sol Morphiæ Chlor ʒii Mist Camph ʒii M ½ st et repetatur post horas quatuor	Take 2 drachms Solution of Morphine Chloride, Camphor Mixture 2 ounces. Mix. Half to be taken immediately and repeat after 4 hours.
22	℞ Ol Ricini ʒſs st sumatur et repetatur 3^{tiis} horis si opus	22. Take ½ ounce Castor Oil. Let it be taken immediately and repeat in three hours if needed.
26	℞ Liq Ammon Fort ʒv	May 26. Take 5 drachms Strong Solution of Ammonia.

---

175   See Appendix II.

176   Castor was described as 'the peculiar matter found in bags, near the rectum of the beaver'; it was occasionally used in hysteria, as in this case. See Appendix V.

	Tinct Camphor ʒii	*2 drachms Tincture of Camphor.*[177]
	Spirit Rosmar ʒi M	*1 drachm Spirit of Rosemary. Mix.*
	ft liniment regione intra	*Make a liniment, [apply] between*
	scapulari	*shoulder blades.*
27	℞ Strychniæ gr i̶f̶s̶ ii	*27. Take 1̶ ½̶ 2 grains Strychnine,*[178]
	Ext Colocynth C Əi̶v̶ Əii	*4̶ 2 scruples Compound Extract of Colocynth,*
	Ext Hyos Əiv M	*2 scruples Extract of Henbane. Mix*
	divide in pil xx i 4^tis	*Divide into 20 pills. One [to be taken] every 4*
	horis	*hours.*
	Rep Mist Castor [*illeg.*]	*Repeat Castor mixture [illeg.].*
June 1	Rep pil sine Colocyn	*June 1. Repeat the pills without Colocynth.*
	Common dieta pint of beer	*Common diet. [To have] a pint of beer.*
2	Arrow root daily	*June 2. [To have] arrowroot daily*
	instead of common diet	*instead of common diet.*
	A pint of beer	*[To have] a pint of beer.*
	Rep^r Liniment Ammon	*Repeat Liniment of Ammonia.*
	Omitte [*illeg.*]	*Leave off [illeg.]*
24	Pil Aloes c Myrrhæ gr x o nocte	*June 24. [Take] 10 grains Aloes with Myrrh*
		Pills [to be taken] every night.
	℞ Ferri Iodide Əi	*Take 1 scruple Iron Iodide,*
	Extract Gent ʒiʃs	*1½ drachms Extract of Gentian.*
	Mf mass divide in	*Mix. Make a mass. Divide*
	pil xx capiat unam ter die	*into 20 pills. Let her take one three times a day.*

[p.138]

John Sharpe [*age not recorded*]

[*Stutter did not record a medical history for this patient and so it is difficult to guess at a diagnosis. However, it seems likely that he had a fever because of the prescription of the febrifuge mixture. In addition, it is known that digitalis was used in inflammatory disease as well as in heart conditions. John was bled twice and given antimony tartrate ointment (which caused blistering). The only other comment one can make is that bleeding was thought to be especially useful in pleurisy and pneumonia.*]

[p.139]

May 20	V S ad ʒxii	*Venesection up to 12 ounces [of blood]*
		withdrawn.

---

[177] The compound tincture of camphor contained opium and was sometimes used externally as an analgesic.
[178] In the nineteenth century strychnine was considered to be an excellent addition to purgative pills as it aided the relief of constipation by improving the tone of the muscular wall of the intestine. *Guide*, p. 215.

	℞ Pil Aper C ii nocte sumendas	Take Compound Aperient Pills. Two to be taken at night.
	℞ Mist Febrif ℥viii Tinct Digit ♏ lxxx cochlear ii magna 4^tis horis	Take 8 ounces Febrifuge Mixture,[179] 80 minims Tincture of Digitalis. Two tablespoonfuls [to be taken] every 4 hours.
	℞ Ung Ant Pot Tart ℥i	Take 1 ounce Antimony and Potassium Tartrate Ointment.
25	Rice & milk for dinner	May 25. [To have] rice & milk for dinner
27	Applica cucurbitulas cruentas et ditrah^r ℥x sanguinis	May 27. Apply wet cups and withdraw 10 ounces of blood.
Jun 2	Omitte Mist Febrif	June 2. Leave off the Febrifuge Mixture.
	℞ Potass Nitratis ℨii Tinct Digitalis ♏ xL Tinct Hyoscyan [sic] ℨiii Aquæ ℥vii Mist Acaciæ ℥i M cochlear ii magna ter in die	Take 2 drachms Potassium Nitrate, 40 minims Tincture of Digitalis, 3 drachms Tincture of Henbane, 7 ounces Water, 1 ounce Acacia Mixture. Mix. Two tablespoonfuls [to be taken] three times a day.
Jun 8	Common diet	June 8. Common diet.
June 15 [blank]		June 15. [blank]

[p.140]

W. Leech [age] (38)

[Only two prescriptions were recorded for this patient and both were consistent with Stutter's diagnosis of 'rheumatism'. They were a medicine containing guaiacum, and a pain relieving liniment of colchicum, opium and soap to be applied to the painful joints. Tincture of guaiacum had been popular for the treatment of rheumatism since the eighteenth century. With a preceding chill and flitting joint pains this sounds very much like an attack of rheumatic fever (see Appendix II).]

1840
10 June
A blacksmith. Has enjoyed robust health all his life till 11 weeks ago when he was seized with a cold chill, succeeded by fever and Rheumatism in several joints, particularly the left knee. The febrile attack and pains in the joints continued until a week ago, when the former disappeared entirely. Slight pain still in the left knee, which is larger than the right and slightly hot.

A blacksmith. [He] has enjoyed robust health all his life [until] eleven weeks ago when he was seized with a cold chill. This was succeeded by fever and rheumatism in several joints, particularly the left knee. The febrile attack and pain in the joints continued until a week ago, when the former disappeared entirely. [He still has] slight pain in the left knee, which is larger than the right and slightly hot.

---

[179] 'Febrifuge' means 'fever reducing'.

Pulse 84, small. Skin cold. Bowels open and tongue pretty clear. Appetite good, sleeps well.

Pulse [rate] 84 [per minute]. Skin cold. Bowels open and tongue pretty clear. [His] appetite [is] good [and he] sleeps well.

Common diet

Common diet.

[p.141]

Rheumatismus

Rheumatism.

June 10

    ℞ Tinct Guaiaci Amm ℨiii
    Mist Acaciæ ℥i
    Mist Camphor ℥vii
    cochlear ii ter in die

    ℞ Tinct Colchici ℥ſs
    Linimenti Saponis
    Liniment Opii a a ℥ſs

June 10.
Take 3 drachms Ammoniated Guaiacum Tincture
1 ounce Acacia Mixture,
7 ounces Camphor Mixture.
Two spoonfuls[180] [to be taken] three times a day.

Take ½ ounce Tincture of Colchicum,
½ ounce each of Soap Liniment and
Opium Liniment.

June 15 Cucurbitulis cruentis
        genu sinistro ditrah^r
        ℥v sanguinis

June 15. With wet cups
on the left knee, let
five ounces of blood be withdrawn.

---

180 Almost certainly Stutter intended to prescribe a dose of two tablespoonfuls but omitted to write *magna* after cochlear.

APPENDIX I

Brief Biographies of Doctors and Nurses Mentioned in the General Introduction

Bayne, William Joseph, JP
Dr Bayne was a Cambridge MD, being a fellow of Trinity College Cambridge. He was made Physician to the Suffolk General Hospital on 28 April 1831. Members of the Hospital Committee voted for him unanimously, largely because of his written promise that he was 'ready, if elected, not only to attend inpatients but also to attend in their own houses those outpatients residing in Bury whose state of health prevents their coming to the hospital'.[1] He resigned his post on 1 Jan. 1839,[2] just before Stutter became House Apothecary. With his letter of resignation he sent a donation of £10 to the hospital. Between 1831 and 1839 Dr Bayne played an active part in the medical and wider community. In 1831 he became a member of the Suffolk Medical Benevolent Society.[3] He was elected vice president of the Eastern Medical and Surgical Association in October 1835[4] and was made a JP for Bury in February 1836.[5] He married Alicia Pryme on 1 April 1837.[6]

Catton, George (–1829)
George Catton was house apothecary and surgeon to the Suffolk General Hospital from 1827 to 1828. Like his predecessor James Mornement, he suffered from ill health, and resigned his post in October 1828. He died on 2 June 1829.[7] Life was a risky business for medical students and young doctors in the nineteenth century. In 1869 Sir James Paget published a short essay in the St Bartholomew's Hospital Reports entitled 'What becomes of medical students?' With the help of others he had traced the careers of 1000 of his old pupils up to fifteen years after entering medical school. Of the thousand, it was discovered that 41 had died during pupilage and a further 87 within twelve years of practice. Among the 41 students who died, 4 had succumbed to fevers caught in the hospital. Of the 87 who died in practice, 21 died of diseases 'incurred in their duties'.[8]

Clayton, Benjamin Lane (–1819)
Benjamin Lane Clayton was apprenticed to Robert Purvis of Beccles on the 7 August 1781, at a premium of £50 for seven years. He was in practice in Norton by 1791, because on 5 October 1791 the *Bury and Norwich Post* recorded that he had

---

1   Minute books of Committee and Board Meetings of the Suffolk General Hospital: SROB ID 503/3.
2   *Ibid.*: SROB ID 503/5.
3   The van Zwanenberg papers: SROI q s 614.
4   *Ibid.*
5   *Ibid.*
6   *Ibid.*
7   *Ibid.*
8   Stephen Paget (ed.), *Memoirs and Letters of Sir James Paget*, London, 1901, p. 241.

attended the delivery of a child monster. This event was also mentioned in the diary of William Goodwyn of Earl Soham:

March 1793

A female child born at Langham in Suffolk with two distinct heads, necks and backbones, was shown here in a large glass of spirits. The features of its faces were very similar. It was a full-grown foetus and alive at the birth but died at that period. It was the woman's first child who now travels the country with it. All the viscera were single. The heart laid immediately under the bases of the necks in the middle & at the top of the thorax. All the other parts as legs, hands, arms etc were well form'd & in number only as belonging to one child.[9]

Benjamin Clayton married Anna Chambers on 4 April 1796 but his wife unfortunately died at the age of thirty on 29 September 1805, the year Clayton was elected a member of the Suffolk Medical Benevolent Society. He married Ann Midson on 22 January 1810. He seems to have been an active and capable surgeon, as the following report may illustrate:

An accident happened at the funeral of the late Mr Stedman which took place at Thurston on Friday last. During the part of the service over the grave, E. Byford, a nurse of Ixworth, in stepping back, fell over a grave and fractured both bones of her leg; she was conveyed into the church and fortunately Mr Clayton and Mr Chinery, surgeons, being present, they immediately set the limb and she was afterwards conveyed home in a fair way of doing well.[10]

Benjamin Clayton had several apprentices, including Woodward Mudd (1801–05), Joseph Fiott Hodgkin (1815–20), and Charles Chambers Hammond (1811–18).[11] Plowman Young, who, along with Hammond, was apprentice to Clayton from 1811 to 1818, married Clayton's daughter and went into partnership with his father-in-law in February 1819.[12] Benjamin died on 27 May 1819 and was buried in Norton churchyard.[13]

Crabbe, George (1754–1832)

George Crabbe is, of course, more famous as a poet than a medical man. However, he did originally intend to become a doctor. He was apprenticed to a Mr John Smith of Wickhambrook in 1768.[14] Smith was a farmer as well as an apothecary and it is said that his apprentice resented working on the farm and sharing a room with the ploughboy. He hated the position so much that he implored his father to obtain an apprenticeship for him elsewhere. His father complied with his wishes, and George spent the years 1770–5 in Woodbridge as apprentice to a Mr John Page. He then worked in Aldeburgh from1775–6, as assistant to a Mr James Maskill. In 1776 Crabbe went to London to try to further his medical studies. Whilst there he

---

[9] The diary of William Goodwyn: SROI HD 365/2.
[10] *Bury and Norwich Post*, Wed. 8 March 1815, p. 2, col.1.
[11] This information comes from the signatures on some dispensary drawers which are still in existence at Stanton House, Norton. This was Benjamin Clayton's house. The business of general practice was carried on in this dwelling until 1973 when it became a private residence.
[12] *Bury and Norwich Post*, Wed. 17 Feb. 1819, p. 2, col. 3.
[13] C. Partridge, *Suffolk Churchyard Inscriptions*, Suffolk Institute of Archaeology, Pt 1 in 1913, Pt 2 in 1920 and Pt 3 in 1923.
[14] van Zwanenberg: SROI, q s 614.

narrowly escaped being dragged in front of the Lord Mayor as a resurrectionist because it had been discovered that he had the body of a child in his room. He had obtained the corpse for dissection. How is not related, but his landlady accused him of digging up her own child, who had died the week before. Fortunately for George, he had not yet touched the face of the corpse and so he was able to prove that the child was not his landlady's. This event, and his chronic shortage of money, forced him to return to Aldeburgh where he practised on his own from 1777 to 1780 (Maskill having conveniently left town). However, he was not a success as an apothecary and he gave the job up in 1781. He appealed to the politician Edmund Burke, and through his influence was encouraged to join the Church. George passed the examination and was admitted to deacon's orders in London. He returned to Aldeburgh briefly as a curate, but then in June 1782 he was appointed domestic chaplain to the duke of Rutland. Crabbe henceforth remained a churchman and a man of letters and had no further truck with the apothecary trade.[15]

Creed, George, JP (1799–1868)

George Creed was the son of John Stevens Creed, a Bury surgeon. He was educated at Bury School and was then apprenticed to his father from 1816 to 1822. Following this he spent a year at St George's Hospital. In July 1824 he was appointed surgeon to the West Suffolk militia, a position he held for forty-four years. He was elected surgeon to the new Suffolk General Hospital in November 1825, an appointment that he relinquished in May 1847. He was elected FRCS in 1844. George was a justice of the peace, and from 1838 to 1839 he was mayor of Bury St Edmunds. In his early years he had an extensive practice, but later on he was often absent from the town because he was engaged in agricultural pursuits. Towards the end of his life he developed severe heart disease and congestion of the lungs. He died on 28 November 1868, aged sixty-nine.[16]

Crosse, John Green (1790–1850)

John Green Crosse was a famous Norwich surgeon. He was born at Boyton Hall, Great Finborough, Suffolk, on the 6 September 1790. As a boy he broke his leg and was attended by Thomas Bayly from nearby Stowmarket. The next year (1806) he was apprenticed to the said Thomas Bayly for five years. He appears to have enjoyed his apprenticeship and found it useful, because he defended the system of apprenticeship when he was asked to give evidence before a select commission of the House of Commons on medical education in 1834. John Crosse kept a diary, journal and casebook throughout his career, giving details of all he saw and did. In 1811 he attended Charles Bell's Great Windmill School of Anatomy, and then in 1812 he went to St George's Hospital as a student for a year. He became a member of the Royal College of Surgeons (MRCS) on 16 April 1813. Later that year he went on to Dublin and then to Paris in 1814 (having failed the examination for Membership of the Irish College of Surgeons on two occasions). He returned from Paris in 1815 and settled in Norwich, being appointed assistant surgeon to the Norfolk and Norwich Hospital in 1823. He was made a full surgeon in 1826 and became a renowned lithotomist (i.e. one who removes bladder stones). He was awarded the Jacksonian Prize by the Royal College of Surgeons in 1833 and an honorary MD from the

15 N. Blackburne, *The Restless Ocean: The Story of George Crabbe, the Aldeburgh Poet 1754–1832*, Lavenham, 1972; *Life of George Crabbe, by his son*, 1834.
16 van Zwanenberg: SROI q s 614.

University of Heidelburg in 1835. Crosse was made a Fellow of the Royal College of Surgeons (FRCS) in 1843 (the year the fellowship was introduced) and in the same year he was elected Member of the Medical and Chirurgical Society of Calcutta. He received an MD (by examination) from St Andrews University in 1845. In 1846 he was made a fellow of the University of New York College of Physicians and Surgeons and in 1848 he became an Honorary Member of the Medical and Chirurgical Society of Bombay. Towards the end of his career it is estimated that Crosse was earning £3500 a year, which was not bad for a provincial surgeon, although it came nowhere near the £21,000 a year which the renowned English surgeon Astley Cooper was said to have earned in London in 1815.

John Green Crosse married Dorothy, the daughter of his old master Thomas Bayly in 1816. They had eight children. Crosse died in 1850 aged fifty-nine, and is buried in Norwich Cathedral. His papers are divided between the Norfolk Record Office and the Royal Society of Medicine.[17]

Dalton, John, Jnr (1803–59)
John Dalton junior spent most of his professional life in Suffolk. He was apprenticed to his father, John Dalton senior (1771–1844), of Bury St Edmunds, from 1819 to 1824. He then spent nine months at St George's and St James' dispensary. He obtained the MRCS in 1820 and the LSA in 1824. He was appointed third surgeon to the Suffolk General Hospital in December 1825. His appointment was carried by 178 votes to 148. He assisted at the dissection of William Corder, the murderer, in 1828,[18] and on 26 February 1829 the Committee thanked him for his 'beautiful preparation' of the skeleton. William Scarfe, who was a woodsman living at Thorpe Morieux, recorded in his diary in February 1830 that 'John Treasy from Bretenham was cut in the new Horsptill at Bury and was cureaud. He was cut for the gravel by Dr Dalton at Bury [sic].'[19] Despite his successes, Dalton resigned as surgeon to the Suffolk General Hospital on 6 May 1843 following a complaint by the Hospital Committee that he had not visited the wards for a week.[20] He continued in private practice in Bury St Edmunds and died in 1859.

Dunthorn, Dr J. (1791–1856)
Dr Dunthorn obtained his MRCS in 1808 and was a naval surgeon before he went into practice at Wickhambrook in Suffolk. In October 1832 he diagnosed cholera in a family of nine who lived at Wickhambrook. Cholera was sweeping the country at the time and it seems that Dr Dunthorn's diagnosis may have been correct, because four members of the afflicted family died. He took W.G. Stutter into partnership in 1841 and retired in 1849. Two years before that (in 1847) he obtained an MD from Erlingen in Germany. Unfortunately, Dr Dunthorn had an accident with a twelve bore gun in 1856 when he was aged sixty-five. One barrel of his two-barrelled shotgun went off when he was reloading the other. The shot penetrated his axilla and smashed the head and shaft of his humerus. He lived in agony for another twenty-one weeks.[21]

---

[17] Mary Crosse, *A Surgeon in the Early Nineteenth Century*, Edinburgh and London, 1968.
[18] van Zwanenberg: SROI q s 614.
[19] *The World According to William Scarfe*, ed. Pip and Joy Wright and Levine Robinson. Manuscript seen by Dr Cockayne before publication.
[20] Hospital minute book: SROB ID 503/7.
[21] van Zwanenberg: SROI q s 614.

Fuller, Harry (1835–1900)

The son of Robert Osborn Fuller, Harry was educated at Bury School. From 1852 to 1857 he was apprenticed to Thomas Coe of Bury St Edmunds. He then spent eighteen months at the London Hospital, becoming house surgeon to the Suffolk General Hospital in 1860. He remained in this post until 1890, and when he resigned the Committee awarded him a pension. He practised in Bury for a short time after leaving the hospital, but died in 1900. His incredible length of tenure as house surgeon meant that he dealt with a multitude of emergency cases over the years and came to have the respect of his hospital colleagues.[22]

Hake, Dr Thomas

Dr Hake had previously been Physician to the Brighton Dispensary. He canvassed for the post of Physician to the Suffolk General Hospital in April 1840, but was defeated by Dr Ranking on a count of 266 votes to 233.[23] However, three months later, in July 1840, he was unanimously elected as Physician to the hospital.[24] Hake became a member of the Suffolk Benevolent Medical Society in 1840 and became vice president in 1841. Like Dr Probart he was a magistrate and together with many of the rest of the medical fraternity in the area he attended the first operation under ether at the Suffolk Hospital in 1847. He attended the Suffolk Branch of the Provincial Medical and Surgical Association in June 1844, and became chairman at a meeting of that association in 1848. He lectured to the Young Men's Institute in Bury St Edmunds and the Ipswich Mechanics Institute from 1851 to 1853. The subjects included 'Climate viewed in relation to the welfare of man', 'Anatomy and its application to Science and Art', 'Sources and Prospects of Science psychologically considered' and 'Growth and Decay of Living Beings'.[25] Dr Hake resigned from the hospital in November 1853[26] and was replaced by Dr Marnock in January 1854.[27] His wife died at Racine in the United States of America on 15 March 1855, when Thomas Hake was described as 'late of Bury St Edmunds'.[28]

Hubbard, George Prettyman (1822–72)

The eldest son of the Bury surgeon George Hubbard II (1785–1860), George Prettyman went to Bury School in 1830–36. He was apprenticed to his father in 1841, but it seems likely that he worked as dispenser and secretary to the Suffolk General Hospital from April to September 1841, either before or even after he became an apprentice. After the apprenticeship he went to St Thomas's Hospital for eighteen months. He obtained his LSA in 1847 and returned to practise in Bury St Edmunds. He died at the age of fifty.[29]

Jackson, Alexander Russell, MD

Dr Jackson was appointed physician to the Suffolk General Hospital in June 1839. In his petition to the governors, which was published in the local newspapers, he mentioned that had served for eighteen years with the Bengal Establishment of the

---

[22] *Ibid.*

[23] *Ibid.*

[24] *Ibid.*

[25] *Ibid.*

[26] Hospital minute book: SROB ID 503/9.

[27] Hospital minute book: SROB ID 503/10.

[28] van Zwanenberg: SROI q s 614.

[29] *Ibid.*

East India Company.[30] In September 1839 he wrote to the Committee with his suggestions for the enlargement of the dispensary and other matters.[31] It is not clear whether or not his ideas were accepted, but Dr Jackson resigned from the staff of the hospital in March 1840.[32]

Jardine, Henry (1820–)
Henry Jardine was the son of J.H. Jardine of Stoke by Clare.[33] He was apprenticed to Mr William Ward, House Apothecary and Surgeon at The Suffolk General Hospital on 2 October 1838.[34] His father had paid the £40 for his first year's apprenticeship the day before.[35] Henry is not mentioned in the hospital minutes after October 1838 but he must have continued his training, because when he had completed his apprenticeship he went to St Bartholomew's Hospital for eighteen months.[36] In 1854 he was in practice in Goswell Street, London, where he was also Druggist to the Royal Maternity Charity.[37]

Jeaffreson, William (1790–1865)
William Jeaffreson was born in Wickham Market in 1790 and went to school in Bury St Edmunds. In September 1807 he was apprenticed to G.D. Lynn of Woodbridge at a premium of £157 for five years. He went to the Borough Hospitals (i.e. Guy's and St Thomas's) to complete his education, obtaining the MRCS in 1812.[38] He then returned to Framlingham where he practised for the rest of his life. On 8 May 1836 he performed a successful ovariotomy,[39] and on 6 June 1836 he read a paper on ovariotomy to the Eastern Provincial Medical and Surgical Association.[40] The very first ovariotomy is thought to have been done by Ephraim McDowell (1771–1830) of Danville, Kentucky, in 1809. The patient was a 47-year-old woman called Jane Todd who sang hymns through the twenty-five minute operation. But McDowell removed the 15 pound tumour without complications and the patient lived for another thirty-one years. McDowell did thirteen ovariotomies in all, and eight of the patients recovered. Nevertheless, the operation was slow to catch on, especially in England, due to the natural conservatism of the medical profession and their fear of sepsis.[41] So Jeaffreson's operation in 1836 was among the earliest to be done in this country. He is said to have done four further ovariotomies, and his temerity certainly aroused the criticism of some London surgeons, who were no doubt jealous of his success.[42] But it is true to say that the cards were stacked in favour of country surgeons at that time. They usually operated in the patient's house, away from hospital theatres where wounds were at great risk of becoming infected. Jeaffreson also became skilled in the removal of bladder stones using the lithotrite

---

[30] *Ibid.*
[31] Hospital minute book: SROB ID 503/6.
[32] *Ibid.*
[33] van Zwanenberg: SROI q s 614.
[34] Hospital minute book: SROB ID 503/5.
[35] Hospital minute book: SROB ID 503/6.
[36] van Zwanenberg: SROI q s 614.
[37] *Ibid.*
[38] *Ibid.*
[39] Ovariotomy is the operation of removing an ovarian tumour, now usually called an oophorectomy.
[40] van Zwanenberg: SROI q s 614.
[41] R. Porter, *The Greatest Benefit to Mankind*, London, 1997.
[42] J.A. Shepherd, 'William Jeaffreson (1790–1865), Surgical Pioneer', *British Medical Journal*, 6 Nov. 1965, p. 1119.

(an instrument for crushing the stones within the bladder), and he performed this operation quite frequently. His first successful case took thirty-seven sittings before the stone was removed![43] All his surgical operations were done as part of his work as a busy general practitioner, and his election as a fellow of the Royal College of Surgeons in 1844 was no doubt well deserved.

William married Caroline Edwards on 30 October 1816. They had eleven children, of whom three became doctors. Unfortunately, Jeaffreson had a severe attack of whooping cough when he was forty-nine years old. The paroxysms did him an irreparable injury and after that he was seldom seen on horseback. But he remained bright until his seventy-first year, when his powers declined, and he died at Framlingham on 8 November 1865.[44]

King, Robert Carew (1781–1842)

Robert Carew King was born on 14 July 1781. His father was headmaster of Ipswich School and three of his brothers also became doctors. Robert did his apprenticeship with Alexander Bartlet of Ipswich, and in 1805 he went into partnership with Mr Denny of Saxmundham. At first King lived in Yoxford, but when Denny died the following November, he moved to Saxmundham. He was a noted lithotomist (performing two successful operations of that nature in 1822). His chief claim to fame is that in 1836 he helped William Jeaffreson do a successful ovariotomy. In the fullness of time this gave him the courage to do a similar operation himself. Robert Carew King had at least seven apprentices and he died in harness at the age of sixty-one. There is a memorial to him in Witnesham church which says that he gained great eminence by his skill in both surgery and medicine.[45]

Mornement, James (1804–27)

James was an apprentice with Robert Camell and Frederick Morris, both of Bungay, from 1820 to 1825. He subsequently spent six months at St Bartholomew's Hospital, and then in November 1825 he was elected as the first House Apothecary to the Suffolk General Hospital. Unfortunately he had to resign from his post due to ill health. When he reached the point at which he could no longer perform his duties, his mother was allowed to stay with him and nurse him in his room, and it was she who attended a Committee Meeting to present her son's resignation on 1 March 1827.[46] James died on 2 July 1827 at his father's house at Lopham Park. He is said to have had a long and painful illness.[47]

Mudd, Barrington Richard (1822–)

Barrington was the son of Mrs Elizabeth Mudd (widow) of Gedding, Suffolk. His father, Francis David Mudd, a surgeon, died on 24 February 1835. Francis and Elizabeth's second daughter Emily married William Middleton White in October 1838.[48] White (1813–76) was his father-in-law's successor in the Gedding practice. In 1838 Barrington Mudd became his brother-in-law's apprentice.[49] He officially

---

[43] *Ibid.*
[44] van Zwanenberg: SROI q s 614.
[45] *Ibid.*
[46] Hospital minute book: SROB ID 503/1.
[47] van Zwanenberg: SROI q s 614.
[48] *Ibid.*
[49] *Ibid.*

held this post until 1845, but he must have been seconded to the Suffolk General Hospital to gain more experience. When his apprenticeship came to an end, he went off to the Royal Infirmary in Aberdeen for eighteen months, obtaining his LSA in 1845. He tried to get a job as House Surgeon to the East Suffolk Hospital in 1845, but failed.[50]

Mudd, Woodward

Woodward Mudd of Hunston was bound apprentice to Mr Clayton of Norton on 8 January 1801.[51] He was Clayton's apprentice until 1805 and seems to have been a turbulent youth. In May 1803 a Susan Barrell appeared before James Mingay and George Stone, justices of the peace, at Norton, charged with having had a bastard child. Susan swore that on 8 March 1803 she had given birth to a male child at the house of Widow Sparham in the parish of Norton and the father was Woodward Mudd of Norton.[52] On 24 May 1803 Woodward Mudd himself appeared before the two JPs and accepted that he was indeed the father of the bastard child. He was ordered to pay 6s to the parish of Norton for lying-in costs plus maintenance of 1s 6d per week. Susan Barrell was ordered to pay 6d per week to the parish.[53] This episode does not seem to have deterred Woodward one bit. On 11 April 1806 there was a further successful bastardy order against him. On 11 March 1806 a girl called Mary Leech had been delivered of a female bastard child, once again chargeable to the parish of Norton. It was judged that 'Woodward Mudd of Norton, aforesaid, surgeon, did beget the said child on the body of her, the said Mary Leech'.[54] But however much of a scandal these births created at the time, Woodward seems to have continued in practice without any undue censure, and on 3 April 1811 he was obviously considered respectable enough to be elected a member of the Suffolk Medical Benevolent Society.[55] Whatever his faults, he also seems to have made an effort to keep himself up to date in his profession, because he was recorded as a member of the Suffolk Medical Book Club when the first anniversary meeting was held at The Angel Hotel, Bury St Edmunds on Wednesday 6 July 1813.[56]

Newham, Samuel (1820–67)

Samuel Newham was born in King's Lynn. He was a student at Guy's Hospital and obtained his MRCS and LSA in 1840. From 1841 to 46 he was House Surgeon and Secretary to the Suffolk General Hospital. In December 1848 he canvassed to be elected Surgeon to the hospital. No doubt to his great disappointment, John Kilner was appointed to the post instead of him in January 1849. Despite this setback, Newham did very soon join the staff as a surgeon. George John Hinnell was his

---

[50] *Ibid.*
[51] This information comes from the signatures on some dispensary drawers which are still in existence at Stanton House, Norton. This was Benjamin Clayton's house. The business of general practice was carried on there until 1973 when it became a private residence.
[52] Bastardy order: SROB FL 54612/7/34/1.
[53] Bastardy order: SROB FL 612/7/33/2.
[54] Bastardy order: SROB FL 612/9/2/1.
[55] The Commonplace Book of Sir Thomas Gery Cullum: SROB 317/1. The Suffolk Medical Benevolent Society had been instituted in 1787, the patron being the duke of Grafton. The benevolent fund was supported by charitable donations and was intended to benefit widows, orphans and indigent members of the profession. However, it also ran an annuity scheme. Those who had paid their dues were awarded a pension of at least £50 a year for life from the age of sixty.
[56] *Bury and Norwich Post*, 30 June 1813, p. 2, col. 2.

apprentice at the hospital from 1843 to 1848, as was Henry Taylor, who was bound to him from 1844 to 1849. Samuel died in 1867 at the age of forty-seven.[57]

Paget, Sir James (1814–99)

Sir James Paget was a very eminent surgeon indeed. In later life he had many honours heaped upon him including that of Serjeant Surgeon Extraordinary to Queen Victoria, Fellow of the Royal Society and President of the Royal College of Surgeons. He also had no less than two diseases named after him (Paget's disease of the breast and Paget's disease of the bones).

In 1830, when he was sixteen years old, Paget started his medical career as an apprentice surgeon and apothecary to a Mr Costerton in his home town of Great Yarmouth. Although in later life James felt that the time he had served with his master had been too long, he also acknowledged that he had gone to London with a better knowledge of medical practice than those students who went there later in the century without the benefit of a preliminary apprenticeship. He went to St Bartholomew's Hospital in 1834 and passed the examination for membership of the Royal College of Surgeons (MRCS) in 1836. James had decided that he would like to be a London surgeon, but the path to promotion was long and tortuous. His first job was as curator of the hospital museum, becoming demonstrator in morbid anatomy in 1839. In 1843 he was appointed lecturer on physiology and Warden of the College at St Bartholomew's Hospital, and he stayed in this post until he was finally elected to the staff as assistant surgeon in 1847.

Paget did not seriously go into private practice until 1851, when he was thirty-seven years old. He earned £700 in his first year and from then on his income increased yearly until it exceeded £10,000 per annum. His remuneration only started to fall when he decided to stop operating a few years before he retired. Despite his huge success, Paget was of the opinion that had he died at the age of forty-seven (as he might well have done – he had five attacks of pneumonia during his professional career), his wife and six children would have had a very thin time of it indeed. And that is without mentioning his other relatives. His father had been a brewer, but the business failed, and James spent many years helping to pay off the paternal debts.[58]

Pentney, Nurse

Unlike the doctors, it is very difficult to find information about the nurses who served the Suffolk General Hospital. However, we do know something about Nurse Pentney because she became old and ill in service. It seems that she was one of the nurses who served the institution from its inception, but the first mention of her in the hospital minute book is when she was granted a Christmas gratuity of £1 1s on 29 December 1831. On 29 September 1840, her quarterly wage was noted. She and two other senior nurses (Smith and Buckle) received £2 12s 6d a quarter (i.e. £10 10s a year, plus board) whilst Nurse Arbon, a more junior nurse, received £1 11s 6d (£6 6s a year). The unnamed 'girl assisting' was paid £1 1s (£4 4s a year). In May 1842 Nurse Pentney was ill and the Committee ordered Matron to procure 'efficient assistance during Nurse Pentney's illness'. It seems that this help took the form of a charwoman who was employed three days a week. In April 1843 Dr Hake was requested to give his opinion as to the necessity of continuing the extra diet to Nurse Pentney, and on 16 May 1843 she came before the Committee to say that she still

---

57 van Zwanenberg: SROI q s 614.

58 S. Paget (ed.), *Memoirs and Letters of Sir James Paget*, London, 1901.

wanted to work as a nurse at the hospital. It was then unanimously resolved 'that Matron be directed to procure (subject to the approval of the Committee) a strong and efficient Assistant to Nurse Pentney'. But it was all to no avail. On Tuesday 26 September 1843 it was reported that 'Pentney was incapable from age of the duties of her situation'. So on the 17 October 1843 the Committee agreed that 'a gratuity of £10 be given to an aged Nurse Pentney, who had been a most effective servant of the establishment for upwards of seventeen years'. She was to leave two weeks later. The last note about her in the minute book was made on the 7 November 1843. Apparently she still had not left the hospital, and so the gratuity of £10 was presented to her and she was asked to go on the following Saturday.[59] Ten years later, a similar fate was to follow for Nurse Arbon, who in April 1853 was given two month's notice because she had become 'incapable from age of attending to her duties' and after a service of 'upwards of twenty years' she too was discharged with a gratuity of £10.[60] We do not know what became of either of these nurses when their gratuities ran out. They did not receive pensions from the hospital.

Pott, Percival (1714–88)

Percival Pott was born in 1714 in Threadneedle Street, London. At fifteen he was apprenticed to Edward Nourse of St Bartholomew's Hospital. He was to maintain his connection with this hospital for the rest of his life.

In 1756 Pott was riding his horse in Southwark when the animal slipped and threw him off. He suffered an open fracture of the lower leg, with the bone ends protruding. Pott got himself home by persuading helpers to use a detached door as a stretcher. The treatment in those days would normally have been amputation of the limb, but Edward Nourse advised conservative management. The fracture healed and Pott retained a usable leg. Fractures of this type have been called 'Pott's fractures' ever since. Also there is 'Pott's peculiar tumour', a swelling on the roof of the skull due to inflammation. Insufficient blood supply in the legs has been called 'Pott's gangrene' and Pott's disease of the spine is caused by tuberculosis of the vertebrae. Pott used the convalescence from his own fracture to write a treatise on ruptures, which appeared in 1757. Later he wrote *Observations on the Nature and Consequences of Wounds and Contusions of the Head*. This was well received, but what sealed his reputation was an essay published in 1775 linking cancer of the scrotum in chimney sweeps to their exposure to soot. He wrote:

> It is a hard fate that afflicts these people. During their early childhood, they are usually treated with the greatest brutality, freezing and nearly starving to death. They have to squeeze themselves up through narrow and sometimes hot chimneys where they tear and burn themselves, and on reaching puberty they become peculiarly sensitive to a troubling deadly illness which apparently results from deposits of soot in the skin folds of the scrotum.

This was a brilliant observation, but it would take another 140 years before it was put to the test. In 1915 Yamagiwa and Ichikawa in Japan showed that coal tar caused cancer when it was repeatedly brushed on the ears of rabbits.[61]

[59] Hospital minute books: SROB ID 503/1–7.
[60] Hospital minute books: SROB ID 503/10.
[61] K. Haeger, *The Illustrated History of Surgery*, London, 1988, p. 151.

Probart, Francis George JP (1782–1861)

Born in Thorsby, Lincolnshire, Dr Probart was an Edinburgh graduate. He qualified MD in 1825.[62] He was a member of the Linnean society and author of a prize essay on the chemical composition and physiology of bile. He was elected third physician at a special board meeting of the Suffolk General Hospital on 2 November 1826.[63] He quickly established a good reputation. As Sir Thomas Gery Cullum noted in a letter dated 27 November 1827 to his son, the Reverend Thomas Gery Cullum who was then residing in Nice:

> Our new Dr Probart seems to be almost universally consulted. He has been at Ickworth lately for some advice for some ladies from Paris, and I believe he has been consulted by Lord Hervey himself.[64]

Probart's income for his first year in practice was £898 4s, although set against this he had to count the expenses of hiring a chaise and postillion (usually from the Six Bells or the Angel). The hire charge depended on the distance. It was 13s 6d to go to Ixworth, for instance, while it cost £1 5s 6d to travel to Stowmarket. His total expenditure on chaise hire for the year 1827 was £51 11s 0d. The good doctor also recorded the presents of game he was given in 1827 – pheasants, partridges, hares etc. – amounting to nineteen items. His usual visiting fee was one guinea but he scaled this up for the aristocracy. Lord Bristol, for instance, was invariably charged three guineas.[65] He was elected a member of the Suffolk Benevolent Medical Society in April 1829, became a trustee of the same in July 1830 and its President in July 1849.[66] Probart was for a time secretary of the Suffolk Medical Book Club that had originally been founded in 1816.[67] He attended the Suffolk Branch of the Provincial and Surgical Association in 1844 and 1847,[68] and was elected a magistrate in February 1836.[69] In January 1847 he witnessed the first operation under ether at the Suffolk General Hospital,[70] and in February 1855 Dr Probart attended the Reverend Sir T.G. Cullum in his fatal illness.[71] He was married twice. His first wife, Elizabeth, died on 18 April 1833.[72] He then married Anne Cocksedge on 9 July 1834. She died on 14 April 1854.[73] His only daughter, Agnes, married Walter Scott, MD, on 29 June 1863.[74] His son, Colonel Francis Probart, died at the age of forty-nine on 18 February 1885.[75] Dr Probart himself died in his eightieth year on 25 April 1861. He apparently had a stroke and fell from his horse whilst out riding along the Newmarket Road in Bury St Edmunds.[76] He had been working up until the time of his death. On 16 April 1861 Dr Probart was recorded as 'Physician of the

62 van Zwanenberg: SROI q s 614.
63 Hospital minute books: SROB ID 503/1.
64 SROB E2/21/2.
65 Dr Probart's accounts: SROB 2753/4/21.
66 van Zwanenberg: SROI q s 614.
67 Suffolk Medical Book Club: SROB 2753/4/25.
68 van Zwanenberg: SROI q s 614.
69 *Ibid.*
70 *Ibid.*
71 *Ibid.*
72 *Ibid.*
73 *Ibid.*
74 *Ibid.*
75 *Ibid.*
76 *The Gentleman's Magazine*, June 1861, p. 706.

week' in the hospital minute book. Two weeks later his death was recorded in the same volume. A note was made that:

> Dr Probart, as senior physician, had been of great value to the suffering poor, who had been the objects of his care for the space of more than 34 years.[77]

Pyman, Francis Charles (1805–38)

Francis Charles Pyman was apprenticed to James Bedingfield of Stowmarket from 1819 to 1826. He then went to the City Dispensary for nine months, obtaining his LSA and MRCS in 1826. For a time he was assistant to a Mr Peck of Newmarket, but then became House Apothecary to the Suffolk General Hospital in October 1828. He resigned this position in January 1833 because he had accepted a post with the East India Company. He married Sophia Catherine Rainey in 1836, but unfortunately he died in Bury St Edmunds in March 1838.[78]

Ranking, William Harcourt, MD (1814–67)

Dr Ranking was a Cambridge man, having been admitted to St Catherine's College in 1831. He was elected Physician to the Suffolk General Hospital on 22 April 1840, beating Dr Hake by 266 votes to 223.[79] He was said to have been an able physician, who translated a number of French medical works into English. Dr Ranking presented a paper on 'The Coexistence of Disease of The Heart and Chorea' at the first meeting of the Suffolk Branch of the Provincial Medical and Surgical Association in 1843. He described 'a Case of Dissecting Aneurysm of the Aorta' in the *Journal of the Provincial Medical and Surgical Association* in 1846, and in January 1847 he wrote a letter to *The Lancet* detailing how he had treated a case of tetanus with ether.[80] Dr Ranking was appointed as Physician to the Norwich Hospital in March 1847 and he resigned his post at the Suffolk General Hospital on the thirtieth day of that month.[81]

Ross, Andrew

Andrew Ross was elected Physician to the Suffolk General Hospital at a Special General Board meeting on 6 February 1839.[82] He replaced Dr Bayne, but his tenure was a short one, for he resigned on 16 June 1840, being replaced by Dr Hake.[83]

Stedman, Foster (1818–)

Foster Stedman was born on 10 April 1818. He was apprenticed to Henry Woodruffe Bailey of Thetford from 1834 to 1839 and then spent fifteen months at Guy's Hospital.[84] He was practising in Pakenham, Suffolk by 1840, and was still there in 1849.[85]

---

[77] Hospital minute books: SROB ID 503/12.
[78] van Zwanenberg: SROI q s 614.
[79] Hospital minute books: SROB ID 503/6.
[80] van Zwanenberg: SROI q s 614.
[81] Hospital minute books: SROB ID 503/8.
[82] Hospital minute books: SROB ID 503/5.
[83] Hospital minute books: SROB ID503/6.
[84] van Zwanenberg: SROI q s 614.
[85] *Ibid.*

Steggall, John Heigham (1789–1881)
This man is interesting in that his autobiography *A Real History of a Suffolk Man* was published in 1857.[86] The editor was the Reverend Richard Cobbold, of Wortham, the author of *Margaret Catchpole*. Steggall's father was rector of Westhorpe and Wyverstone and John Heigham was sent to school in Walsham le Willows at the age of seven. A year later he ran away from school and lived for a time with some gypsies. By doing this he made his point, and his father took him away from the unpopular school in Walsham and sent him to another establishment in Botesdale. When he left school he became apprentice to a surgeon in Bacton. Then, 'on a bachelor uncle's persuasion', he joined a whaler as a ship's surgeon. He saw service in New Zealand and the South Seas. In 1810 he sailed in an Indiaman as an ensign in the 15th Madras Regiment. Although the ship was a merchantman, it was acting as a cruiser when it became involved in action against the French near Mauritius. Steggall was injured in this action. A splinter of wood went into his thigh and it became infected. He was invalided out of service in 1811 with three years' sick pay. He decided on a career in the church and went to Corpus Christi College, Cambridge, becoming a priest in 1815. He was curate in the parishes of Badingham and then Wyverstone. But he felt that he was getting nowhere so he decided to go back to his old profession of medicine. He went to live in Rattlesden and set up practice. Then in 1823 Lord Thurlow appointed him perpetual curate of Great Ashfield, a small village about five miles from Rattlesden. He continued in his medical practice as well as carrying out his parochial duties (which were probably not great). His presence in Rattlesden aroused the jealousy of local doctors who maintained that he was unqualified.[87] But Steggles was able to contest this because he had done an apprenticeship and been a ship's surgeon long before the Apothecaries Act of 1815. However, on Friday 23 March 1838 Steggall was called to a girl aged nine who lived in Rattlesden. The child had been wearing boys' boots when she had been planting corn in the fields that morning. She had walked a quarter of a mile home just before midday and had complained of pain in her leg when she arrived. There was a sore place on the top of one of her feet. Steggall dressed this but the wound became infected and over the next week or two things went from bad to worse. It seems that the bones of the foot had become infected. Steggall suggested sending the patient into hospital to have the leg amputated, but when this was broached the patient's father decided to consult another surgeon. Mr William Middleton White (1813–76) from nearby Gedding (who incidentally was Barrington Mudd's brother-in-law) was called in on 19 April 1838. He in turn consulted two more surgeons (Mr Spencer Freeman (1804–83) and Mr Charles Robert Bree (1811–86) from Stowmarket) and, aided by them, Mr White amputated the leg at the patient's house on Saturday 21 April 1838. The child survived, but at the Suffolk Lent Assizes on 2 April 1839 White brought a civil action against Steggall on behalf of the young patient. The *coup de grâce* for Steggall probably came when the bones from the amputated leg were produced in court.[88] They were extensively diseased, almost certainly by osteomyelitis. The case went against him and he was fined £10. Soon after the trial John Steggall gave up the practice of medicine. Lord Thurlow built him a parsonage

---

86   R. Cobbold (ed.), *A Real History of a Suffolk Man*, London, 1857.
87   *The Lancet*, 13 Jan. 1838, 27 Jan. 1839 and 6 April 1839.
88   *The Bury and Norwich Post*, 3 April 1839: report of trial Gladwell v. Steggall which had taken place on 2 April 1839.

at Great Ashfield and he retreated there to minister to his congregation until he died in 1881. Thanks to his biography, we know something of what he felt about it all:

> She obtained a verdict of £10 damages, and of course a hue and cry was raised against me, although I was recognised to be a regularly educated practitioner. I say nothing against surgeons. I well know the hacking work they have and the responsibility attached to their profession. But I know that if it were not for the very fearful amount of ignorance and the dependence which ignorant people place upon them, the profession would not be as good as it is.

Ward, William

Ward was Stutter's immediate predecessor as House Apothecary to the Suffolk General Hospital. He was elected to the post on 13 February 1833[89] and resigned on 18 December 1838.[90] In December 1840 he gave evidence at an inquest into the death by scalding of an inmate at Thingoe Union,[91] but there is no other evidence that he might have practised in Suffolk after he left the hospital.

Woodroffe, Mrs Ann

Mrs Woodroffe was elected Matron of the Suffolk General Hospital at a special Board Meeting on 12 February 1834. She defeated a Mrs Wales by 315 votes to 114. Like the House Apothecary, she was resident and had to ask the Committee's permission to be absent, even for a couple of nights, as she did on 26 December 1834. Naturally she had to make sure that there was someone fit to superintend for her. Mrs Woodroffe was directed to purchase a washing machine on 21 July 1840. Whether this innovation was her idea or came from a member of the Committee we shall never know, although we may assume that she was not against it. Mrs Woodroffe gave notice of her resignation on 7 May 1844. She originally said that she would like to remain until the 29 September, but she came back to the Committee on the 11 June 1844 to say that she would like to leave a week later, which she did. It very much sounds as if she had another position lined up. She drew her final quarterly salary of £7 10s on 18 June 1844.[92]

Young, Plowman (1796–1840)

Plowman Young was the eldest son of William Young, who was a builder in Mildenhall. He was apprenticed to Benjamin Lane Clayton from 1811 to 1818, and then went to Guy's for six months. He joined his old master in partnership in Norton in February 1819,[93] only three months before Clayton died on 27 May 1819. Plowman Young married Benjamin Clayton's daughter Anna Maria on 27 November 1819.[94] He carried on the Norton practice for about ten years, but by 1830 he had moved to Bury St Edmunds. On 3 June 1830 the Committee of the Suffolk General Hospital received a letter from him enclosing £10 (later increased to £10 10s) in which he said that he had recently become a resident of the town. He also mentioned that, 'If now or at any future period you can impose on me any professional labours by which I can further your beneficial plans it will be my great pleasure to

---

[89] Hospital minute books: SROB ID 503/3.
[90] *Ibid.*
[91] van Zwanenberg: SROI q s 614.
[92] Hospital minute books: SROB ID 503/1–7.
[93] *Bury and Norwich Post*, Wed. 17 Feb. 1819, p. 2, col. 3.
[94] van Zwanenberg: SROI q s 614.

contribute my feeble quota of service to the general good'. But there is no indication that the members of the Committee were keen to take up his offer, even when he sent another donation of £100 in July 1830.[95] Reading between the lines, one has the feeling that Plowman fancied himself as a consultant physician. In fact, he went off to Pisa and obtained his MD (which was the recognised qualification for a physician) in 1837. His wife must have been in Pisa with him, because their youngest son was born there in that year. But there may have been another reason for Young being in Italy in 1837. He may have been advised to go there for the good of his health, because there is little doubt that, like his old master Benjamin Clayton, he suffered from tuberculosis. He died in Lucca on 15 July 1840 at the age of forty-four,[96] and was buried at Livorno.[97] More than a year before his death, his books were auctioned at a sale in Bury on 25 January 1839. The house in which he had lived, 90 Northgate Street, Bury St Edmunds, was put up for rent at the same time. The domicile was well set up for a large family. It had ten bedrooms, dining, drawing, and breakfast rooms, a study, water closet, kitchen, cellar, and offices as well as a coach house and a five-stalled stable.[98] Young had definitely needed a big house. He had eight sons, although only five of them survived to be adults. The eldest, Benjamin Clayton Young, died at the age of thirteen, while the sixth and seventh sons also died in infancy. The second child, William Chambers Young (1822–86) together with the third son James Hammond Young (1823–1905) left England with Major Bunbury in 1841 to settle in Australia. William took part in an expedition to central Australia and afterwards settled in the Tonga Islands, becoming the adopted son of King George of Tonga. He died in January 1886 and was buried at Eua, Tonga Islands. Meanwhile his brother James went to Queensland, the Tonga Islands and New Zealand. James died in November 1905 and was buried at Auckland, in New Zealand. The fourth son, Frederick John (1828–1908) had a more conventional career. He went to Cambridge, and then entered the church. He was Rector of South Milford, Yorkshire, from 1859 to 1908. The fifth son, Henry Charles (–1906) went into the Navy but he too ended up in New Zealand. The eight son, Augustus Warren Young (the one born in Pisa in 1837), went to Trinity College Dublin and obtained his BA in 1860, later moving to Paignton in Devon. He was still living there in 1908.[99] In addition to his large family, Young had four apprentices. They were Nathaniel Collyer, who was an apprentice from 1828 to 1833, Robert Day, 1830–35, William Gaskoin Stutter, 1832–37, and Edward Chinery, 1833–38.[100] Collyer and Day followed their master's example in going on to Guy's to complete their studies, whereas Stutter, as we know, went to St George's. Only Stutter and Day ended up practising in Suffolk. Collyer joined the Indian Medical Service and died of a fever in Cawnpore on 27 June 1857, whilst Chinery migrated to Lymington in Hampshire.[101]

95   Hospital minute books: SROB ID 503/2.
96   *The Gentleman's Magazine*, September 1840, p. 335.
97   S.H.A. Hervey, *Biographical List of Boys Educated at King Edward VI Free Grammar School in Bury St Edmunds*, 1550–1900, Suffolk Green Books no. 13, Bury St Edmunds, 1908.
98   *Bury and Norwich Post*, 16 Jan. 1839, p. 2, col. 6.
99   Hervey, *Boys Educated at King Edward's*, II, p. 441.
100   van Zwanenberg: SROI q s 614.
101   *Ibid.*

APPENDIX II

Diseases Mentioned in the Casebook and Introduction

[Note: in Appendices II to V the page numbers following the names of Stutter's patients are those used in the original casebook.]

Anaemia

Anaemia can be defined as a reduction in the amount of blood in the body. This makes sufferers look pale and causes them to be tired and breathless. In Stutter's day there was insufficient knowledge to classify the various causes of anaemia but it was recognised that chlorosis seemed to be due to iron deficiency. The two terms were therefore almost synonymous. In his book *The Principles and Practice of Medicine*, published in 1892, Sir William Osler (1849–1919) classified chlorosis as a 'primary or essential anaemia' and devoted several pages to its description. He did, of course, know that anaemia was also secondary to other diseases like cancer, renal failure and tuberculosis. By 1892 Addisonian anaemia had also been described, but in 1839 that was very much in the future.

Bronchitis

Bronchitis may be defined as an inflammation of the larger and medium-sized air passages in the lungs. It can be the result of infection or the inhalation of irritating fumes, and may be acute or chronic. The chronic state is much encouraged by tobacco smoking.

   Robert Nelson, aged sixty (p. 130), was in hospital with bronchitis from 15 April to 19 May 1840. Unfortunately Stutter did not record a history, but it is the likely that the patient had an acute exacerbation (i.e. worsening) of his chronic bronchitis.

Bubo post ulcus venerium

A bubo is an infected swelling of the neck, groin or armpit. It is usually secondary to a superficial infection in the area of the body served by the lymphatic drainage system of that particular region. Thus an infected finger might cause a bubo in the axilla, whilst an infected bite or cut on the leg might be the harbinger of a similar lesion in the groin.

   William Downey (p. 8) aged twenty-three, whose care Stutter took over from Dr Bayne, had a bubo secondary to a venereal ulcer, presumably on his penis. It may well have been syphilitic in nature. He was discharged 'cured' on 22 January 1839. If the diagnosis were syphilis, the 'cure' would only represent resolution of the primary chancre in the first stage of the disease. William Downey might have had a lifetime of illness before him.

Chlorosis

Chlorosis literally means 'the green sickness' and it became a common diagnosis sometime in the seventeenth century. Thomas Sydenham (1624–89) recommended iron filings suspended in wine as a treatment. This was very perceptive of him since we now know that most cases of chlorosis were likely to have been the result of iron-deficiency anaemia. The condition was commonest in young women, who were not taking enough iron in their diet to replace the blood lost in menstruation. The usual source of iron would have been meat, but this may not have been available to the poor. At higher levels of society it was thought that refined young women should not eat too much meat because it was 'too stimulating'. Doctors did not help much either, since many of them tended to bleed their patients for nearly everything.

In fact, this is what happened to Caroline Clark, aged nineteen (p. 24), who was admitted to the Suffolk General Hospital from 19 March to 30 April 1839. She was thought to be suffering from chlorosis, and although she was sensibly prescribed an iron mixture on 4 April, on 27 April 1839 ten ounces of blood were taken from her by wet cupping. The very same day she was pronounced 'cured'.

Cholera

This is a water-borne disease caused by a bacterial organism called Vibrio cholera. The infection causes severe diarrhoea, and death, when it occurs, is usually due to an overwhelming loss of body fluids. The rapid expansion of towns and cities in the wake of the industrial revolution, with their overcrowding, deficient drainage and contaminated water supplies, favoured the spread of the disease. During a cholera epidemic in London in 1854, a medical practitioner called John Snow (1813–58), carried out a systematic investigation involving the consumers of water in an area of London where several private water companies supplied the drinking water. Snow showed that the number of fatalities in each street corresponded to the degree of pollution in that stretch of the Thames from which each company extracted its water. People drinking water from the Broad Street pump were more likely to die than those who consumed water from elsewhere. This seemed to prove that cholera was indeed water-borne. But the end of the story did not come until 1883, when the German doctor, Robert Koch (1843–1910) finally identified the causative organism. The early Victorians thought that 'bad air' or miasmas caused infectious diseases like cholera. Fortunately, some of the steps which they took to remove bad air, like installing sewers and arranging for streets to be cleared of rubbish, made it more difficult for water supplies to become contaminated by human excrement, thus greatly reducing the incidence of the disease. Although the last indigenous cases of cholera occurred in the United Kingdom in 1893, epidemics continued to occur in India and Pakistan throughout the twentieth century. According to the *Ipswich Journal*, in October 1832, Dr J. Dunthorn (1791–1856) of Wickhambrook (who was to take Stutter into partnership ten years later), made a diagnosis of cholera when he attended a family of nine in that village. Of those nine people, four died. There is no record of Dr Dunthorn's treatment, but the standard remedy at the time was calomel, a purging agent that would only have served to make the patient's dehydration worse. If he had wanted to send his patients to hospital Dr Dunthorn would not have been able to do so. The management did not regard such diseases to be its responsibility (see the General Introduction).

Chorea

Chorea, or more properly Sydenham's chorea, after the famous English physician Thomas Sydenham (1624–89), usually affects children between the ages of seven and fourteen who have been living in poor social circumstances. The condition is commoner in girls than boys by a factor of three to one. It is a disorder of the central nervous system, and it occurs in association with rheumatic fever. In fact it may be the *only* manifestation of rheumatic fever. The onset is usually gradual with general tiredness and lack of sleep. The patient may become very nervous and the speech incoherent. Commonly, the sufferer develops purposeless movements of the arms and legs and muscular weakness is usual. Fortunately, chorea is usually self-limiting and mild cases may subside within a few weeks, although the average time to complete recovery is normally about three months. The regime of good diet and rest that existed in the Suffolk General Hospital in 1839 would have been very beneficial to this condition. In October 1841, Dr Babington MD, FRS, published a review of chorea in the *Guy's Hospital Reports*. Nine cases of chorea had been admitted to Guy's in the previous year. Most were purged and given zinc sulphate. Blistering of the neck and spine with emplasters of lytta seemed popular with those ordering the treatment, and so were electric shocks to the spine. Dr Babington mentioned that there had 'probably never been so complete an opportunity for trying the effects of electricity and galvanism, in all their varieties and in all diseases, as in the Electrical Apartment at Guy's Hospital'.

Three cases of chorea are mentioned in Stutter's casebook. They are Maria Cousins, aged sixteen (p. 32) (inpatient from 9 April to 11 June 1839), Matilda Rumble, aged eleven (p. 30) (inpatient from 9 April to 30 April 1839) and Elizabeth Payne, aged twelve (p. 112) (inpatient from 17 March to 31 March 1840). None of them seems to have been given zinc sulphate. Maria Cousins had leeches applied, but emplasters of lytta do not seem to have been used in any of Stutter's three cases. Nor is there any mention of the use of galvanism.

Disease of the ovaries

Whole tracts could be written on the diseases which affect the ovaries, but in the context of this volume it is almost certain that Susan Warren, aged fifteen (p. 47), was suffering from cancer of the ovary. She was admitted to hospital from 30 July until the 15 October 1839 and again from 18 February until 10 March 1840. It seems almost certain that she died on the second occasion.

Eczema

This is a common problem. Eczema is the term used to describe a characteristic itchy, red, scaly rash which usually has a very poorly defined edge. Blistering may also occur. Eczema can be inherited or set off by contact with irritant or allergic substances.

Even in the twenty-first century sulphur is used in the treatment of eczema when the main purpose is to remove scale. An ointment containing 2 per cent sulphur and salicylic acid is still prescribed by many dermatologists.

Susan Banham (p. 17) is recorded as suffering from eczema in Stutter's case-book. She was an inpatient from 1 January until 5 March 1839.

Epilepsy

Epilepsy is a group of disorders characterized by unprovoked, recurrent seizures that are caused by sudden disturbances of electrical activity in the brain. These in turn disrupt normal neurological functioning. Symptoms depend on the type of epilepsy and the location of the disturbance in the brain. They may be very mild with no more than a transitory absence, or violent with generalised seizures and unconsciousness. In a review of the condition published in the *Guy's Hospital Reports* in April 1841, Dr B.G. Babington MD, FRS, admitted that doctors of his day knew as little about epilepsy as his predecessors had done in ancient times. This was because medical scientists were as yet ignorant of the normal workings of the brain. As to treatment, he felt that bleeding and evacuants were sometimes necessary in those patients of a plethoric nature, but on the whole he favoured preparations of bark (i.e. quinine), iron, arsenic, silver and zinc. He especially liked zinc sulphate, which he considered to be safe, even in large doses.

Erysipelas

This is an infection of the skin and soft tissues caused by the bacterium strepto-coccus pyogenes or more properly, the Beta-haemolytic streptococcus, Lancfield Group A. It can spread rapidly, and before sulphonamide drugs came on the scene in the late 1930s it often caused fatal infections of the bloodstream. The bacterium can easily be transferred from patient to patient on inadequately washed hands, unsterile instruments and in the nasal secretions of medical attendants and nurses. It made surgical wards and operating theatres in nineteenth-century hospitals very dangerous places, and if you could afford it, it was far safer to have your operation done at home. In 1839 the bacterial cause of infections was still undiscovered and the response to an outbreak of erysipelas at the Suffolk General Hospital was to stop admitting new patients and discharge as many as possible of those remaining. The floors of the wards were then thoroughly scrubbed and the walls were whitewashed in an attempt to rid the building of the contagion.

It was not until the year 1878 that Louis Pasteur (1822–95) presented his case for the germ theory of infection to the French Academy of Medicine. Although this was a breakthrough, it took many more years before his ideas were accepted. For instance, it has been said that Florence Nightingale (1820–1920), never gave credence to the theory.

Erythema multiforme

Erythema multiforme is the name given to an acute sensitivity reaction of the skin characterised by symmetrically distributed lesions which look like the targets on shooting ranges. These are the so-called 'target' lesions. The condition is rare after the age of fifty. It is often preceded by a herpes infection and it is more common in the spring and autumn. The rash is usually not itchy, but there can be bleeding into the spots. Most people make a complete recovery in two to four weeks.

Stutter's patient John Scott (p. 74), could well have had erythema multiforme. He was a fit young man who had herpes of the lips in autumn. The rash appeared on his arms and legs and spared his trunk. It seems that there was bleeding into the lesions, which Stutter described as 'purpuric'. The patient recovered spontaneously, despite the treatment.

Hepatitis

These days we would understand hepatitis to mean an infection of the liver with viruses A, B or C. Hepatitis A is caught by ingesting the faeces of someone with the disease, whereas hepatitis B and C are caught from sharing hypodermic needles and from infected blood products. They can also be transmitted sexually. In Stutter's time the term 'hepatitis' may have covered a basketful of conditions, from chronic disease of the gall bladder to cirrhosis of the liver, syphilis and cancer of the head of pancreas.

Isaac Carter, aged seventy-six (p. 28), was admitted to the Suffolk General Hospital from 9 April to 30 April 1839 with 'hepatitis chronica'. No history was recorded in the casebook and his treatment was largely confined to preparations for his bowels, so it is difficult to make a modern diagnosis. We can perhaps get a little closer with Mary Death, aged forty-one (p. 114), who was admitted from 17 March to 21 April 1840 with 'hepatitis rheumatica'. She had had pain in the right side of her abdomen radiating to her shoulder. In addition she was jaundiced, with tender-ness over the liver. This suggests disease of the gall bladder. She was given mercury pills (despite the fact that she had lost all her teeth but one due to excessive saliva-tion – presumably with mercury – thirteen years before), magnesium sulphate and carbonate, and bled twelve ounces on admission. The next day she was cupped in the region of the right hypochondrium (i.e. just below the right ribs) and ten ounces of blood were withdrawn. This was followed by the application of a cataplasm in the same anatomical position. She was ordered a low diet on admission but this was upgraded to a common diet on 1 April. On 12 April she was allowed rice and milk. A large cataplasm was applied to the left side on the 26 March. She was prescribed some tincture of opium on 15 April, which is the last entry made before she was discharged on 30 April. Perhaps she had an obstructive jaundice due to gallstones, which were eventually passed through her common bile duct into the bowel, relieving her jaundice. At forty-one she was certainly the right age for gallstones. Generations of medical students have repeated the little ditty for remembering the characteristics of those who most often suffer from that condition. They are fair, fat, fecund, flatulent females of forty.

Hypertrophy of the heart (or hypertrophia cordis)
The muscles of the heart usually enlarge when they have more work to do. In Stutter's time rheumatic heart disease was very common. Leaky or obstructed heart valves certainly gave the heart muscle more work to do, as would high blood pressure (a concept totally foreign to the doctors of the early nineteenth century). However they would recognise the increasing breathlessness, swelling of the legs and heart murmurs associated with advanced cardiac problems.

James Arnold, aged sixty-eight (p. 15), was admitted to hospital on 19 February 1839 but discharged himself on 26 February. John Chinery, aged forty-five (p. 38), stayed longer. He was admitted on 18 June 1839 and discharged on the 16 July.

Hypertrophy of right side
This may mean quite literally enlargement of the right side of the body, a congenital condition, or it my have been enlargement of the right side of the heart. This seems to be more likely in the case of George Talbot, aged fifty-eight (p. 40), whose prescriptions suggest that he was indeed a cardiac case.

Hysteria
Hysteria may be defined as a condition in which the symptoms or signs of illness are reproduced by a patient for some advantageous purpose, without the sufferer being fully aware of his or her motive for doing so. It is always dangerous for doctors to attach psychological labels to patients who apparently suffer from physical illness. This must have been especially so in the nineteenth century, when there were few investigations available to confirm or confute a clinical diagnosis.

Leucorrhoea and Gastralgia
Leucorrhoea is an excessive white vaginal discharge, which in the nineteenth century was thought to be due to a 'relaxed condition of the system'. In the *Family Physician*, published in 1887, readers were reminded that leucorrhoea was often associated with anaemia and general debility and in these cases 'nothing did so much good as a course of quinine or iron'. In the twenty-first century doctors would search for a more specific reason for the discharge, such as a vaginal infection, an erosion of the neck of the womb or even a foreign body in the vagina. But when these causes have been excluded, there remain not a few cases in which diagnosis remains a mystery.

Elizabeth Canham, aged forty-two (p. 26), was in hospital for two weeks with 'Leucorrhoea et Gastralgia'. The latter term simply means pain in the stomach, which, as we all know, can have many causes.

Leprosy

It is astonishing to find this disease mentioned in the Suffolk General Hospital's minute book, albeit two years after Stutter had departed. On 22 August 1843, Mr John Kemp, an exciseman, appeared before the Committee to make an application for his daughter Emma Kemp to be admitted to the hospital because she had leprosy. Dr Probart confirmed the urgency of the case and she was admitted, her father agreeing to pay the hospital ten shillings a week throughout her stay.[1]

Nowadays, leprosy is known as Hansen's disease. This is after Armaeur Hansen (1841–1912) who discovered the causative organism, Mycobacterium leprae. In Europe, leprosy was at its height in the eleventh to thirteenth centuries with numerous hospitals being built for the reception of those affected. Sufferers might have scaly rashes, and thickened and ulcerated skin. They could also suffer the loss of fingers, toes and nasal bones. They were often ostracised by society. But by the mid-fourteenth century leprosy was in decline in Europe, probably because the causative organism had become less virulent. The disease still occurs in developing countries, but in Bury St Edmunds in the 1840s it would have been just as rare as it is today.

Measles

Measles is a viral illness which is spread from person to person by droplet infection. Ten to twelve days after contact with a case the newly infected person feels unwell with a headache. A dry cough, runny nose and inflamed eyes follow. Then there is a high fever and a red blotchy rash starts on the face. It moves downwards over the next three days and covers most of the body. Ultimately it subsides and the symptoms pass, although the cough may persist for another week. Ear infections and bronchopneumonia are common complications and in poorly fed youngsters measles can cause severe diarrhoea. This in turn can result in extreme malnutrition from which sufferers may lose their sight or die. Others may die of encephalitis. In well-nourished children the mortality rate is less than 1 in 10,000 cases, but in poverty-stricken East Anglia in the early nineteenth century malnutrition was common and the death rate must have been much higher. One has to say too that the doctors may have contributed to the high mortality rate with their treatment (although, of course, this was not their intention).

In his diary, Thomas Giordani Wright, who was apprenticed to a Mr McIntyre in the colliery district of Newcastle, described a measles outbreak in the practice in 1829. On 7 April he recorded that two children had died of measles. The same day he bled another severely ill young measles-sufferer using the jugular vein. He then prescribed an emetic, followed by a warm bath and a blister, but despite his efforts his patient died three days later.[2]

In October 1842 Dr H. Marshall Hughes writing in the *Guy's Hospital Reports* described his treatment of a child aged three whom he had first seen as a patient at the Surrey Dispensary on 23 July 1840. He does not give the sex of the child calling him or her 'it' throughout. He mentions that two of the child's brothers had died of chest complications following measles two years before. They were treated with mercury (which may have speeded their deaths). There were still several brothers and sisters left and the whole family lived in a small and close room behind a small

---

1   Hospital minute book: SROB ID 503/7.
2   A. Johnson (ed.), *The Diary of Thomas Giordani Wright, Newcastle Doctor 1826–1829*, Woodbridge, 2001, p. 312.

retail shop where the parents sold bull's eyes, gingerbread, stay-tapes and 'bobbings' [*sic*]. When Dr Hughes saw the child it had had measles for two days. The patient was feverish and although the chest was resonant it was unusually obstructed by mucus in the small and large tubes. He ordered three leeches to the chest, a hot bath, an ipecacuanha emetic and twenty minims of antimonial wine every six hours, in a saline aperient mixture. The next day he found that the leeches had bled well, but the ipecacuanha had not caused sickness as intended. The respiratory rate was 84 per minute and the pulse rate 130 per minute. The face was flushed and purplish, and the physical signs much as before. He ordered five grains of ipecacuanha and a sixth of a grain of tartar emetic, but as this did not produce vomiting, an ounce of antimonial wine was prescribed, a quarter of which was to be given every five minutes till vomiting resulted, and then a quarter of a grain of tartar emetic, with a little sugar, every four hours. The next day he found that neither fluid nor the powders had caused vomiting, but the child was marvellously improved. The breathing was easy, the rate of respiration about 30 per minute, pulse rate 120 per minute. Although some diarrhoea persisted a dose of castor oil was now given, followed by chalk mixture – the powders being repeated night and morning. The next day, progress was satisfactory and the diarrhoea less, but on the day after that broad vesicles appeared on the lips and tongue, and the back of the throat was covered with a thick grey excretion. The conjunctiva of one eye was inflamed and the cornea hazy.

> The next morning the larynx became obstructed and on the succeeding day there existed considerable depression and collapse of the features. Tonics, eggs, beef tea and tea and milk were now freely administered, but the child died exhausted in six days.

The above case-histories make depressing reading to the modern reader. Most of the treatments used were either useless or positively harmful, and perhaps those families who could not afford a doctor fared best when the measles was in town. Of course, people suffering from measles were not admitted to the Suffolk General Hospital and so the House Apothecary did not have to deal with any. Nevertheless, Susan Reeve, aged twenty-three (p. 108), was blind in the left eye due to an attack of the disease when she was aged ten or eleven.

Opthalmia scrofulosa
Mary Motte, aged fifteen (p. 34), was admitted from 9 April to 30 April 1839. It seems that she had a skin infection around her eyes. We would probably call it impetigo and conjunctivitis. She was cured with tincture of Iodine applied with a brush and silver nitrate eye drops.

Paraplegia
This means loss of the use of the lower limbs and is commonly caused by severe injuries to the spinal cord. William Malt, aged twenty (p. 5), was discharged 'cured' in March 1839, having been admitted under Dr Bayne with this diagnosis. Unfortunately, there is no clinical history and so we can only assume that perhaps he was cured of a subsidiary complaint and not the paraplegia itself.

Phthisis (i.e. Consumption or Pulmonary tuberculosis)
The German doctor Robert Koch (1843–1910) identified the tubercle bacillus in 1882, but in 1839 the cause of phthisis was a mystery. We now know that pulmonary

tuberculosis is passed from person to person by coughs, sneezes and spitting. It is a disease that is inexorably linked to poverty, with its consequent overcrowding and poor diet. These conditions were very prevalent in Victorian England. Tuberculosis can be very infectious, and middle- and upper-class people (whose houses were full of servants) often caught the disease. Doctors were particularly at risk because of their contact with patients. In its early stages it was and still can be difficult to diagnose. When it first occurs the disease usually attacks one or other or both of the upper lobes of the lungs. The patient has a persistent cough, has usually lost weight, feels very debilitated and may or may not complain of night sweats. The pulse rate may be increased slightly, but apart from that, physical signs can be few and if there is no history of the patient having coughed up blood-stained sputum (which tends to be a giveaway), the medical attendant may be perplexed. Listening to the chest with a stethoscope may reveal no abnormality. It is only in the later stages of the disease that more pronounced physical signs develop. Cases of phthisis were not supposed to be admitted to the Suffolk General Hospital in 1839, but without the benefit of chest X-rays (not discovered until 1895) it would have been very difficult to tell which patients had the infection. Since it was a common disease, it is certain that many of the patients who were admitted had pulmonary tuberculosis.

The only case recorded as having phthisis in Stutter's casebook was Samuel Burman, the shoemaker aged twenty (p. 76), who had a tuberculous cavity in his right upper lobe. But from their histories and physical signs Sarah Bryant, aged twenty-five (p. 96), and Frances Baker, aged thirty-four (p. 100), almost certainly had the disease too. Mary Willingham, aged thirty-five (p. 132), was admitted with tuberculous peritonitis on 28 April 1840. From Stutter's notes it is pretty obvious that she also had advanced pulmonary tuberculosis. She died on 19 May 1840.

It is perhaps interesting to note that Dr H. Marshall Hughes MD, writing in the *Guy's Hospital Reports* of April 1842, reported that of 250 cases of phthisis who had died in Guy's Hospital, the Surrey Dispensary and the Marylebone Infirmary, 8 per cent were under twenty years old, 43 per cent were aged twenty to thirty, 19 per cent were aged forty to fifty and only 4 per cent were over fifty. He also observed that fewer females than males affected with phthisis reached the age of forty.

Pneumonia
In the days before antibiotics the diagnosis of pneumonia was as much feared as that of cancer today. We now know that pneumonia is caused by infection of the lungs. Nineteenth-century doctors did not know this, believing it to be an inflammation caused by exposure to cold or the cessation of menstruation. They did, however, realise that it might be precipitated by other diseases like measles and also that it could be associated with malnutrition, debilitating conditions like cancer or phthisis, and prolonged bed rest in old age. In the *Guy's Hospital Reports* of October 1842 Dr H. Marshall Hughes gave a summary of his views on pneumonia and its treatment. He described in some detail the physical signs to be demonstrated in the chest by percussion, palpation, and the noises to be heard on listening with the stethoscope. He then went on to mention treatment of acute pneumonia. For many years the plan adopted at Guy's Hospital had been to bleed the patient until they nearly fainted and then administer a pill containing half a grain of opium and a quarter of a grain of tartarized antimony with one or two grains of calomel, every three or four hours, according to the severity of the symptoms. This was usually combined with a saline mixture containing twenty or thirty minims of antimonial wine. If the symptoms had not improved in a few hours bleeding was repeated, and sometimes, though not often, repeated again. Should the patient be thought to be too

weak for venesection, he or she was cupped until six or twelve ounces of blood had been extracted. As the patient improved the medicines were repeated less frequently 'even though the mercury had not produced its specific effect on the mouth'. Sometimes blistering was tried in the later stages of the disease, although Dr Hughes doubted its usefulness.

James Clark (p. 86), was admitted to the Suffolk General Hospital with pneumonia on 10 December 1839 and died on the same day. He was not bled, perhaps because he was judged to be too weak. But he was given opium, which no doubt eased his symptoms.

Psoriasis

A common rash characterised by chronic, dull red, scaly patches. The patches are often described as a 'salmon pink' colour, having silvery scales. These usually have a very well-defined edge to them, and may particularly affect the scalp, elbows and knees. The condition is often inherited. For many years preparations containing coal tar were the basis of treatment. These are still used, although they would no longer be the first choice because of the risk of provoking skin cancer.

Abraham Orris, aged forty-three (p. 17), was admitted to the Suffolk General Hospital from 19 February to 23 April 1839 suffering from psoriasis.

Purpura and Urticaria

Urticaria is commonly known as nettle-rash or hives. Hives are caused by the leakage of blood plasma out of small blood vessels under the skin, and this in turn is precipitated by the release of a chemical called histamine from cells called mast cells. The condition can be caused by food allergies or an allergy to medication. It can also be the result of infection or exposure to excessive heat or cold.

In the case of John Scott (p. 74), the eruption followed a head cold some nine days previously. The cold had been accompanied by a cold sore on his lip (herpes labialis). On 23 October 1839 the rash was pretty florid and was associated with some purpura (i.e. purple blotches under the skin). The rash had almost disappeared by the 28 October 1839, but the patient was not discharged until 26 November 1839. Many of the features of this illness suggest that the patient did, in fact, suffer from erythema multiforme, and not simple nettle-rash (see section on erythema multiforme above).

Rheumatism

This can be taken to mean aches and pains in the muscles and joints. 'Rheumatism' is a general term that results from a number of pathological causes, some of which are as elusive today as they were in 1839. According to *Buchan's Domestic Medicine*, first published in 1769, 'rheumatism prevails in cold, damp, marshy countries. It is most common among the poorer sort of peasants, who are ill clothed, live in low damp houses, and eat coarse and unwholesome food, which contains but little nourishment, and is not easily digested.'

The symptoms were said to be commoner in middle age, and William Mulley, aged forty-six (p. 19), certainly fitted that bill. He was in hospital for just over two months.

Rheumatic fever and rheumatic heart disease

This disease was and is primarily one of childhood and adolescence. Its incidence is highest amongst poor people who live in bad social conditions. In 1839 nobody knew anything about the bacterial cause of disease, but there is now a strong case for thinking that rheumatic fever is the late result of infection with the Beta-haemolytic streptococcus, Lancefield Group A. This microbe causes severe pharyngitis or tonsillitis, both of which were untreatable before the days of penicillin. A few weeks after the initial invasion by the bacteria, the patient becomes lethargic, develops a fever and suffers from quite severe joint pains. This is rheumatic fever. It can go on for weeks or months. But even when the sufferer has recovered from their initial illness, they may not be completely out of the wood, because a late effect of the disease is damage to the heart valves. The valve most commonly affected is the mitral, but the aortic and tricuspid valves may sometimes be damaged too. Before cardiac surgery, nothing could be done about defective heart valves and sufferers usually developed heart failure and died prematurely. Since the advent of cardiac surgery in the twentieth century, however, it has become possible to replace faulty valves and give patients a normal life expectancy.

Rheumatoid arthritis

In his book *The Principles and Practice of Medicine* published in 1892, William Osler still called rheumatoid arthritis 'arthritis deformans'. By that time it was recognised that the disease was separate from rheumatism and gout, but earlier in the century the distinction seemed less clear and doctors thought that the three conditions were intimately related. Rheumatoid arthritis is commoner in women than in men, and (as Osler noted) affects the rich as well as poor. It often begins with pains and swelling in the hands and feet gradually spreading to other joints, causing severe deformities. Sometimes the disease burns itself out and this is the constant hope of both sufferers and their carers. In the nineteenth century morphia was used to relieve the pain with some abandon because there was little else. Hannah Pratt (p. 126), almost certainly had rheumatoid arthritis but she seemed to get by without the prescription of an opiate.

Scabies or 'the Itch'

Scabies is caused by a tiny mite which is just visible to the naked eye. The animal burrows into the skin and causes a severe itch, which the sufferer cannot help scratching. These scratches may then become secondarily infected, and the patient can end up being covered in small boils. The mite has favourite sites for burrowing, namely the fronts of the wrists, the web and sides of the fingers, the backs of the elbows, the genitals, the front of the armpits, the buttocks, the front of the knees, the ankles and the top of the feet. Infestation results from close contact with other people who already harbour the mite and the condition is associated with over-crowding and poor personal hygiene. Scabies must have been rife in nine-teenth-century gaols and workhouses. The traditional treatment for 'the Itch' was sulphur ointment, which was probably reasonably effective.

Smallpox

Smallpox had been the number-one killer disease in England from the mid-seven-teenth century until the late eighteenth century. The first ray of hope towards a possible end to the scourge came when Lady Mary Wortley Montague brought news of the procedure that came to be known as 'variolation' back to England from Turkey, where her husband had been the British Ambassador. She had observed how the Turks successfully prevented smallpox, and so she had her son Edward variolated on 18 March 1718. The operation was done by taking some matter from a vesicle belonging to an existing case of smallpox and introducing it into the body of the recipient by means of a small scratch or scratches with a needle. The hope was that this would then induce a mild form of smallpox, which in Turkish hands it usually did. But when British surgeons adopted the procedure, variolation became a far more severe affair. Instead of using the Greco-Turkish method of superficial scarification, operators made deep incisions in several sites. This method caused severe reactions and no doubt secondary infections too. The procedure fell into disrepute until Robert Sutton (1707–1788) of Kentford in Suffolk developed a new method of treatment between the years 1755 and 1761. He seems to have reverted to the much milder method practised by the Turks. He was very successful, but one of his sons called Daniel (1735–1819) was even more so. At the age of twenty-eight he moved to Ingatestone in Essex where his inoculation practice is said to have earned him £6,300 in the year 1765.[3]

The real breakthrough, however, came in 1796, when Edward Jenner (1749–1823) proved that inoculation with cowpox conferred immunity to smallpox. The advantages of cowpox over smallpox lymph were that it was safer to use and generally caused a much less severe illness. What is more, cowpox was not transmitted aerially and the use of the cowpox virus did not entail the risk of spreading disease among unprotected members of the community. The method slowly caught on and by the 1830s it was the accepted method of prevention. But this did not stop people dying of the disease. An epidemic in 1837–40 caused the deaths of more than 42,000 victims, chiefly babies and young children. It started in the west and south-west in the summer of 1837, spread through Wales the following winter and was widespread in the eastern counties by 1838. Vaccination was made compulsory in 1853, but this law was revoked in 1907. Smallpox continued to occur throughout the nineteenth century but ceased to be endemic in Britain. The final chapter came in 1977, when, after a ten-year global eradication programme carried out by the World Health Organisation, the last case of natural smallpox occurred in the town of Merka in Somalia.

Syphilis
In 1905 Fritz Schaudinn (1871–1906) and Erich Hoffman (1868–1905) discovered the protozoan parasite which causes this venereal disease. They called it *Spirochaeta pallida* but it has since been renamed *Treponema pallidum*. It may be that Columbus brought the disease back from the Americas. What is certain is that an epidemic of the disease broke out in 1493–94 in Naples, where the French and Spanish had been waging war. Sufferers had genital sores, rashes, swollen glands and abscesses which ate into the bones. It was often fatal and was obviously much more vigorous than the chronic disease it became in later centuries. By the nineteenth century syphilis was rarely immediately fatal, but the disease caused much morbidity, because, left to its own devices, the organism affected almost every system in the body. The treatment was still mercury, which in itself is very toxic. So much so that it must be wondered if the treatment was not sometimes worse than the disease. Known cases of syphilis were not usually admitted to the Suffolk General Hospital in 1839–41, but William Downey (p. 8) may well have had it.

Trigeminal neuralgia
Robert Gladwell (p. 45) was admitted to the Suffolk General Hospital on 30 July and discharged on 27 August 1839. He was readmitted on 22 October and discharged cured on 10 December 1839. Although Stutter did not enter the patient's

---

3   J.R. Smith, *The Speckled Monster*, Chelmsford, 1987, p. 74.

age or a diagnosis, it seems likely that Robert Gladwell was suffering from trigeminal neuralgia, or tic douloureux. This is a disorder of the fifth cranial nerve, which causes severe stabbing pains in the areas of the face where the branches of the nerves are distributed – the upper and lower jaws, lips, eyes, nose, scalp and fore-head. It usually affects one side of the face only but it can sometimes be bilateral. A further possibility is that Robert Gladwell was suffering from shingles, which can also affect the fifth cranial nerve, and is every bit as painful as trigeminal neuralgia. However, the diagnosis is unlikely in view of the application of an emplaster of lytta behind the ears on 6 November 1839. This was itself designed to cause blistering and it seems unlikely to have been used if the patient already had blistering from shingles. Morphia was probably the most useful drug used, although no doubt the meat, beer and porter were appreciated too. In the twenty-first century anticonvulsant or antidepressant drugs are given for their analgesic properties and sometimes acupuncture is tried. The use of leeches has long been out of fashion in the treatment of trigeminal neuralgia.

Urticaria, see *Purpura*

APPENDIX III

Diagnostic Methods

In the early and middle nineteenth century doctors had very few diagnostic tools at their disposal, although things were just beginning to change.

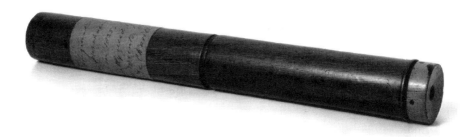

6. Monaural stethoscope of the Laennec type. The instrument was 9 inches long and 1½ inches in diameter. Reproduced by permission of the Wellcome Library, London.

Auscultation using the stethoscope

René Théophile Hyacynthe Laennec (1781–1826) of Paris published his *Traité de l'Auscultation Médiate* in 1819. This introduced the stethoscope to the world, but although it was a real advance, English doctors were reluctant to use the new invention since many of the older generation regarded it as a new-fangled bit of French frippery. The instrument, which at this time was a simple wooden tube, did not really come into more general use until around 1828. In George Eliot's novel *Middlemarch*, set in the early 1830s, Dr Lydgate was regarded as being very *avant-garde* because he used a stethoscope to examine his patients. The majority of physicians still thought they were doing their job properly if they took a careful clinical history, cast an eye over the patient's countenance, observed the tongue and looked at the condition of the sputum, faeces and urine. To the old guard, physical examination of the patient's body was utterly superfluous. But obviously things were changing by Stutter's era, because he listened to the patient's heart and chest, palpated the abdomen for masses and tested the urine for albumen (see below). So he was doing almost everything expected of a modern doctor at the time.

Measurement of body temperature

The famous Dutch physician, Hermann Boerhaave (1668–1734) of Leiden, had experimented with the use of a thermometer to measure his patients' temperatures, but his instrument was fifteen inches long and had to be inserted into the rectum for at least twenty minutes before a reliable reading could be taken. Although some interest in the technique was later shown in centres of medical excellence like

118

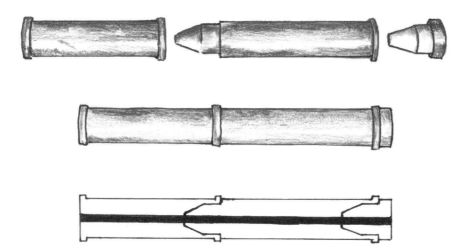

7. Diagram of a monaural stethoscope. The instrument was made divisible so that it was easier to carry in a pocket. Laennec had observed that a tube with a funnel-shaped depression at one end was more suitable for exploring breath sounds and râles – hence the detachable cone-shaped piece at the distal end of the instrument. A tube of uniform diameter with thick walls all the way was better for exploring the voice and heartbeats. Drawing by Frances Ridsdill Smith.

Edinburgh and Vienna, the thermometers of the late eighteenth and early nineteenth centuries were still too cumbersome for normal use. It was not until 1867 that Clifford Allbutt (1836–1925) developed a short clinical thermometer that was six inches long and produced a reading in five minutes. Only then did the routine measurement of patients' temperatures become practicable.

Microscopy
Like most medical innovations, microscopy was slow to be accepted. In his memoirs, Sir James Paget (1814–99) described how in 1835 he had discovered some specks in the muscles of a body he was dissecting. These later turned out to be the cysts of *Trichinella spiralis* (the small parasitic worm that humans catch by eating improperly cooked pork). He wanted to look at the specks under a microscope, but St Bartholomew's Hospital did not have such an instrument (or at least not one that was available to students). The problem was solved when Paget took the specimens to Robert Brown at the Natural History Department of the British Museum.

There is no evidence to show that Stutter was using a microscope at the Suffolk General Hospital in 1839–40. In fact, it was not until November 1860 that the Hospital Committee put aside £21 for one to be purchased.[1]

Measurement of blood pressure
Stutter could never have taken a patient's blood pressure because the means to do so

---

[1]   Minute books of the Committee and Board Meetings of the Suffolk General Hospital: SROB ID 503/11.

were not invented until 1896, when Scipione Riva-Rocci (1863–97) produced his revolutionary instrument, the sphygomanometer.

Percussion

In his book, *Inventum novum*, published in 1761, Leopold Auenbrugger (1722–1809) of Vienna had described how the chest could be tapped or 'percussed' like a barrel to determine whether or not there was enlargement of the heart or dullness due to lung disease. As usual, the discovery was very slow to be accepted, but Stutter was certainly using the method in 1839.

Urine testing

In the 1830s you diagnosed diabetes by tasting the urine for sweetness or observing its sticky property when it was dropped on a piece of linen. Fehling's chemical test for sugar in the urine was not introduced until 1848. Albumen, however, could be detected by boiling a sample of urine, and in 1827 Richard Bright (1789–1858) of Guy's Hospital had clearly demonstrated the association between nephritis and albumen in the urine. He taught his students to boil a small amount of urine in a spoon held over a lighted candle. If albumen was present the fluid would become opaque before the boiling point was reached. But despite the teaching of pioneers like Bright, routine urinalysis was very slow to catch on, although obviously some urine testing was being done in the Suffolk General Hospital in Stutter's time. Here and there he recorded that his patients' urine had been tested for albumen[2] and sometimes the specific gravity was entered too. The latter is a measure of the concentration of the urine. It is done with a simple calibrated instrument called a hydrometer (or urinometer) that sits in the urine specimen glass like a fisherman's float. The test is used as a pointer to the presence or absence of renal disease. Poorly functioning kidneys cannot concentrate the urine satisfactorily and so the specific gravity remains low.

---

[2]   This test was normally done by heating the urine, although on one occasion – see Leah Cross, age twenty-two (p. 41), 19 July 1839 – drops of nitric acid were added to a specimen to see if a cloud of albumen formed.

APPENDIX IV

Physical Treatments

Bleeding (otherwise known as phlebotomy or venesection)
This had been practised since ancient times. It consisted of opening a vein (usually at the elbow) with a knife and allowing the blood to drain into a bowl. The amount of blood extracted was usually about twenty ounces. In medieval monasteries such as that at Bury St Edmunds, bloodletting was practised routinely because the authorities thought it was a good way to control the monks' libido and preserve them from impure thoughts.[1] Whether or not it worked for that indication we shall never know, but in the treatment of the sick, bloodletting came to be considered especially useful in the management of fevers and inflammatory conditions. This medical orthodoxy began to be questioned in the seventeenth century by the Flemish physician

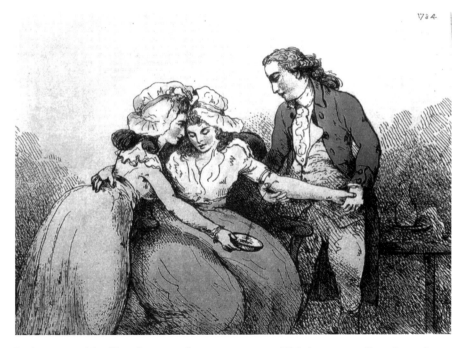

8. A surgeon bleeding the arm of a young woman. This is a copy of a coloured etching by T. Rowlandson, dated 1784. Although fashions in dress had changed by Stutter's time, the procedure had not. Reproduced by permission of the Wellcome Library, London.

---

1   C. Rawcliffe, ' " On the Threshold of Eternity": Care for the Sick in East Anglian Monasteries', in. C. Harper-Bill, C. Rawcliffe and R. Wilson (eds), *East Anglia's History*, UEA, 2000, p. 66.

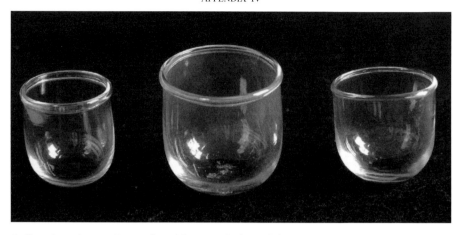

9. Cupping glasses. Reproduced by permission of the Wellcome Library, London.

Johannes Baptista van Helmont (1579–1644) and his followers. And in 1835, Pierre Louis (1787–1872) of Paris also came to the conclusion that bloodletting was a waste of time. He published a paper in which, using a statistical approach, he demonstrated that patients with inflammatory conditions, including pneumonia, derived no benefit at all from bleeding. But doctors continued to use the treatment. Louis' rival F.J.V. Broussais (1772–1838) bled every patient in sight, and was very popular for doing so. Patients wanted something done and those doctors who stood by and waited for nature to do her work tended to be unpopular (and sometimes poor to boot). In his memoirs, written in the early 1880s, Sir James Paget (1814–99) described how in the early 1830s, when he was serving his apprenticeship with Mr Costerton of Great Yarmouth, many country people deemed it a good thing to be bled once or twice a year as a safeguard or help to health. They usually came in on market days in spring and autumn and were bled until they fainted. Paget had no recollection of any evidence that either good or harm came of the practice, but the procedure was certainly deeply embedded in folklore. More than twenty years later, in *The Lancet* of 3 February 1855 there is a report of the famous Dr Addison of Guy's Hospital having treated a case of pneumonia by bleeding the patient. By that time the popularity of the treatment was certainly in decline, although in 1892 Sir William Osler (1849–1919) in his book *The Principles and Practice of Medicine* offered the opinion that 'during the first five decades of the nineteenth century the profession had bled too much, whereas in more recent times doctors had certainly bled too little'. He still felt that timely venesection could well be life-saving in cases of pneumonia.

Cataplasm (or Poultice)[2]
Poultices were commonly used to promote suppuration (i.e. the discharge of pus) They could be made of barley meal and lead acetate, mashed turnip or even bread and milk.[3]

---

[2] See also 'poultices' in Pharmaceutical Introduction.
[3] See also under 'capsicum' and 'mallow' in Appendix V.

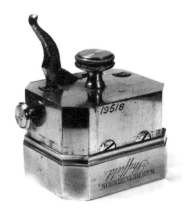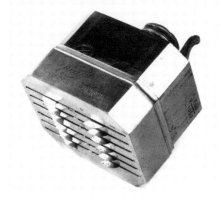

10. Automatic scarifier showing spring mechanism.

11. Automatic scarifier showing blades.

Illustrations 10 and 11 are photographs by W.H. Hutchison and are reproduced by permission of the Wellcome Library, London.

Cupping
Both wet cupping and dry cupping were practised and are described below.

i. Wet cupping
Wet cupping was a complex procedure. It necessitated the use of glass cups and a scarifier. The scarifier (sometimes called a scarificator) was a spring box containing up to seven rows of little lancets which projected from the face of the box to a distance of up to one quarter of an inch.[4] After the spring of the scarifier had been set and the site of application selected, both the site and the cups were heated using warm water. With a torch (i.e. a candle) in one hand and the glass in the other, the operator placed the cup on the patient's skin with one edge raised by about one and a half inches. The lighted torch was then placed under the glass towards the centre for two seconds and then quickly withdrawn, creating a vacuum. When the glass was fully applied to the sufferer's skin, the flesh would rise slowly into the small chamber, occupying one third of the volume. The glass was left in position for one minute and then removed. Next, the scarifier was applied to the area of skin previously covered by the glass. Its lancets were sprung, causing multiple small lacerations. Following this the instrument was quickly removed. A vacuum was created in the cup with the lighted torch in the same manner as before and the vessel was reapplied to the skin so that blood would be sucked into it.

ii. Dry cupping
Dry cupping or vesication was the production of a blister by the application of the cup alone. Various ingenious modifications of the plain glass cup were produced in the early nineteenth century, including those that could be evacuated by a pumping

---

4 Scarifier blades were graduated according to the site of application. For the chest, back and abdomen quarter inch blades were used but behind the ears, blades that only protruded one seventh of an inch were recommended. For the temple it was one eighth of an inch and for the scalp one sixth of an inch.

syringe. These instruments would avoid the use of double evacuation by means of the lighted torch.

Wet cupping seems to have been discontinued about the same time as venesection, but dry cupping as a counter-irritant continued to be used in the treatment of pneumonia and rheumatic conditions until well into the first half of the twentieth century.

Enemas

Constipation was regarded almost as a sin so, like their medical ancestors in previous centuries, most doctors of the early nineteenth century were ever ready to use an enema (or clyster) to relieve the problem. The instrument cases of ships' surgeons always contained at least one impressive looking large metal syringe that was used for the purpose. And given the high meat and low fluid diet of sailors in the early nineteenth century, no doubt medical attendants were often called upon to administer clysters to their nautical charges. Enemas had been developed for uses other than evacuation of the bowel, and all sorts of solutions were introduced into the rectum with therapeutic intent. In 1828 a Dr Alexander reported to the Liverpool Medical Society that he had successfully treated a case of tetanus with an infusion of tobacco smoke given via the rectum.[5]

Galvanism/galvanic troughs

Galvanic electricity is the direct current that is created when certain metals, usually zinc and copper, are put in contact with each other along with a solution such as saltwater. Luigi Galvani (1737–98) first noticed this effect during his famous experiments with frogs' legs, starting in 1791. He described how he suspended the legs of skinned dead frogs by copper wiring from an iron balcony. When the feet touched the iron uprights they twitched and the muscles contracted, which seemed to show that electricity could stimulate life. Alessandro Volta (1745–1827) did further studies on this effect. In 1800 he invented his 'Voltaic pile' or battery that consisted of disks of silver, copper and cardboard (moistened with a salt solution) stacked into a column. If a wire were connected from one end of the column to the other, a direct current would flow through the wire. In the early part of the nineteenth century great advances were made in the scientific knowledge of electricity, but in the 1830s the use of electrotherapeutics in medicine was still very limited. One of the earliest proponents was Dr Golding Bird (1814–54) who ran the electrical room at Guy's Hospital. In an article published in the *Guy's Hospital Reports* of April 1841, he stated that nearly all public medical charities had had an electrical machine and a galvanic pile for many years, but that most physicians tended to use the apparatus available to them in a haphazard fashion and usually as a last resort. In his work he had tried to be more scientific and he gave an account of the cases he had treated successfully. These included patients with chorea, paralysis, amenorrhoea and skin complaints.

In February 1834[6] Dr Bayne (see Appendix I) suggested that two galvanic troughs should be purchased by the Suffolk General Hospital 'as a therapeutical agent in the treatment of nervous diseases' at a cost of approximately thirty shillings each. Their purchase was agreed, but there is no reference to the use of galvanic troughs in Stutter's casebook.

---

5   J. Shepherd, *A History of the Liverpool Medical Institution*, Liverpool Medical Institution, 1979, p. 57.
6   Hospital minute books: SROB ID 503/4.

Issue

This was an artificial ulcer caused by making an incision through the skin and keeping it open by the insertion of metal 'tents' or peas to form a drain to carry off noxious humours. They were often used in fevers and in the treatment of leg ulcers in which they formed an alternative drain for humours while the ulcer was being healed. There is no record of Stutter using an issue on any of his patients.

Leeches

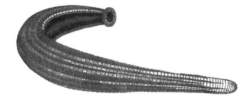

12. This drawing of a medicinal leech was taken from Harter, *Images of Medicine* – see Bibliography.

The medical leech *Hirudo medicalis* can ingest up to five times its own weight in blood. Its use in medicine goes back to ancient times and it is said that Nicander of Colophon was one of the first recorded users in the second century BC. The leech is native to Europe and Asia, and was introduced into North America by European immigrants. In the nineteenth century it was extensively cultivated for its medicinal uses and was still regarded as a cure-all. For instance, some doctors felt that a dozen leeches around the temples would help a headache, while fifty on the abdomen would cure anything from tumours to obesity. When they were placed in the mouth or nose it was recommended that a thread should be passed through the tail of each leech to prevent the patient from accidentally swallowing them.[7]

In the contracted state, each leech is about 3 to 3.5 cm long and 1.5 to 1.8 cm wide. The body is formed of ring-shaped segments, of which there are from 90 to 100; it tapers towards its ends, each of which has a disc shaped sucker. The saliva of the leech contains hirudin, a polypeptide that has anticoagulant properties. Leeches were used in the treatment of pericarditis[8] as late as 1950. To this day they are still sometimes employed to reduce post-operative haematomas.[9]

In the 1840s the chief supplier of leeches to the Suffolk General Hospital was Mr Teasdale the Chemist.[10] He probably obtained them from importers in London, who may in turn have turn shipped them in from producers on the continent.[11]

Paracentesis abdominis

This was a method of drawing off excess fluid from the abdomen using an instrument like the one in Illustration 13. The patient was encouraged to empty his or her bladder. Then a small nick was usually made in the skin of the abdominal wall with a scalpel. The pointed metal trocar with its surrounding cannula (or tube) was thrust

---

7   J.L. Turk and E. Allen, 'Bleeding and Cupping', *Annals of the Royal College of Surgeons of England* 65, 1983, pp. 128–131.
8   Pericarditis means inflammation of the sac around the heart.
9   A haematoma is a blood clot under the skin.
10   Hospital minute book: SROB ID 503/7.
11   Advertisement in the *British Medical Journal*, 2 May 1857: Bechade and Co., Fleet St., London – 'breeders of leeches and owners of extensive marshes in France and Hungary. A regular supply of fresh leeches received twice a week.'

13. This engraving of a trocar and cannula dates from the twentieth century. However, the design is probably much the same as the one used by Stutter. Reproduced from Harter, *Images of Medicine* – see Bibliography.

through the abdominal wall at the site of the scalpel incision. Following this, the trocar was removed and the fluid was allowed to drain into a dish through the cannula.

Susan Warren, aged fifteen (p. 47), had the procedure performed on at least two occasions. It must have been painful.

Plaisters or Plasters[12]

Common plaster was made by boiling lead acetate and olive oil together to produce a putty-like material that could be used for covering small wounds.

Adhesive plasters were manufactured by rendering common plaster and Burgundy pitch together. Not surprisingly, they were used for keeping other dressings in place.

Anodyne plasters were made of adhesive plaster mixed with camphor and powdered opium. They were used for treating painful joints, etc.

Blistering plasters were usually made of turpentine, yellow wax, mustard and powdered Spanish flies (Lytta). These plasters would provoke a blister when applied to the skin and were thought to aid recovery by extracting poisons from the body.[13]

Seton

The seton consisted of pinching up a fold of skin and inserting through it a large cutting needle armed with several threads which were left through the skin and pulled back and forth to cause suppuration. The principle was the same as in an issue but the results more drastic. It was inflammatory and painful and Stutter does not seem to have used the method.

Vapour baths

In the early years of the nineteenth century both warm and vapour baths became very popular, the latter being constructed in such a way that steam from boiling water, either plain or medicated, was passed through pipes to flow around the patient. The heat was moderated by moisture diffused through the air; consequently the patient's temperature was raised much less than when using a hot bath, and a vapour bath was considered to be safer and in most cases more effective. Many conditions, including fevers, liver complaints, dropsy and gout, were thought to benefit from using the steam which could be applied either to the whole body or part of it. The temperature and length of time of the bath was adjusted according to the purpose for which it was being used.

In 1821, Sir Thomas Cullum, a surgeon of Bury St Edmunds, in a letter[14] to his

---

[12] See also 'plasters' in Pharmaceutical Introduction.
[13] See also under 'cantharides' in Appendix V.
[14] Letters of Sir T.G. Cullum, to his son: SROB E2/21/2, 2 May 1821.

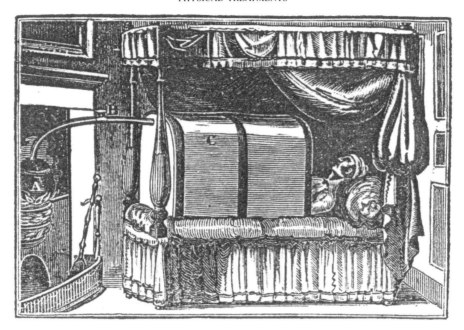

14. This is a copy of an illustration appearing in *An Essay on Bathing*, by Sir
A. Clarke, 1819. It represents a steam, or vapour, bath. Steam baths became very
popular during the early nineteenth century and one was installed in the Suffolk
General Hospital. Reproduced by permission of SROB.

son said 'Your mother thought the Steam Bath the most comfortable thing and did
not experience any faintness; perhaps Mrs Cullum will try the Steam Bath near
Downing St, Westminster, recommended by Sir Wm. Adams.'[15] Two years later, in a
letter dated 15 June 1823, Cullum wrote 'Gall,[16] the druggist in Abbeygate Street is
fitting up Steam Baths which seem now to be much recommended in the stead of
common warm baths'.[17] He repeated this information in a further letter dated
January 1824, adding that Lady Cullum had used it several times and found 'much
benefit by preventing the return of the little teasing Fever, which you know she is
much subject to'.[18]

Mr Colvile, a local clergyman, first suggested the installation of medical vapour
baths at the Suffolk General Hospital at a Committee Meeting on 1 November
1836.[19] At the next meeting on 8 November this suggestion was approved by the
Medical Committee, who on 29 November 1836 said that they thought that sulphur
baths would be the most suitable, but they had no experience in advising on their
construction. The following March the minutes reported that 'the offer of Rev.

[15] Sir William Adams (1783–1827), surgeon to the West of England Infirmary.
[16] Abraham Gall, chemist and druggist at 52 Abbeygate Street, Bury St Edmunds, 1813–38.
[17] Letters of Sir T.G. Cullum, to his son: SROB E2/21/2, 15 June 1823.
[18] Letters of Sir T.G. Cullum, to his son: SROB E2/21/2, 4 Jan. 1824 (no. 3).
[19] Hospital minute book: SROB ID 503/5.

Colvile of procuring and fitting sulphur vapour baths in the present accident ward for £150 be accepted'.[20]

On 15 March 1839 Stutter ordered that Morris Bird (p. 9) should have a sulphur vapour bath every other day, but as there is no medical history for this patient we do not know why – although scabies is a possibility. It may be pure coincidence, but three weeks following Morris Bird's treatment the Committee ordered that the sulphur bath be repaired.[21]

---

[20] *Ibid.*
[21] Hospital minute book: SROB ID 503/6.

APPENDIX V

Drugs and Chemicals

The original definition of drug was a medicinal substance of vegetable or animal origin, and it is in that sense the term is used here. Of the drugs and chemicals used by Stutter, 75 per cent came from the roots, barks, woods, leaves, flowers and seeds of a wide variety of plants, shrubs, bushes and trees which occurred naturally or were cultivated. Today, in the twenty-first century, 25 per cent of the world's medicines are plant-based, and the search continues for plants that might have medicinal properties. Some of those in use in the early nineteenth century were indigenous to this country, while others came from all over the world. Just three of the drugs were of animal origin; these were cantharides from the Spanish beetle, castor from the North American beaver and honey from our native bee. Leeches were also used, although it is difficult to classify them as a 'drug'. They were reared locally in ponds and streams or imported from France or Germany.

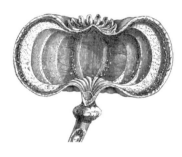

15. A section through the capsule of the opium poppy, the source of one of the most important drugs available in Stutter's era.

In the late eighteenth and early nineteenth centuries the two most important drugs were cinchona and opium. The former was one of the first drugs to have a recognised beneficial effect and to be clearly associated with a specific set of symptoms, namely those of malaria, whilst opium was the only effective pain reliever and narcotic available.

In 1816 a German chemist[1] obtained morphine in a pure state from opium; this was later shown to belong to a group of chemicals known as alkaloids.[2] Four years later two French chemists[3] isolated the alkaloid quinine from cinchona bark. The implications of this work were enormous. For the first time ever, the active ingredients of two crude drugs were available in standardised amounts. For example, it is now known that crude opium contains about twenty-five different alkaloids, the most important, morphine, being present in amounts varying from 10 to 20 per cent. Similarly, about thirty alkaloids have been reported as occurring in cinchona barks, the quinine content varying from 2 to 8 per cent. With the pure active principle now available it was no longer necessary to boil up the crude drug with water to extract an unknown amount of active alkaloid. Furthermore, crude drugs had often been adulterated by the deliberate addition of cheaper material. The *London Pharmacopœia* of 1836 commented that 'Quinine Disulphate is a prominent example of the advantage

---

[1]   Freidrich Serturner.
[2]   Physiologically active, and frequently poisonous, substances containing nitrogen in their structure and occurring in some plants, although the term now applies to synthetic chemicals having similar structures to those occurring in nature.
[3]   J. Caventou and J. Pelletier.

which medicine has derived from Chemistry. It possesses all the virtues of the cinchona, unmixed with inert or superfluous substances, such as the woody fibre or resin.'[4] For the patient the advantage was that the pure alkaloid could be made into pills or dissolved in small quantities of pleasantly flavoured mixtures instead of large amounts of unpleasant tasting liquids.

By 1840 practically all the important medicinal alkaloids had been isolated, including (in addition to morphine and quinine), strychnine, codeine, atropine and colchicine. Today, over eight hundred alkaloids have been recognised, but only some twenty-four are in common use, chiefly in medicine. In addition to alkaloids, physiologically active chemicals known as glycosides[5] are present in some plants. Digitalis is the crude drug provided by the dried leaves of the purple foxglove and has been in use since the eighteenth century, but it was not until the twentieth century that the glycoside digitoxin was obtained. Today the faster acting digoxin, derived from the white foxglove, is a vitally important cardiac glycoside used to treat congestive heart failure by causing the heart muscle to work more efficiently. Amongst other glycosides is salicin, the active constituent of the willow bark (*Salix*), which had a long history of use as a remedy against fever and rheumatism. It is from this bark that aspirin eventually evolved.

Iodine was first isolated from seaweed in 1812 and a few years later a method of manufacture for the chemical was perfected. Hydrocyanic acid, obtained from cherry laurel leaves, was introduced into British medical practice in 1815. Ether, resulting from the action of sulphuric acid upon alcohol, was at that time already well known and considerable quantities were being made, but it was not used as an anaesthetic until 1846.[6]

But although there had been some advances in therapeutics by the early nineteenth century, doctors continued to practise medicine as it had been practised for centuries, with an emphasis on blood letting (see Appendix IV), purging and blistering. As far as the doctor was concerned, the main advantage of these traditional treatments was that for the most part they enabled him to do something for the patient without causing any immediate harm. Of Stutter's patients, two-thirds were given laxatives – mercury, colocynth, senna and castor oil being the drugs frequently used for this purpose.

Stutter used a total of seventy-eight drugs.[7] The most popular was mercury, which he prescribed on fifty-six occasions (Table 3) whilst nine drugs were used only once. These included castor, obtained from the North American beaver, and the dangerously drastic purgative, croton oil. The staggering thing is that approximately half of these early nineteenth-century drugs were still being used in the 1940s.

---

[4] *Translation*, p. 116.
[5] The active constituent of the plant is combined with a sugar; if the sugar is glucose it may be termed a glucoside.
[6] J.C. Hanbury, 'The Use of Fine Chemicals in Pharmacy, 1700–1900', *Pharmaceutical Journal*, 3 Sept. 1951, pp. 321–2.
[7] This was a very small proportion of the total number of drugs described in Thomson's *London Dispensatory* of 1830.

Table 3. Drugs and chemicals prescribed by Stutter: their frequency of use

Drug	Times prescribed	Drug	Times prescribed
Mercury	56	Turpentine	5
Camphor	55	Strychnine	5
Potassium salts	40	Peppermint	5
Iron	35	Iodine	5
Colocynth	27	Chalk	5
Antimony	23	Orange	4
Hyoscyamus	23	Hops	4
Nitrous ether spt.	21	Ginger	4
Magnesium	20	Guaiacum	4
Cantharides	20	Cinnamon	4
Ammonia	20	Cinchona	4
Sodium	19	Chiretta	4
Rose	19	Capsicum	4
Digitalis	18	Tartaric acid	3
Ipecacuanha	15	Sulphuric acid	3
Colchicum	15	Sulphur	3
Castor oil	15	Fever mixture	3
Aperients	15	Asafoetida	3
Opium	14	Silver nitrate	2
Quinine	13	Pitch	2
Acacia	13	Gamboge	2
Aloes	13	Common enema	2
Gentian	12	Ergot	2
Squills	11	Dandelion	2
Rhubarb	11	Conium	2
Morphine	11	Bismuth	2
Hydrocyanic acid	10	Senega	2
Galbanum	10	Yeast	1
Soap	9	Vinegar	1
Jalap	9	Spearmint	1
Senna	8	Aluminium	1
Sarsaparilla	6	Nux Vomica	1
Lead	6	Mallow	1
Nitric Acid	6	Croton oil	1
Calumba	6	Castor	1
Wild cucumber	5	Cascarilla	1
Valerian	5		

Drugs of vegetable and animal origin

The stem of the African acacia tree exudes a gummy substance, which when collected and dried in the sun was known as **Acacia** gum or gum Arabic. It possessed no therapeutic action except to act as a demulcent, and in order to stop tickly coughs it was recommended that a piece of the gum should be allowed to dissolve slowly in the mouth. The mucilage, prepared by dissolving the gum in water, was very useful pharmaceutically because it was used to suspend insoluble drugs in mixtures. Matilda Rumble's (p. 30) mixture of acacia with decoction of rose petals made a very pleasant-tasting demulcent preparation which the eleven-year-old girl would have found vastly preferable to the mixture of castor oil and turpentine that she had had to take five days previously. For home use one ounce of the gum in a pint of barley water was said to be an excellent lubricating beverage in cases of inflammation of the kidneys or bladder.

Evaporating the juice from the large leaves of various species of *Aloe*, imported from the West Indies and Africa, produced **Aloes**. This was a popular drug in the nineteenth century, recommended 'to increase menstrual flow and destroy worms'.[8] Pills of aloes were used for their powerful purgative action, whilst the decoction was considered to be rather gentler and was used in chronic constipation, jaundice and chlorosis;[9] Caroline Clarke (p. 24), who had the latter condition, was prescribed the decoction. Aloes was also a home remedy for constipation; in 1840 a chemist at Bury St Edmunds[10] prepared an aloes pill mass to the recipe of a Reverend Armstrong at a cost of 2s 4d (about 11 new pence);[11] from this he was able to hand-roll pills as needed.

Asafoetida, an oily gum resin, was collected from the roots of a large plant growing in the Middle East and Afghanistan;[12] it was colloquially known as 'Devils Dung' because of its unpleasant smell and foul taste. In Stutter's day it was given for its reputed antispasmodic, stimulant and expectorant actions in cases of hysteria, asthma, whooping cough and intestinal worms.[13] It was difficult to mask its unpleasant taste. One suggestion was to add a small amount of aromatic solution of ammonia to each dose; Stutter followed this recommendation in the case of Maria Cousins (p. 32). Sir T.G. Cullum[14] in a letter to his son in 1825, concerning his daughter-in-law's illness wrote 'you should ask Dr Vacca to prescribe some medicine for Mrs Cullum, that in case any sudden and more violent spasm in the chest than usual should happen a medicine should be ready at hand to take immediately; I should think a solution of Asafœtida would be a useful addition to the camphor or other draught'.[15] Towards the end of the century asafoetida's supposed effect in nervous disorders had been largely rejected, but its use in intestinal flatulence and as an expectorant in bronchitis was still being recommended. By the mid-twentieth century the drug had no place in medicine, although sometimes it was prescribed as a last resort in cases of hypochondria. Today there is little scientific evidence to justify the use of asafoetida.[16]

---

[8] *Consp.*, p. 9.
[9] An anaemia once common in young girls.
[10] John Nunn, Chemist & Druggist, Abbeygate Street, Bury St Edmunds.
[11] Nunn, vol. 3, p. 554.
[12] *Ferula foetida.*
[13] *Consp.*, p. 17.
[14] Sir T.G. Cullum (1741–1831) was admitted a member of the Corporation of Surgeons on the 7 May 1778, and for many years practised as a surgeon in Bury St Edmunds.
[15] Cullum, 15 Feb. 1825.
[16] *Herbal*, p. 39.

Broom tops were obtained from a shrub[17] native to Britain and Europe. Decoctions of the tops were frequently dispensed as heart tonics and diuretics until late in the nineteenth century.[18] Stutter prescribed the tops for Susan Warren (pp. 47–8) and Frances Baker (p. 101); their diagnoses and other medication suggest that in both cases Stutter was using it for its diuretic action. Broom is one of the herbal medicines that have been studied in recent years, with its chemistry being well documented. The active constituent is an alkaloid[19] named sparteine, which has been used to treat abnormal rhythms of the heart. Unfortunately it is also toxic and has been reported to depress the action of the heart, possibly resulting in cardiorespiratory collapse. Nowadays it is considered inappropriate to use broom in herbal medicine.[20]

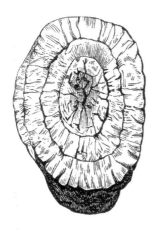

16. Calumba root, *Jateorhiza palmate*.

Calumba came from the root of a climbing plant growing in the forests of Zambezi where it was much used as a remedy for dysentery and for the yellow colouring matter it contained. It was brought to Europe towards the end of the seventeenth century, coming into medical use to check the vomiting of cholera and pregnancy, and also to treat diarrhoea. By the 1880s it was considered to be just a good tonic when the patient complained of loss of appetite and/or dyspepsia. Stutter prescribed calumba six times; John Chinery (p. 38) was possibly given it to counteract any nausea caused by the digitalis he was taking. In two other mixtures containing the root, sodium bicarbonate was also present, suggesting that they were intended to relieve dyspepsia.

Camphor is a crystalline substance obtained from the steam distillation of the wood of a tree[21] native to China; it is now also prepared synthetically. The *London Pharmacopœia* of 1836 contained a description of Camphor Mixture which concluded by stating 'as very little camphor is dissolved, the mixture is generally used only as a vehicle for more important medicines'.[22] Doubtless that is the reason why Stutter used the mixture in fifty of the prescriptions he wrote. Camphor's therapeutic uses included the relief of irritation, spasm and pain and the treatment of hysteria and asthma. Cullum wrote in 1829 of its beneficial action, 'your Mother's irritating Cough was so violent last night that I was obliged to call upon her Maid Servant Ann to get her hot water, to three glasses of which I put one of Camphor Julep,[23] & drinking it as warm as she could bear it, it took off the cough immediately'.[24]

Later in the nineteenth century camphor was believed to be useful in the early

---

17 *Cytisus scoparius*.
18 *Guide*, p. 173.
19 A physiologically active and frequently poisonous substance contained in some plants.
20 *Herbal*, p. 50.
21 *Cinnamonum camphora*.
22 *Translation*, p. 323.
23 Julep: a sweet drink consisting of syrup, flavouring and water; in this case made by suspending camphor in a solution of gum Arabic sweetened with sugar. See p. xxxvi.
24 Cullum, 29 Nov. 1829.

stage of the common cold,[25] and its use for this purpose in the twentieth century is mentioned, whilst a camphorated tincture of opium long retained its popularity as a cough remedy. As late as the first half of the twentieth century there was an official formula for an injection of camphor to be given as a restorative in case of collapse, especially in pneumonia.[26] Stutter prescribed liniments of camphor for five patients; similar preparations were extensively used both in medical practice and as a home remedy ('camphorated oil') until their withdrawal from sale in the 1970s.

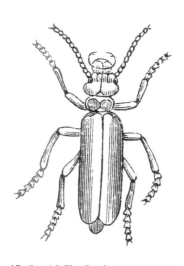

Cantharides, also known as Spanish Flies, were actually dried beetles. They were (and are) widely distributed over southern Europe.[27] Early nineteenth-century physicians used the crushed beetles to raise skin blisters. The site of application varied according to the symptoms – on the forehead for palsy, for example, or behind the ear in cases of severe inflammation of the eye. The main use of cantharides was as a 'counter-irritant', relieving the patient by diverting attention from the primary source of pain. Plasters were also applied in cases of pneumonia, hepatitis and gastritis, being placed immediately over the painful area. Thankfully, it was considered advisable to 'avoid applying plasters to debilitated patients or those suffering from smallpox, measles or dropsy as they were apt to cause a very painful and dangerous erysipelas and gangrene'.[28] Cantharides plasters could cause adverse reactions, including retention of urine; such reactions were more likely to occur if the plaster was over a newly shaved part or kept in place too long after the blister had formed. Placing gauze wetted with vinegar, or a piece of silver paper moistened with oil, between the skin and plaster was said to reduce the chances of these problems occurring.[29] In the twentieth century it was recommended that cantharides plasters should be no larger than one inch in diameter.[30] Twelve of Stutter's patients had cantharides plasters applied. William Shepherd (p. 93) had one placed in the region of his heart on three occasions. Internally, cantharides was little used. Adverse reactions included urinary bleeding and incontinence with abdominal pain and vomiting; in severe cases convulsions, coma and death might occur. Stutter prescribed a mixture containing tincture of cantharides for Abraham Orris (p. 17). It was popularly believed that cantharides was an aphrodisiac. During the 1950s a worker in a drug wholesaler's added cantharidin[31] to some coconut ice, which was eaten by two young women who subsequently died of cantharidin poisoning.[32]

17. Spanish Fly, *Cantharis vesicatoria.*

---

[25] *Guide*, p. 238.
[26] *BPC*, p. 264.
[27] *Cantharis vesicatoria.*
[28] *London*, p. 222.
[29] *London*, pp. 226–7.
[30] Martindale, *The Extra Pharmacopœia*, 24th edn, vol. I, 1958, p. 353.
[31] Cantharidin is the active ingredient present in the dried beetles.
[32] Martindale, *The Extra Pharmacopœia*, 24th edn, vol. I, 1958, p. 353.

Capsicum,[33] a spice commonly known as chillies or cayenne pepper, also had a traditional use as an herbal remedy for colic, dyspepsia, laryngitis (as a gargle), externally for neuralgia including rheumatic pains, and as a lotion or ointment for unbroken chilblains.[34] In the early nineteenth century the medical opinion of capsicum was that it acted as a stimulant and could be successfully given in gout, dyspepsia and with cinchona in fevers. Stutter's prescriptions for Samuel Chinery (p. 36), and William Mulley (p. 20), included quinine, which suggests that both these patients may have been feverish. It was also said to be most useful in quinsy[35] when given internally or used as a gargle, whilst poultices acted as rubefacients without causing blistering.[36]

Infusions of the bark of **Cascarilla**[37] combined with squill and camphor were considered useful in chronic lung conditions;[38] Stutter prescribed it for Robert Nelson (p. 131), who had bronchitis.

Castor was described as 'the peculiar matter found in bags near the rectum of the beaver',[39] most being obtained from the Canadian beaver. In an Oxfordshire village in the 1650s, Dr Thomas Willis visited a father and son suffering from henbane poisoning and prescribed for them 'tincture of castor, with a spoonful of trea-cle-water (which remedies I had about me) to be given them at every turn all night'. The two patients survived, which prompted the doctor to write, 'Castor is deservedly esteemed to be contrary to the venom of Opiates'.[40] Nearly two hundred years later castor was prescribed for hysteria, epilepsy and fevers and was believed to be useful in amenorrhoea[41] and chlorosis;[42] but owing to 'its scarcity and the high prices of good specimens it was seldom ordered'.[43] However, in 1911 it was believed that castor had an important action on the circulation, increasing the output from the heart and raising blood pressure, being used in certain conditions that were not improved by digitalis.[44] Caroline Wayfield (p. 137) had a history of hysteria and was prescribed a mixture containing tincture of castor and asafoetida. Thus Stutter conformed to contemporary medical thinking, since both drugs were recommended for the treatment of hysteria. In 1839, Lady Blake had a prescription dispensed in Bury St Edmunds for a mixture containing tinctures of castor and hops, of which she took a teaspoonful in water when her heart palpitations were troublesome.[45]

The oil obtained by pressing the seeds of the **Castor Oil** plant has a very long history of use in medicine, the plant being illustrated in a copy of Dioscorides' *Herbal*, made in Constantinople *c.* AD 512. Castor oil was a mild, effective purgative, which worked rapidly but was unpleasant to take. Suggestions to overcome this included adding a little peppermint water, whisky or brandy to the oil and swallowing it as it floated on the top. Another was to emulsify the oil with egg yolk

[33] For medical use the fruits obtained from *Capsicum minimum*, a shrub cultivated in many parts of the world, especially in Africa.
[34] *Herbal*, p. 60.
[35] Acute inflammation of the tonsils.
[36] *London*, p. 891.
[37] A small shrub, *Croton eleotaea*, growing in the Bahamas.
[38] *Translation*, p. 323.
[39] *Consp.*, p. 23.
[40] K. Dewhurst, *Willis's Oxford Casebook (1650–1652)*, Oxford, 1981, p. 44.
[41] Absence of menstruation.
[42] An anaemia, common in young girls.
[43] *London*, p. 241.
[44] *The British Pharmaceutical Codex*, London, 1911.
[45] Nunn, vol. 2, p. 127.

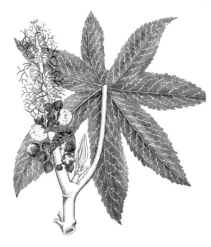

18. The castor oil plant, *Ricinus communis.*

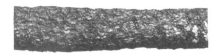

19. Cinchona bark, *Cinchona officinalis.*

and peppermint water. It was recommended in cases of habitual constipation, piles and spasmodic colic. Stutter prescribed the oil for eight patients in doses ranging from a quarter to one fluid ounce.

The leaves, root and stems of the **Chiretta** herb of the mountainous districts of northern India had a long history of use in that country, where it was highly esteemed for its bitter and tonic properties and was prescribed for dyspepsia and to improve appetite.[46] As it was not introduced to European medicine until about 1830 it would have been a relatively modern drug to Stutter, who prescribed the infusion for Thomas Ruddock (p. 89), William Shepherd (p. 93) and Phoebe Horrex (p. 99). Chiretta was not fashionable in this country for very long, probably because of its very disagreeable bitterness. Gentian (q.v.) had a similar action and was very much more pleasant to take.

The bark from various species of **Cinchona** trees which grew in South America, produced one of the two most important drugs available to western medicine at the beginning of the nineteenth century. It was known and used by the natives of Peru and Bolivia to successfully treat malarial fever, a disease that was claiming millions of lives worldwide each year. The bark was brought to Spain as early as 1632, probably by the Jesuits, and became known as Jesuit's bark or Peruvian bark. It was introduced into medical practice for the cure of intermittent fever (malaria) and soon acquired a great reputation as a remedy for that disease. This led a Professor of Medicine at the University of Padua to claim that cinchona bark did for medicine what gunpowder had done for war.[47] The active principal of the bark, **Quinine**, was isolated in 1820,[48] with commercial production of quinine sulphate quickly following. It was one of the first drugs to have a recognised beneficial effect and to be clearly associated with a specific set of symptoms. By 1836 physicians were advised that sulphates of quinine could be successfully used in all cases in which cinchona was indicated.[49] Stutter following this recommendation by using quinine disulphate on ten occasions compared with four for cinchona. The bark was also used for other fevers, like typhoid, gaol fever, scarlet fever, smallpox and measles. Some physicians even used it for rheumatism (including Stutter for two of his patients[50] with this diagnosis). Professor Todd of London University only found cinchona useful for this disease

---

[46] Wallis, p. 278.
[47] V. Coleman, *The Story of Medicine*, London, 1985, p. 82.
[48] Quinine was isolated by the two French chemists, J. Pelletier and J. Caventou.
[49] *London*, p. 274.
[50] William Mulley (p. 20) and Susan Plumbe (p. 70).

after giving liberal doses of calomel, antimony, colchicum and opium, and said that adding spirit of turpentine increased the efficacy of the bark.[51] So we must conclude that polypharmacy is not a new phenomenon! Quinine was an expensive chemical, the average wholesale price in the years 1839–41 being £8 per pound; in contrast camphor was 2s 8d per pound, citric acid 4s 0d per pound and tartaric acid 1s 4d per pound.[52]

The bark, or the oil, of the **Cinnamon** tree[53] of Sri Lanka was used principally to impart a pleasant flavour to mixtures of other medicines as, for example, in the formula for Chalk Mixture.[54] In the home the oil had a long history as a treatment for the toothache and was also taken for stomach cramps, colic and hiccough. Langdale's Medicinal Essence of Cinnamon was a very popular patent medicine, reputed by the manufacturers 'to relieve coughs, colds, etc in an incredibly short space of time'.[55] Leah Cross (p. 41) and Ann Copping (p. 62) were both prescribed cinnamon to make their iron powders more palatable.

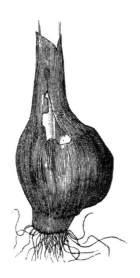

20. Colchicum corm,
Colchicum autumnale.

Colchicum[56] is obtained from the meadow saffron,[57] a plant common in parts of England. The drug was used in dropsy,[58] gout and rheumatism and had a strong purgative action considered to be too violent to be encouraged, although it was sometimes prescribed with other laxatives. Stutter prescribed it in pills on seven occasions, in each case combining it with colocynth; his other prescriptions were for four mixtures, and a lotion and liniment as external applications. *The London Dispensatory* said that 'In gout and rheumatism its efficacy has been fully ascertained, and in allaying the pain, it may be said to possess a specific property.'[59] As far as gout was concerned the statement was entirely correct, for colchicine, the active constituent of the bulb, was isolated in 1820 and eventually became the standard drug for relieving the pain of acute gout.

Colocynth, or Bitter Apple, is the pulp from the fruit of a plant,[60] similar to a vegetable marrow in appearance. When taken internally it caused violent purging accompanied by severe griping; for this reason it was scarcely ever given alone, but used in combination with other purges to quicken the action. It was used in the form of an extract made by boiling down the pulp and was one of Stutter's more popular drugs. He prescribed pills containing colocynth on twenty-eight occasions; in all but three he used the compound extract, which contained two further purgative drugs, aloes and scammony resin. Notwithstanding this, in every prescription Stutter

---

51 *London*, p. 273.
52 The Chemist and Druggist, *Quinine and Camphor*, London, 10 June 1897, p. 974.
53 *Cinnamomum zeylanicum.* The oil was obtained by the steam distillation of the bark.
54 See entry for Chalk under 'Chemicals' in this appendix.
55 *Extra*, p. 406.
56 A corm is a bulblike underground stem.
57 *Colchicum autumnale.*
58 Retention of fluid in the body.
59 *London*, p. 285.
60 *Citrullus colocynthis*, cultivated in Cyprus, Egypt and Spain.

added further drugs, using mercury in twenty-two of them; contemporary opinion was that adding mercury in the form of calomel[61] to colocynth made an excellent purging pill, which did not cause griping. Six of the prescriptions included extract of hyoscyamus, the active principal of which was later identified as hyoscine, which prevents excessive and painful contractions of the intestinal walls. It was thus a sensible addition, as the hyoscine would counteract the griping action of the colocynth. In 1813 Sir T.G. Cullum was prescribed pills containing the compound extract of colocynth by no less a person than the President of the Royal College of Surgeons, Sir Henry Halford. However, after taking two of the pills each night Sir Thomas wrote, 'N.B. After using these Pills a few times I found them too purgative and have since taken only one at bedtime.'[62]

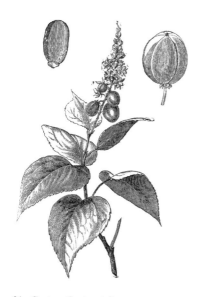

21. Croton, *Croton tiglium*.

Pressing the seeds of a small tree[63] grown in India produced **Croton Oil**. This was another relatively new drug in Stutter's day; it had been introduced to this country in about 1819. Its internal use was described as a 'very rapid, drastic cathartic, given in certain cases of apoplexy and of obstinate constipation; when applied externally produces a burning sensation and redness followed by severe pustules'.[64] Stutter resorted to its internal use on one occasion for Susan Welch (p. 58), prescribing a pill containing one minim of the oil and five grains of the compound extract of colocynth; the combination of these very strong purgatives must surely have had a very drastic effect. A fortnight later, the same patient had to use an ointment of the oil combined with antimony and potassium tartrate on her abdomen each night; both these substances would have acted as counter-irritants. The prescription ledgers of John Nunn, chemist of Bury St Edmunds for the years 1837–41 record numerous prescriptions for croton oil.[65]

Both the leaves and roots of the common **Dandelion**[66] were well known as traditional herbal remedies for gallstones, jaundice, dyspepsia and rheumatism. In the early part of the nineteenth century dandelion was used for chronic inflammation, liver and stomach conditions, dropsy, jaundice and tuberculosis of the lung.[67] Modern animal studies have shown that dandelion does have some diuretic and anti-inflammatory effects.[68] Stutter used this drug for one patient only, George Brame (p. 84), prescribing him the extract made from the juice of the fresh root, once in a mixture with gentian and sodium bicarbonate and again as a pill mixed with lead acetate.

---

61 Calomel is mercurous chloride.
62 Commonplace book of T.G. Cullum: SROB 317/1.
63 *Croton tiglium*.
64 *London*, p. 301.
65 Nunn, vols.1–4.
66 *Taraxicum officinale*.
67 *Consp.*, p. 100.
68 *Herbal*, p. 96.

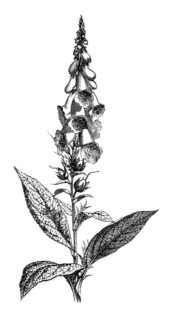

22. Foxglove, *Digitalis purpurea.*

Digitalis is the crude drug provided by the leaves of the purple foxglove,[69] a herb common in England and throughout Europe; it joins cinchona bark and the opium poppy as being one of the most useful drugs available to Stutter. Whilst both quinine and morphine had been chemically isolated, and had become commercially available and in regular use by the 1830s, it was to be more than one hundred years before digoxin, the active principle of the foxglove, was introduced into medicine. It is an important cardiac drug used to treat congestive heart failure by causing the heart muscles to work more efficiently, thus improving the action of the kidneys in reducing fluid retention in the body. In 1785, William Withering had shown in 'An Account of the Foxglove', that dropsy might be due to cardiac disease, for which 'digitalis, if carefully used, was an excellent remedy' and it was much used for this reason in Stutter's day. With less logic it was also recommended for inflammatory diseases, haemorrhages, particularly from the uterus, and as a narcotic in mania, 'soothing the nervous system and procuring sleep for the patient'.[70] Digitalis is a potent drug and relatively small overdoses can cause adverse reactions. In 1820 these were listed as vomiting, purging, vertigo, delirium, convulsions and death. As there was no means of measuring the amount of active drug in the tincture or infusion, dosage was uncertain at best and dangerous at worst. This situation prevailed until the early 1900s when a somewhat crude method (involving the use of fifty live frogs) of assaying digitalis was introduced.[71] Stutter prescribed digitalis on nineteen occasions, using the tincture in mixtures or powdered leaves in pills; three of the patients – George Talbot (p. 40), James Arnold (p. 15) and John Chinery (p. 38) – were suffering from enlargement of the heart. Susan Plumbe's history (p. 69), showed her to be subject to palpitations accompanied with pain in the region of the heart, and Susan Warren (p. 48) had fluid retention. In each of these cases administration of digitalis was logical.

Elaterium is dried sediment from the juice of the fruit of wild cucumber,[72] a trailing plant which was once cultivated to a limited extent in England. It was a little used drug, described as a powerful cathartic and hydragogue,[73] used for very obstinate constipation and ascites[74] where other remedies had failed. It seems that Susan Warren (pp. 46–48) was suffering from the latter condition, most probably due to cancer of the ovary. The casebook records that liquid was drawn off from her abdomen and she was prescribed pills containing elaterium.

The flowers of the common **Elder** were used to make Elder-flower Water, a lotion intended for the eyes and the skin. The flowers were also mixed with melted

---

69 *Digitalis purpurea.*
70 *London*, p. 323.
71 *Extra*, p. 171.
72 *Ecballium elaterium.*
73 A purgative causing copious liquid evacuations.
74 The presence of free fluid in the peritoneal cavity.

lard to make a cooling ointment; this was often used as a base for other medicaments as in the case of Abraham Orris (p. 38). A small amount of dilute hydrocyanic acid was added to soothe his psoriasis.

A decoction made by boiling the fresh bark of the common **Elm** with water was said to act as a diuretic[75] and 'had been given with benefit in herpetic eruptions'.[76] Abraham Orris (p. 38), mentioned above, was given this decoction to be taken in place of the arsenic solution previously prescribed for him.

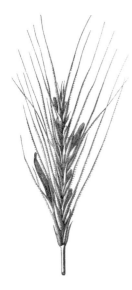

Ergot was obtained from a parasitic fungus[77] which attacks the kernels of some cereals, particularly rye. Prolonged ingestion of contaminated rye bread leads to ergotism, a condition that results in agonising pain, and ultimately gangrene, in the extremities due to the contraction of the peripheral arteries. There is little reference to the use of ergot in Stutter's day, although by 1877 it was said to be a valuable remedy in pupura,[78] a condition characterised by the escape of blood into the skin and mucous membranes causing purple spots. John Scott (p. 74), who had this condition, was prescribed ergot powder. Mary Cook (p. 103) was given a mixture containing ergot but unfortunately there is no case history for her. In later years the chief use of ergot was to contract the uterus and check haemorrhage after childbirth. The alkaloid, ergotamine, was isolated from the fungus in the twentieth century, and became the drug of choice for the treatment of migraine. A combination of ergotamine, cyclizine[79] and caffeine, known as Migril, gave relief to countless migraine sufferers.

23. Rye attacked by ergot, *Claviceps purpurea.*

A gum resin known as **Galbanum** was obtained from large plants[80] growing in the Middle East. It was used in a similar way to asafoetida and was reputed to be of value 'in hysteria, particularly that which attends irregular and deficient menstruation'.[81] Towards the end of the nineteenth century it was said to have no special therapeutic value,[82] but as late as 1932 its use was listed as a stimulant expectorant for chronic bronchitis.[83] On account of its disagreeable taste and odour it was administered in pills; externally it was applied as a plaster to joints affected with rheumatic pains. Kezia Atkins (p. 67), had absence of menstruation, hysteria and a pain in her side, for which she was prescribed galbanum pills and plaster. In all, eight patients received prescriptions containing this drug.

Gamboge, another gum resin, was obtained from moderate sized trees[84] growing in Cambodia and China. It was a drastic cathartic used in severe constipation. Susan

---

75 *London*, p. 626.
76 Herpes is a viral disease causing inflammatory skin eruptions.
77 Especially *Claviceps purpurea*, which attacks rye.
78 *Guide*, p. 261.
79 An antihistamine used as an anti-emetic.
80 *Ferula galbaniflua.*
81 *London*, p. 219.
82 *Guide*, p. 189.
83 *BPC*, p. 476.
84 *Garcinia hanburii.*

Warren (p. 47) was the only patient to receive it; she had already been taking other strong laxatives.

Extracts, infusions or tinctures of the dried roots of yellow **Gentian**[85] were given as tonics, although in large doses it had laxative properties. It acted as a bitter tonic 'improving the appetite and beneficial in dyspepsia, gout and hysteria'.[86] A standard mixture of gentian and sodium bicarbonate retained its popularity well into the twentieth century. Five of Stutter's patients received mixtures having basically the same formulation, whilst another four patients had pills of the extract. A home recipe for tonic pills containing gentian appears in Sophia Barnardiston's notebook of medical recipes.[87]

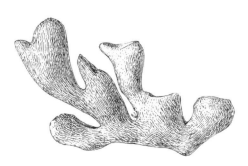

24. Roots of Jamaican ginger, *Zingiber officinalis*.

Ginger consists of the rhizome[88] of a plant[89] cultivated in many tropical countries; the most highly valued were those imported from Jamaica. It was well known as a natural food flavouring and was traditionally used as a herbal remedy for colic and dyspepsia. Some studies in the 1980s suggested that ginger was effective as a prophylactic against seasickness, although more recently its use for this condition has been disputed.[90] In Stutter's day it was recommended for 'flatulent colic, dyspepsia and gout; when chewed a considerable flow of saliva is produced, useful in relaxation of tonsils'.[91] A home medical guide suggested that ginger often relieved the irritation of piles.[92] Susan Welch (p. 57), and Frances Steggles (p. 125), took powders containing ginger, which served to mask the metallic taste of iron in the prescription. Similarly its presence in mixtures for Samuel Chinery (p. 36), and Susan Reeve (p. 108), helped to cover the bitter taste of quinine. Mary Cook (p. 103) had a powder of ginger, rhubarb and bicarbonate of soda, a combination of drugs that retained its popularity as a general stomach mixture until the late twentieth century.

Guaiacum wood, introduced into Europe in 1508 by the Spaniards as a remedy for venereal disease, was obtained from two species of evergreen trees[93] growing in South America, Florida, the Bahamas and Cuba. It gained such a reputation that the use of mercury for this complaint was discontinued for a considerable length of time. In later years it was found to be more useful in skin diseases and a tincture made from the gum of the same tree was of benefit in chronic rheumatism. Of the four patients prescribed guaiacum, two[94] had a diagnosis of rheumatism and the

---

85 *Gentiana lutea*, growing on the lower slopes of mountains in central Europe.
86 *London*, p. 345.
87 Barnardiston, p. 20.
88 An underground stem usually lying horizontally in the ground.
89 *Zingiber officinale*.
90 *Herbal*, p. 136.
91 *London*, p. 632.
92 *Medical*, p. 54.
93 *Guaiacum officinale* and *G. sanctum*.
94 Hannah Pratt (p. 127) and W. Leech (p. 141).

records for the other two[95] suggest that they were suffering from the same condition. In the early twentieth century, tincture of guaiacum was used in one of the first chemical forensic tests to detect bloodstains.[96]

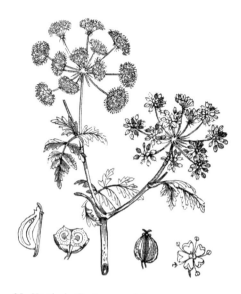

25. Hemlock, *Conium maculatum.*

Hemlock, or Conium, was obtained from the leaves of a plant[97] growing throughout Britain and Europe. In Stutter's day it was known to be a narcotic and since it caused less constipation than opium it was sometimes used for the relief of pain in cancer.[98] Tetanus, chorea, epilepsy, asthma and whooping cough were other conditions for which it was recommended.[99] Samuel Burman (p. 77), and Mary Cook (p. 102), were the only two patients who were prescribed conium; Samuel had a diagnosis of tuberculosis, and the conium was possibly intended to relieve his cough.

Henbane was obtained from a plant[100] growing throughout Europe. It was used in ancient Greek and Roman medicine as a sedative and painkiller.[101] In Stutter's day henbane was considered to have a narcotic action very similar to opium, but without causing constipation. It was given in cases of hysteria, rheumatism and gout, and with colocynth or other purgatives for colic.[102] Some of these uses were justified when, in the early 1900s, it was shown that the chief constituent of henbane leaves was the alkaloid hyoscyamine, described as 'a cerebral and spinal sedative, used in insomnia, especially when opium can not be given; and to relieve the griping caused by drastic purgatives'.[103] Stutter used it for the latter purpose on six occasions by adding the extract to colocynth pills. Mixtures containing the tincture of hyoscyamus leaves continued to be given to relieve the discomfort of cystitis, until the treatment of urinary tract infections was revolutionised by the advent of antibacterial chemicals in the later decades of the twentieth century. It was also known in 1830 that dropping a solution containing hyoscyamus into the eye dilated the pupil, and it was used in cataract operations.[104] This use was vindicated in the next century by the isolation of a further alkaloid, hyoscine, which proved to be an efficient

---

95   Susan Jackson (p. 11) and William Mulley (p. 19).
96   *Extra*, p. 683.
97   *Conium maculatum.*
98   *Consp.*, p. 45.
99   *London*, p. 287.
100 *Hyoscyamus niger.*
101 C. Stockwell, *A History of Plants and Healing*, London, 1988, pp. 74, 83.
102 *London*, p. 368.
103 *The British Pharmaceutical Codex*, London, 1911.
104 *London*, pp. 863–4.

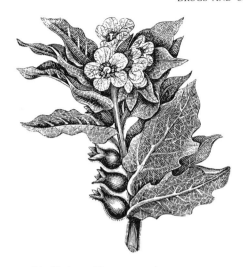

26. Henbane, *Hyoscyamus niger.*

mydriatic.[105] Henbane was at one time used as a domestic remedy for toothache, the seeds of the plant being 'thrown on hot coals and the vapour given off allowed to enter the mouth'.[106]

Honey, described 'as a saccharine fluid made by the hive-bee from the nectar of flowers' was sometimes used in enemas or added to gargles for quinsy and ulcers of the mouth. The use of purified or clarified honey was preferred; this was prepared by melting the honey, then allowing it to stand before straining off the impurities that rose to the surface. Honey and acetic acid were combined to make Oxymel, which was frequently used as a basis for Oxymel of Squills, a popular and long surviving ingredient of cough mixtures. Leah Cross (p. 41), had a mixture of spirits of turpentine made slightly more palatable by the addition of honey to the formula.

Hops, the fruits of the well known climbing plant,[107] cultivated in England for use in the brewing industry, were also frequently used in medicine during the first part of the nineteenth century. The purpose was to improve the patient's appetite. The fruits contained a volatile oil, which produced a sedative and soporific effect. It was also suggested that hops would relieve the pain of rheumatism, but confidence in its action lessened and it was not included in the *London Pharmacopoeia*. Nevertheless, Stutter prescribed hops for five patients;[108] contemporary records show the frequent use of tinctures and extracts of hops in mixtures ordered by Dr Probart (see Appendix I) and others in Bury St Edmunds.[109]

Ipecacuanha came from the dried roots of a small plant growing in the forests of Brazil.[110] The ingestion of small doses of the powdered root caused patients to perspire profusely. An eighteenth-century physician, Thomas Dover,[111] added a little opium to the ipecacuanha and this combination of the two powders became known as Dover's powder, extensively used for rheumatism, dropsy, gout, fevers, dysentery and even diabetes. Stutter used compound ipecacuanha powder[112] on nine occasions; a side effect of the powder was that it was liable to cause vomiting. Cullum wrote in 1822 that 'I have formerly taken Dover's powder, it is a good medicine but

105   A drug that dilates the pupil of the eye.
106   Wallis, p. 294.
107   *Humulus lupulus.*
108   The synonyms for *Humulus lupulus* were Hops, Humulus and Lupuli. Stutter prescribed hops on five occasions, twice referring to it as Humulus and three times as Lupuli.
109   Nunn, vol. 5, pp. 49 and 62.
110   *Cephaelis ipecacuanha*, subsequently cultivated in Malaysia, Burma and Bengal.
111   Thomas Dover (1660–1742) began practice as a physician in Bristol; in 1708 he sailed on a privateering voyage around the world, returned and practised in London, becoming known as the 'Quicksilver Doctor' because of his exaggerated opinion of the value of mercury.
112   This had virtually the same formula as Dover's powder.

it makes one feel sickish and takes away one's appetite'.[113] An 1800s home medical guide recommended rheumatic patients to take ten to twenty grains of the powder saying that 'the patient should lie between the blankets or in a flannel shirt and take frequently, as soon as he begins to perspire, some warm liquid'.[114] Tablets containing aspirin and Dover's powder remained a popular remedy for colds until the 1950s. In larger doses ipecacuanha acted as an emetic and was given at the commencement of fevers, dysentery and diarrhoea.[115] It also acted as an expectorant, being a traditional ingredient of cough mixtures both for adults and children, either as the tincture or wine.[116] Four of Stutter's patients took mixtures containing this wine; in two cases[117] a further ingredient was syrup of poppies, frequently used as a sedative in coughs. In all, Stutter prescribed ipecacuanha on seventeen occasions.

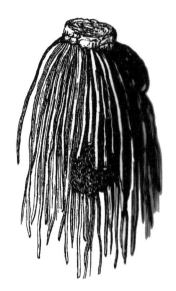

27. Roots of jalap, *Ipomoea purga*.

Another drug brought into Europe by the Spaniards was **Jalap**, obtained from the roots of a plant[118] growing in the Mexican Andes. In small doses it had a laxative action but larger doses caused purging sometimes accompanied by severe griping. In the early 1800s it was thought that if you added it to prescriptions for calomel (mercurous chloride) it quickened the action of that chemical.[119] Stutter followed this advice in four of the eight prescriptions that he wrote for jalap.

The common **Mallow**[120] boiled in water and sweetened with syrup of violets was an ancient herbal remedy for painful urination.[121] In the early nineteenth century it was used in enemas, poultices and fomentations as a demulcent and emollient, whilst the decoction was recommended for dysentery, and urinary complaints.[122] Abraham Orris (p. 17), a patient suffering from psoriasis, was given a decoction of mallow and chamomile flowers to use as a fomentation; this was the only prescription for mallow in the casebook.

Nux Vomica seeds come from a small tree that grows in India[123] and they contain the alkaloid strychnine. However, the extract and tincture of nux vomica had been in use long before the isolation of pure strychnine in 1818, and they continued to be prescribed for many years after that date. They were regarded as excellent tonics, greatly improving the appetite; a mixture of the tincture with potassium bromide was an extremely popular twentieth-century tonic,

[113] Cullum, 21 July 1822.
[114] *Guide*, p. 28.
[115] *London*, p. 246.
[116] Ipecacuanha wine was made in a similar manner to the tincture, the alcohol in the latter being replaced by sherry-type wine.
[117] Thomas Ruddock (p. 89) and Kezia Atkins (p. 90).
[118] *Ipomoea purga*. Jalep should be distinguished froim the medicine julep; see p. xxxvi.
[119] *London*, p. 291.
[120] The common mallow, *Malva sylvestris*, was considered inferior to the marsh mallow, *Althaea officinalis*.
[121] D. Potterton, *Culpeper's Colour Herbal*, Slough, 1983, p. 118.
[122] *London*, p. 413.

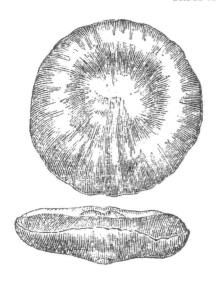

28. Nux vomica seeds, *Strychnos nux-vomica*.

the formula still being included in the *British National Formulary* of 1960. Stutter used nux vomica on one occasion only, for Samuel Chinery (p. 36), who took pills containing the extract combined with gentian. Prescriptions for the pure alkaloid are discussed under Strychnine in the chemical section of this appendix.

Opium, the source of Morphine, is the dried latex from capsules of the opium poppy.[124] At the beginning of the nineteenth century, Professor Thomson[125] considered the drug, 'when properly administered, to be the most valuable medicine available to the medical profession, having wonderful properties of mitigating pain and inducing sleep'.[126] An addictive narcotic, opium contains several alkaloids, including morphine, one of the most powerful natural painkillers and addictive narcotics known, and codeine, a milder painkiller. Heroin is a synthetic derivative of morphine and an even more powerful narcotic. Morphine was isolated from opium in 1816, and the pure substance was available to the medical profession by 1821. There appears to have been some reluctance among physicians to use it, *The Lancet* having to remind the profession in 1854 that it was preferable to prescribe the pure substance rather than opium.[127] Opium was administered using the tincture or powder, the latter usually incorporated into pills. The tincture, commonly known as laudanum, could be purchased from pharmacies without any legal restriction and a potent opium-based proprietary medicine, known as Kendal or Lancaster Black Drop, was freely available. In addition to opium being mainly used for its narcotic and analgesic properties, there were many other conditions for which it was considered valuable, including rheumatism, dropsy, gout, fevers and dysentery. The combination of opium powder with ipecacuanha (Dover's powder) has been discussed under Ipecacuanha. Opium was considered to be a very soothing remedy for coughs of all kinds, particularly those occurring in tuberculosis of the lungs. The tincture of opium and honey of squills in a mixture given to Susan Warren (p. 48), are the basis of a famous cough mixture formulated by a Dr Gee[128] later in the nineteenth century; 'Gee's Linctus' became the most frequently prescribed and sold cough mixture, a popularity which it retained for most of the twentieth century. The use of opium combined with chalk for diarrhoea is mentioned under Chalk. Opium was also added to mercury pills to counteract any ill effects the

123 *Strychnos nux-vomica.*
124 *Papaver somniferum.*
125 Anthony Todd Thomson (1778–1849), physician; MD, Edinburgh, 1799; practised in London, 1800; a founder of the Chelsea Dispensary, 1812, and one of the editors of *The Medical Repository*; appointed professor of materia medica and therapeutics at London University, 1827.
126 *London*, p. 467.
127 *The Pharmaceutical Historian*, vol 18, no. 3, p. 3.
128 Samuel Jones Gee (1839–1911), physician; MB, 1861; MD, 1865; FRCP, 1870; physician and lecturer at St Bartholomew's Hospital from 1868 until his death.

latter would have on the patient's stomach; there are four such instances amongst the patients prescribed mercury by Stutter. Liniments containing soap and opium were applied externally for rheumatic pains, and Stutter chose to prescribe these for four of his patients.[129] Dr Jackson, of Bury St Edmunds (see Appendix I), prescribed a paste of quicklime, opium powder and water for a local saddler, 'a portion the size of a penny piece to be applied to the temple of the patient'.[130] For open cancers, cloths soaked with aqueous solutions of opium relieved the pain and decayed teeth were stuffed with a piece of solid opium. Stutter made use of the pure alkaloid, morphine, on ten occasions; a solution was available making the measurement of small amounts of the drug possible, and this was used in eight of the ten cases. Robert Gladwell (p. 45) was given a powder containing one quarter of a grain of morphine to relieve the pain resulting from the application of a blister. Annie Rands (p. 13) took a draught at night containing half a grain of the same drug.

An infusion made from the peel of the bitter or Seville **Orange**[131] was said, in the early nineteenth century, 'to be good for dyspepsia, particularly that of the drunkard'.[132] The dried peel with fresh lemon peel and some cloves was infused with boiling water for fifteen minutes to produce the infusion. A syrup and tincture were also made; some slight tonic properties were claimed for these preparations but their main purpose was to improve the palatability of bitter mixtures. For example for Sarah Haywood (p. 1), the syrup was added to her iron mixture, and also to the quinine mixture for William Malt (p. 5).

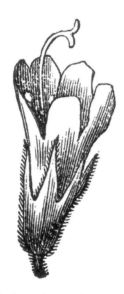

29. Spearmint, *Mentha sativa.*

The oil distilled from the fresh flowering tops of the **Peppermint** plant[133] was used to prepare peppermint water, sometimes used as a carminative, but mostly for covering the taste of other medicaments. **Spearmint**[134] water was given for similar reasons, but it was also thought that the infusion 'allayed sickness and vomiting in a weakened state of the stomach'.[135] Leah Cross (p. 41) had to take turpentine by mouth, and in an attempt make this less unpleasant clarified honey and peppermint water were added.

Pitch, or Burgundy Pitch, is an oily resin from the stem of the Norway spruce.[136] Plaster of Pitch (commonly known as Poor Man's plaster) was applied to the chest for catarrh and to the temples for pains in the head, but for Caroline Clarke (p. 24), the site of application was the left upper abdomen. Stutter prescribed the plaster for only one other patient, Minter Ling (p. 53). Three grains of antimony tartrate were added as a counter-irritant.

Poppy Syrup, made from dried capsules of the Opium Poppy (q.v.), was mildly sedative due to the small proportion of opium it contained. Used for

129   Elizabeth Matthews (p. 49), Ann Copping (p. 63), Kezia Atkins (p. 67) and W. Leech (pp. 140–1).
130   Nunn, vol. 1.
131   *Citrus aurantium.*
132   *Consp.*, p. 58.
133   *Mentha piperata.*
134   *Mentha sativa.*
135   *London*, p. 42.

coughs, as in the cases of Martin Lifley (p. 21), and Kezia Atkins (p. 67), it was also given to children to relieve pain.

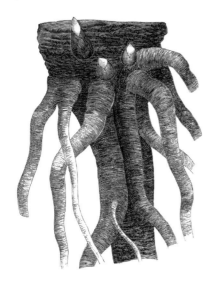

Rhubarb consists of the dried rhizomes of a plant[137] found growing in China and Tibet. It has been used traditionally both as a laxative and an anti-diarrhoeal agent. In six of the eight powders or pills Stutter prescribed, the rhubarb was combined with mercury to increase their laxative affect, and in two of these he also added jalap, which must have resulted in severe purging.

The petals from the red or Provence **Rose**,[138] cultivated throughout the world, were used to make infusion of roses. After they were macerated with hot water containing a small amount of dilute sulphuric acid, sugar was added to the liquid and the result was 'an elegant vehicle for many active remedies, particularly sulphate of magnesium, the nauseous taste of which it covers';[139] Stutter used it for this purpose on four occasions as well as in eight mixtures of quinine bisulphate.

30. Rhubarb rhizomes, *Rheum palmatum*.

Distilling the flowering tops of the ever-green shrub produces **Rosemary** Oil.[140] Well known for its culinary use, rosemary has a long history in herbal medicine, and an infusion was used for nervous head-ache, hysteria and chlorosis. But by the early 1830s it was rarely used except as a pleasant smelling additive. Stutter prescribed it once only – in a liniment of ammonia and camphor for Caroline Wayfield (p. 136). The spirit[141] remained a popular additive in hair lotions, not only for its pleasant odour but also for its supposed effect in stimulating the growth of the hair.

Samuel Chinery (p. 35) was prescribed Confection of **Rue**, prepared from the leaves of a herb usually cultivated in Britain.[142] The contemporary use of the confection was chiefly for hysteria and flatulent colic. Samuel had been a patient since the beginning of June but there is no recorded medical history. Some of his other fourteen prescriptions suggest that he may have been suffering from dyspepsia, in which case the confection may have been of some comfort to him. This is the only occasion on which Stutter prescribed rue.

The ancient Egyptians, Greeks and Romans used the dried stigmas of the **Saffron** crocus[143] as a medicine, spice and dye. Culpeper thought that saffron was 'endowed with great virtues, refreshing the spirits and being good against fainting fits and heart palpitations as well as strengthening the stomach, helping the digestion and

---

[136] The Christmas tree, *Picea abies*, pitch being collected chiefly from trees growing in Finland.

[137] Various species of *Rheum*.

[138] *Rosa gallica*.

[139] *Consp.*, p. 60.

[140] *Rosmarinus officinalis*, growing in Mediterranean regions.

[141] Made by dissolving the oil in alcohol.

[142] *Ruta graveolens*.

[143] *Crocus sativus*.

cleansing the lungs'.[144] By 1830 it was sometimes used for hysteria, but chiefly for colouring and flavouring as in the mixture of camphor and potassium given to David Tweed (p. 116).

The roots of **Sarsaparilla**, a South American plant,[145] were brought to Europe in about 1530. It was introduced as a medicine for the cure of venereal disease. Sarsaparilla fell into disrepute, but was re-introduced in the mid-seventeenth century by William Hunter[146] and Sir W. Fordyce,[147] not as a cure for syphilis but as an adjunct during and after mercurial treatment. It was also recommended for chronic rheumatism[148] and some skin diseases. Recent limited clinical trials using extracts have indicated improvements in some cases of psoriasis,[149] a condition from which Abraham Orris (p. 17) was suffering and for which Stutter prescribed sarsaparilla, as he did for Susan Banham (p. 7), who was suffering from eczema. Other patients receiving sarsaparilla included Mary Wade (p. 43), who was using a mercury iodide ointment and may well have had a skin disease.

Large quantities of the resin **Scammony** were extracted from the root of Orizaba jalap.[150] As a drastic cathartic it was given for chronic constipation. Stutter prescribed it for two patients only – Jonathon Sturgeon (p. 100), and Susan Plumbe (p. 69), when it was combined with mercury, and in the case of Jonathon also with colocynth. Both prescriptions are likely to have caused severe purging.

The Seneca Indians from North America used the roots of one of their native plants[151] as a remedy for snakebite. It was introduced into European medicine as **Senega** in about the middle of the eighteenth century,[152] and came to be regarded as 'a useful expectorant and diuretic'.[153] The only patients to receive this drug were James Clark (p. 87) and George Brame (p. 84).

Senna leaves were collected from two species of a shrub.[154] The dried leaves and pods of both varieties were used for constipation. A popular household remedy for constipation until the mid-twentieth century was prepared by steeping the pods in warm water for six to twelve hours. The resultant strained liquor was then drunk. In 1830 the medical properties of senna were described as 'purgative, generally operating four hours after taking, apt to occasion griping and therefore requires the addition of some aromatic such as caraway or cardamom seeds, or ginger'.[155] The confection,[156] considered to gently relax the bowels, was used by Stutter on six occasions. The laxative action of senna is due to the presence of chemicals known as

---

[144] D. Potterton, *Culpeper's Colour Herbal*, Slough, 1983, p. 160.

[145] *Smilax ornate.*

[146] William Hunter (1718–83), educated at Glasgow, Edinburgh, and St George's Hospital; MD, Glasgow, 1750; physician-extraordinary to Queen Charlotte, 1764; FRS, 1767.

[147] Sir William Fordyce (1724–92), physician; an army surgeon in the war of 1742–48; began to practise in London, 1750; MD, Cambridge, 1770; knighted, 1787.

[148] *London*, p. 568.

[149] *Herbal*, p. 233.

[150] *Ipomoea orizabensis.*

[151] *Polygala Senega.*

[152] Wallis, p. 359.

[153] *London*, p. 502.

[154] *Cassia acutifolia* was known as Alexandrian Senna, grown in Africa, near the River Nile, and *Cassia angustifolia* grown in India and known as Tinnevelly Senna.

[155] *London*, p. 239.

[156] Made from senna leaves, figs, liquorice, tamarinds, sugar and aromatics.

anthraquinones;[157] in modern times the two most active and least toxic of these[158] have been isolated, and preparations containing them are widely prescribed. They are the most frequently used self-administered laxative.

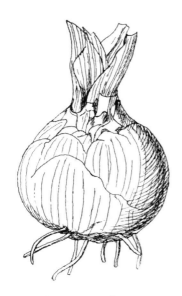

31. Squill, *Urginea scilla*.

Squill, from the bulbs of sea onions,[159] was reputedly known to Egyptian physicians as early as 2000 BC. and was certainly employed in Arabian medicine. It was often formulated with honey and vinegar as 'Oxymel of Squills' and used as an ingredient of countless formulae of cough mixtures,[160] including those for Sarah Bryant (p. 97), and Susan Warren (p. 48). The diuretic properties of squills were also recognised; in 1848 Dr Christison noted that 'Squill is one of the best vegetable diuretics, the effect of which can be increased with mercury.'[161] It was recommended that pills of squill should be used with mercury and digitalis, an edict that Stutter followed in the case of Susan Welch (p. 58). By contrast, Susan Warren (p. 47), was given a mixture of the tincture plus digitalis infusion and decoction of broom, the latter also having a good reputation as a diuretic. In 1783 Samuel Johnson was badly afflicted with dropsy, his legs and thighs being grossly swollen. His doctors initially prescribed squill powder, but later changed to vinegar of squill. Johnson wrote to Boswell on 1 March 1784, 'I have just begun to take vinegar of squills. The powder hurt my stomach so much that it could not be continued.' But the treatment was successful, and his doctors were able to report that the fluid had been removed from his legs and thighs as well as from his chest and that he was as well, if not better, than he had been for the previous seven years.[162]

The distillation of the oily resin of various species of fir trees produced **Turpentine**, which during the nineteenth century was in vogue as a treatment for tapeworms and threadworms. In 1811 Dr Latham of Harley Street wrote that 'An ounce of Rectified Oil of Turpentine may be safely taken at one dose and has proved a cure for worms',[163] for which purpose it was customarily given with castor oil. Stutter gave Matilda Rumble (p. 30), five drachms of turpentine with three drachms of castor oil to take as a single dose. Leah Cross (p. 41) took turpentine made more palatable by the addition of peppermint water and honey; she was also given an enema containing the oil and applied a liniment of turpentine. The latter was widely used as a counter-irritant to relieve the pains of chronic rheumatism and bruises. A liniment was made by emulsifying oil of turpentine with acetic acid and water. Later, a similar substance, known as White Liniment, was probably the most

---

[157] One of a group of hydrocarbons, so named as some are prepared commercially from anthracene and quinone.
[158] Sennosides A and B.
[159] *Urginea scilla*, growing in the Mediterranean coastal areas of Spain, Sicily and Syria.
[160] See also Gee's Linctus, mentioned under Opium in this appendix.
[161] R. Christison, *Dr Christison's Dispensatory*, 2nd edn, 1835, p. 835.
[162] W.E. Court, *The Pharmaceutical Journal*, 10 August 1985, pp. 194–6.
[163] SROB, Common Place Book of Sir T.G. Cullum.

frequently prescribed liniment before the advent of modern gels, such as those that are now formulated with ibuprofen and similar anti-inflammatory substances.

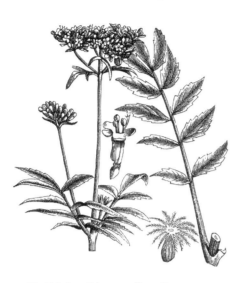

32. Valerian, *Valeriana officinalis*.

The dried roots of wild **Valerian**[164] have a very long history in herbal medicine, Culpeper stating that, 'It is excellent against nervous affections.' In recent years there has been a renewal of interest in the drug as an alternative sedative and hypnotic, and a number of documented studies have described a sedative effect for valerian. Other studies suggested that, in combination with St John's wort, valerian was more effective than diazepam in treating symptoms of anxiety, whilst animal studies indicate that valerian does possess some antispasmodic effect.[165] In Stutter's day valerian was described as being 'antispasmodic, tonic and an emmenagogue[166] that could be used in hysteria, epilepsy and other affections of nervous system'.[167] No diagnosis was recorded for the patients who were given this drug.

Chemicals

Externally, **Aluminium**, in the form of a lotion, was used as an astringent and for cleansing wounds. Matthew Sindall (p. 122) was prescribed a gallon of the compound lotion to apply to tumours and ulcerated skin on both his hips. Diluted with rose water the lotion was also used for the eyes after they had been bathed with a hot solution of vinegar.[168] Sophia Barnardiston recorded a formula for the home treatment of toothache containing 'three drachms of finely pulverized alum mixed with seven drachms of nitrous ether, to be applied with a piece of cotton'.[169]

Ammonia in its natural state is a gas and was consequently used in solution, or as solid salts, particularly the acetate, bicarbonate, carbonate and chloride. In the form of smelling salts and sal volatile,[170] ammonia was a popular household remedy as a first-aid remedy for fainting and collapse. A medicine chest containing both substances for use in church was obtainable at a cost of £1 10s 6d, for 'fainting, or hysteric fits which often occur during divine service'.[171] Solutions of ammonium acetate were given to promote sweating and lessen thirst in cases of fever; Stutter ordered it on five occasions in the casebook, and as late as the 1970s a mixture containing the solution was being used in Suffolk to help the symptoms of the

---

[164] *Valeriana officinalis.*
[165] *Herbal*, p. 261.
[166] A drug that stimulates menstrual flow.
[167] *London*, p. 839.
[168] Nunn, vol. 3, p. 176.
[169] Barnardiston, p. 48.
[170] Aromatic Spirit of Ammonia.
[171] *Guide*, p. xiii.

common cold and influenza.[172] Stutter prescribed fifteen mixtures that included either solution of the acetate or the aromatic spirit of ammonia (sal volatile). Externally, liniments of ammonia, sometimes with the addition of opium tincture, were used to relieve pain, as in the cases of Kezia Atkins (p. 66), and James Carter (p. 81). A contemporary recommendation was for a similar liniment to be spread on a piece of flannel and applied to the throat for tonsillitis and quinsy.[173]

Antimony was considered by early physicians to be too poisonous for internal use. In the fifteenth century a Benedictine monk is said to have given it to the monastery's pigs, causing them to grow vigorously, probably because the antimony had cured them of intestinal worms. When he repeated the experiment on his fellow monks some of them died. This is supposed to be how antimony got its name, because it was originally called antimoine, the French for 'anti-monk'. Taken in small doses antimony caused sweating and nausea; in larger doses it led to vomiting and purging with the danger of causing severe diarrhoea, liver damage, heart failure and possibly death. Despite this, some 'progressive' physicians started to use antimony, and in the early eighteenth century Dr James' 'Fever Powders'[174] became famous. The formula of these was widely known to be very similar to that of the Antimonial Powder[175] of the *London Pharmacopœia*, and was described as 'having the power of restoring bodily functions, inducing sweating, and being an emetic or purgative depending on the dosage used'.[176] The combination of antimony with potassium tartrate was thought to be the most important of the antimonial preparations, recommended not only for fevers and rheumatism but also 'for inflammation of the chest, chorea and apoplexy'.[177] David Tweed (p. 116), who was unable to work because of severe rheumatic pains, was given a mixture containing this preparation, whilst William Mulley (p. 19), who also had a diagnosis of rheumatism, was given a mixture containing antimony wine. In addition to promoting sweating, antimony wine was reputed to be of value as an expectorant, for which purpose it continued to be included in formulae for cough mixtures until the mid-twentieth century. Externally, ointments and plasters of antimony produced 'pustular eruption on the skin which is very useful in mania, white swellings and deep seated inflammations as a counter irritant'.[178] Antimony ointments were prescribed for Frances Steggles (p. 125) and James Sharpe (p. 135), whilst Samuel Chinery (p. 36), was given an antimony plaster.

The only patient for whom Stutter prescribed **Arsenic** was Abraham Orris (p. 17), whose diagnosis was psoriasis, although this was not a condition for which arsenic was recommended at that time. However, later in the century a guide to therapeutics said that 'in dry scaly affections of the skin, such as psoriasis, arsenic acts most admirably'.[179] Stutter appears to have been ahead of current thought. The majority of professionals considered arsenic to be 'a virulent poison, but when properly administered it is a general tonic, also used in chronic rheumatism, dropsy,

---

[172] Compound camphor mixture containing strong solution of ammonium acetate, ammonium bicarbonate and camphorated opium tincture.

[173] *Consp.*, p. 64.

[174] Prepared by Dr Robert James (1705–76), who became a public celebrity.

[175] A mixture of antimony oxide and calcium phosphate.

[176] *London*, p. 736.

[177] *ibid.*, pp. 732–3.

[178] *ibid.*, p. 733.

[179] *Guide*, p. 74.

syphilis etc'.[180] As late as the first half of the twentieth century arsenic was still being recommended as a general tonic and was said to be one of the few substances that really deserved that name, since it increased both the weight and strength of the patient.[181]

Bismuth was sometimes used (as the oxide or nitrate) for its reputed tonic and antispasmodic properties in the treatment of heart palpitations and epilepsy. It was probably more often given for heartburn and dyspepsia, when it was frequently combined with extract of hops[182] as in the cases of both Minter Ling (p. 53), and Elizabeth Canham (p. 26); the former patient complained of nausea with fullness and uneasiness in the region of the stomach after foods.

Chalk, or calcium carbonate, has a long history of internal use as an antacid, and for diarrhoea, when it was often combined with opium. Such a mixture was given to Ann Copping (p. 63), whilst William Mulley (p. 20) was prescribed compound chalk powder, said to be excellent for 'all kinds of fluxes,[183] whether at nose, mouth or belly'.[184] The powder with opium, as well as being used for adults, was considered 'a useful opiate powder for infantile diarrhoea of teething'.[185] Five of Stutter's patients were prescribed mercury with chalk powder, although the chalk used in this had no therapeutic action. The preparation of this powder involved mixing the two ingredients using a pestle and mortar, during which process oxidation of the mercury took place, the chalk helping to keep it in fine globules that did not run together.[186] A simple chalk mixture for children[187] and one with added opium for adults[188] were still being prescribed regularly in the 1950s. In the early nineteenth century it was recommended that chalk powder should be sprinkled over burns when 'the skinning over the sore was much hastened'.[189]

In the early nineteenth century **Citric Acid** was obtained from lemon juice. A solution of the acid sweetened with sugar that had been rubbed with fresh lemon peel was said to produce a beverage resembling lemonade.[190] Citric acid, like tartaric acid, was used to make effervescent powders and draughts. See Effervescing mixtures below.

In the nineteenth and twentieth centuries **Effervescing mixtures** were frequently prescribed. Samuel Chinery (p. 35) was given a mixture of sodium carbonate in water and also twelve powders of tartaric acid. Every four hours one powder was dissolved in two tablespoonfuls of the mixture, the two chemicals reacting to produce carbon dioxide causing and making 'soda water'. Commercial soda water contained carbon dioxide under pressure, causing it to fizz when poured into a glass. In 1815 Thomas Savory[191] had patented Seidlitz Powders, consisting of citric acid, wrapped in white paper, and sodium bicarbonate in blue paper. To use, the bicarbonate was first dissolved in half a pint of water, then the contents of the white

---

[180] *ibid.*, p. 186.
[181] Martindale, *The Extra Pharmacopœia*, 22nd edn, vol. 1, 1941, p. 211.
[182] *London*, p. 743.
[183] Excessive flow of any body secretion.
[184] D. Potterton, *Culpeper's Colour Herbal*, Slough, 1983, p.193.
[185] *London*, p. 35.
[186] *ibid.*, p. 760.
[187] Mixture of Chalk for Infants.
[188] Mixture of Chalk with Opium.
[189] *Consp.*, p. 31.
[190] *London*, p. 542.
[191] Thomas Savory, chemist of New Bond Street, London, founder of the firm that became Savory & Moore Chemists.

paper, tartaric acid, were added and the resulting solution was drunk whilst it effervesced. The powders became hugely popular, widely used for hangovers as 'the morning after powder', and were still available in the mid-twentieth century. Susan Welch (p. 58) had both the alkali and acid ready-prepared in two bottles of mixtures. To take her medicine a dose from each bottle was poured into a glass and drunk whilst effervescing. As late at the 1980s pharmacists in Bury St Edmunds prepared stock bottles of Effervescent Mixtures ready for dispensing, mixture 'A' containing sodium bicarbonate and mixture 'B' tartaric acid.

Although **Ether** is now best known as an anaesthetic, it was being used in medicine many years before it began to be employed as a general anaesthetic in the late 1840s. Rectified ether, prepared by distilling alcohol with sulphuric acid, was said to relieve the paroxysm of spasmodic asthma when taken by mouth or by inhaling the vapour. The danger of the latter was recognised – physicians were warned that 'much caution is required as imprudent inspiration has produced lethargic and apoplectic symptoms'.[192] Stutter did not use this substance but on three occasions he prescribed the less active spirit of sulphuric ether, on one occasion in a mixture for Leah Cross (p. 41), who was having difficulty in breathing. By distilling alcohol with nitric acid instead of sulphuric acid, the more popular spirit of nitric (or nitrous) ether was produced. The general public purchased this as a remedy for fevers and colds. It was called 'sweet spirit of nitre' and was still available well into the twentieth century. The spirit was also used as a veterinary medicine, especially for horses. The *London Dispensatory* said that 'given in a cup of water or any other appropriate liquid it quenches the thirst in fevers and in larger doses reduces nausea and flatulence'.[193] As it was thought to increase the flow of urine, prescribing it with other diuretics in patients who had fluid retention could be advantageous. Mixtures containing the spirit and potassium nitrate were favoured, particularly to reduce temperatures in fevers. Stutter prescribed such for Esther Isaacson (p. 61), James Sharpe (p. 135), Martin Lifley (p. 21) and Susan Welch (p. 59); in all, fourteen patients received the spirit. A home recipe for toothache was to apply the spirit mixed with alum powder on a piece of cotton.[194]

In the eighteenth century a number of physicians in Europe were using water made from the leaves of the cherry laurel to treat chest complaints, because its transitory sedative action reduced persistent coughing.[195] Scheele,[196] in his study of Prussian blue[197] in 1782, obtained a dilute acid, originally called Prussic acid, then, in later years re-named **Hydrocyanic Acid**. Further studies showed that the acid was present in the leaves of cherry laurel and also those of the peach tree.[198] The *London Pharmacopœia* of 1836 gave directions for the preparation of the dilute acid by distilling potassium ferrocyanide with sulphuric acid. Medicinal uses of the acid included the relief of gastric irritation from dyspepsia and other disorders of the stomach, including cancer. It was also used to allay coughs and was recommended for the first symptoms of tubercles in the lungs as well as in whooping cough and

---

192 *London*, p. 910.

193 *Ibid.*, p. 914.

194 Sophia, p. 48.

195 M.P. Earles, 'The Introduction of Hydrocyanic Acid into Medicine', *Medical History* 20, 1976, p. 307.

196 Karl Wilhelm Scheele (1742–86), Swedish chemist and pharmacist who isolated many elements and compounds for the first time, including oxygen.

197 Prussian blue was a synonym for Ferric ferrocyanide, a blue pigment.

198 *Translation*, p. 68.

asthma. The *Pharmacopœia* concluded by warning that 'great caution should be observed in its use, and the dose at first should not exceed five or six minims'.[199] Stutter gave it to eight patients in doses ranging from three to nine minims. By 1820 sales of the dilute acid in London showed that it was being used fairly extensively there; nine quarts of the preparation were sold at Apothecaries Hall over a period of nine months, and another chemist recorded the sale of forty pints over a similar period.[200] Used externally it was said to be the only application that could be relied on to relieve the irritation of impetigo and other skin conditions.[201] Susan Banham (p. 7), who suffered from eczema, was prescribed a lotion of the dilute acid with lead, whilst Abraham Orris (p. 18), was given an ointment of elder flowers containing a small amount of the acid for his psoriasis. Susan Plumbe (p. 69) took a mixture of the acid for palpitations of the heart, and Samuel Burman (p. 77), with a diagnosis of tuberculosis, was also prescribed hydrocyanic acid. Thus, Stutter's use of this relatively recent introduction to medicine was, for each patient, in accordance with the recommendations of the contemporary pharmacopœia.

Iodine was first isolated in 1812. A few years later William Wollaston perfected a production method. Woolaston had practised as a doctor in Bury St Edmunds, but in 1797 he moved to London to further his scientific career.[202] In about 1820, iodine became popular in France for treating wounds. A hundred years later tincture of iodine was a common item in every household. Although it was the first choice anti-septic to be dabbed on all cuts, sores and skin abrasions, iodine was unpopular with children because of the stinging it caused when it came into contact with open wounds.

It was not understood at the time that a dietary deficiency of iodine caused the thyroid gland to become enlarged and visible as a pronounced swelling, or goitre, on the neck. Nevertheless, the conditions for which the internal use of iodine was recommended included 'glandular swellings'. It was noted that 'it succeeds in reducing enlargement of the liver and spleen when mercury has failed'.[203] Potassium iodide was thought to be a very valuable medicine for treatment of the secondary symptoms of syphilis,[204] and it was also prescribed for gout, rheumatism, and to increase the diuretic action of other drugs. John Chinery's diagnosis (p. 38) was hypertrophy of the heart, a condition likely to have caused fluid retention. His drugs included digitalis and potassium iodide. Potassium iodide was sometimes given in cases of asthma and bronchitis, and an expectorant cough mixture of potassium iodide and ammonia remained popular until the late twentieth century. Oral inges-tion of iodine was not without dangers; adverse reactions included reduction of strength, stomach pains, nausea, vertigo and headaches. In addition, disturbances of the nervous system resembling those of Parkinson's disease sometimes occurred. Externally, iodine preparations were extensively used as counter-irritant applica-tions to enlarged glands, swollen joints, chilblains and various forms of skin diseases. Mary Motte (p. 15), had severe inflammation of the eye for which she was

---

[199] *Ibid.*, p. 73.

[200] M.P. Earles, 'The Introduction of Hydrocyanic Acid into Medicine', *Medical History* 20, 1976, p. 310.

[201] *London*, p. 656.

[202] Wollaston later earned a fortune from his discovery of a method of producing pure platinum, from which he constructed vessels for the concentration of sulphuric acid.

[203] *London*, p. 379.

[204] *Translation*, p. 302.

successfully treated with tincture of iodine, applied by brush, with later application of silver nitrate eye drops.

Iron was prescribed for anaemia and chlorosis. The latter was a fashionable diagnosis for a condition that was apparently common in young girls (see Appendix II). It was probably iron-deficiency anaemia. Of the thirty-four prescriptions for iron written by Stutter, eight cases indicate that the patients were suffering from anaemia or from a condition where anaemia was likely to be present. A further two patients were diagnosed as having hysteria, another condition for which iron was recommended. Both the compound iron pill[205] and the compound mixture[206] were frequently prescribed by Stutter. On two occasions senna was added to the prescriptions, to counteract the constipating effects that iron compounds tended to produce. And on one occasion Stutter prescribed a liquid known as 'persesquinitrate of iron', a substance that had been introduced into medicine just two years before the first entry in the casebook. It was described as being astringent and mildly caustic, and said to be a valuable remedy in chronic diarrhoea. Later reports referred to its use in the abdominal haemorrhage of typhoid fever.[207] Contemporary prescription ledgers show that the liquid was being regularly prescribed in Bury St Edmunds.[208]

Although salts of **Lead** were recognised as being poisonous, this did not prevent them being prescribed for internal use. Stutter prescribed pills containing the acetate for two of his patients, Samuel Burman (p. 77) and George Brame (p. 84). The contemporary indication for the chemical was 'in cases of internal bleeding'.[209] Dr Beck of Ipswich prescribed pills of lead acetate for a patient suffering from tuberculosis for 'bleeding from the lungs'[210] and as late as 1934 the same chemical was still being suggested to be used internally for diarrhoea, dysentery and cholera.[211] Externally a solution of the acetate solution diluted with water was a popular lotion used on sprains, bruises, inflammations and even burns, and was prescribed for Susan Banham (p. 7), William Nelson (p. 22), and Anne Rands (p. 13). Ointments containing lead were used to cool inflamed areas.[212] 'Lead Lotion' survived into the second half of the twentieth century and for years was the first-line treatment for bruises and sprains.

Magnesium Sulphate is probably the best-known magnesium compound. In 1675 a Dr Grew evaporated the water from a spring at Epsom and produced what we now know as Epsom Salts.[213] The salts achieved such popularity as a household laxative that by the beginning of the nineteenth century the greatly increased demand induced less scrupulous makers to adulterate their preparations with common salt and Glauber's Salts.[214] Stutter prescribed the salts for ten patients, and a further four of his charges were given either the oxide or carbonate of magnesium; both these substances were used for heartburn. Leah Cross's prescription (p. 41) was labelled 'to be taken if the breathing is difficult'. But it is hard to imagine how

---

205 In addition to iron sulphate this pill also contained myrrh and sodium carbonate, neither of which would have had any discernible therapeutic value.

206 The compound mixture was sweetened with sugar and flavoured with myrrh, nutmeg and rose water.

207 J. Pereira, *Elements of Materia Medica*, 3rd edn, London, 1849, vol 1, p. 787.

208 Nunn, vol. 2, pp. 69 and 84.

209 *Consp.*, p. 89.

210 SROI HA 436/149.

211 *BPC*, p. 818.

212 *London*, p. 971.

213 *London*, p. 411.

214 *Guide*, p. 11.

magnesia[215] could improve her condition. Cullum wrote to his son in September 1822: 'concerning Mrs Cullum's complaint, the Heartburn. I told you I thought a few grains of Magnesia (a small teaspoonful) might be taken two or three times a day.'[216]

In the sixteenth century it was thought that syphilis could be treated with carefully controlled doses of a **Mercury** compound. The medical profession continued to use it enthusiastically for this disease throughout the next three centuries – until the synthesis of organic arsenic compounds[217] in the early part of the twentieth century. Stutter prescribed mercury on fifty-six occasions, principally for its purging action, frequently as Calomel,[218] and often combined with colocynth. The 'Blue Pill'[219] was considered to be the best way to administer the chemical in the treatment of venereal disease because it was much less likely to cause diarrhoea than any of the other forms available. It was prescribed for Isaac Carter (p. 28), Mary Death (p. 115) and William Mulley (p. 19), the first two patients having a diagnosis of chronic hepatitis, whilst the last had rheumatism. Mercury was recommended for all these conditions as well as for some skin diseases and fevers. It was also given as a purgative and 'to assist the diuretic action of squill and foxglove [digitalis]'.[220] James Arnold's diagnosis (p. 15) was 'enlarged heart' (possibly the result of rheumatic heart disease or hypertension); the pills he was prescribed were combined with squill, which had a pronounced diuretic effect, and may well have been beneficial. William Downey (p. 8) had a venereal ulcer and was prescribed pills containing the iodide; the treatment appears to have been successful as the entry is marked 'cured'. Calomel powders were administered to young children for teething well into the twentieth century. This was a very dangerous practice. In 1953 a report in the *British Medical Journal* gave details of thirteen cases of 'pink disease'[221] with two deaths being observed in the children's ward of one hospital. All of the children had been repeatedly given one particular brand of teething powder over long periods.[222] Not before time, the sale of mercury compounds was subsequently banned. The adverse effects of taking mercury could also be serious for adults. Frances Baker (p. 100) was prescribed calomel on 15 January 1840, followed by more two days later; the following week Stutter wrote in her notes 'Mouth affected by the calomel', and instructed that she should stop taking the medicine. Stutter wrote in Mary Death's case history (p. 114), 'has lost all her teeth but one in consequence of excessive salivation [see below] thirteen years ago'. Cullum again thought he had useful advice to give; writing to his son he said: 'You tell me Mrs Cullum is taking the Blue Pill [mercury pill]; she must attend to her mouth & gums, which the mercury will affect more or less, sometimes rather unexpectedly; the Blue Pill is sometimes advised to be taken two nights & then miss the third; [it] sometimes does not affect the bowels, at other times it proves purgative. When Mrs. Cullum finds her gums tender she must leave off taking the pills for a few nights & then begin again.'[223] Syphilis was frequently treated by 'Salivation', so called because it caused

---

215 Magnesium oxide.
216 Cullum, 25 April 1821.
217 These included May & Baker's Stovarsol and Salvarsan made by Bayer.
218 Mercurous chloride, considered to be the most useful of all the mercury compounds.
219 Mercurial pills of the *London Pharmacopœia* were commonly known as blue pills because of their bluish hue.
220 *Consp.*, p. 87.
221 Pink Disease, or acrodynia, was an allergic reaction to mercury in children.
222 W. Martindale, *The Extra Pharmacopœia*, 24th edn, vol. I, 1958, p. 890.
223 Cullum, 18 February 1826.

the patient to salivate profusely. The treatment entailed rubbing ointments, containing a large proportion of mercury, on to the skin, producing the same effects as oral administration without purging. The insides of the thighs were a recommended site for applying the ointment and the patient was encouraged to do this himself. The adverse reactions of the treatment could be severe and unpleasant, the first indication being a faint red line appearing along the gums. This was followed by recession of the gums from the teeth, which then became loose and finally fell out. The increased flow of saliva and debility were further problems for the sufferer. Ointments containing mercury were given to Sarah Haywood (p. 1), and Mary Wade (p. 43); these were not the strong ointments used for salivation but milder preparations widely used in a variety of skin conditions. For two patients Stutter prescribed a liniment of mercury, which, when rubbed on to the affected parts night and morning, was said to relieve swellings and chronic venereal pains.

Concentrated **Nitric Acid** was used in sick rooms where it was hoped that its vapour would destroy contagion. The dilute acid was thought to have tonic and antiseptic properties and was used in cases of chronic hepatitis, to stop severe vomiting, and to relieve dyspepsia and asthma. In 1796 reports from Bombay spoke of it being a remedy for syphilis, and in the early nineteenth century it was suggested that it should be given with mercury in the treatment of venereal diseases.[224] When well diluted with water it made an agreeable and useful beverage for those suffering from fever.[225]

Stutter used the soluble salts of **Potassium** thirty-three times. Most of these salts were reputed to have diuretic properties, especially the iodide and nitrate. The latter was frequently prescribed for its cooling effects in fevers. Other soluble salts used included the acetate, bicarbonate and iodide, whilst the tartrate was sometimes given as a laxative. Solution of potassium hydroxide, being mildly alkaline, was used to neutralise excess stomach acid. It was also used in skin conditions; Susan Banham (p. 7), who suffered from eczema, took a mixture of sarsaparilla and potassium solution every day. After taking it for a week she was declared cured. Potassium carbonate was mainly used in preparing effervescent mixtures (see above) although in common with other potassium salts it was used to reduce fevers. Included in Sophia Barnardiston's recipes is a copy of a prescription containing the carbonate labelled 'Saline draught to allay fever'. This had been prescribed by Sir H. Halford[226] and endorsed, presumably by the patient, 'very good'.[227]

Mary Motte (p. 34), after treatment with iodine, received drops of **Silver Nitrate** dissolved in water for inflammation of the eye, and shortly afterwards was discharged cured. Abraham Orris (p. 17), suffering from psoriasis, was treated with various lotions and ointments including a lotion made of silver nitrate dissolved in water. Eye drops containing silver compounds were still being used in the 1960s, as were silver nitrate 'pencils'[228] for applying as a caustic to warts.

Soap was prescribed to be taken internally in constipation, but was mainly applied externally for bruises and sprains.[229] Stutter made use of soap liniment on five occasions, frequently with tincture of opium added to improve the analgesic

---

224 *Consp.*, p. 5.
225 *Ibid.*
226 Sir Henry Halford, President of the Royal College of Surgeons.
227 Barnardiston, p. 118.
228 Silver nitrate pencils were made by fusing together one part of silver nitrate with two of potassium nitrate.
229 *Consp.*, p. 101.

effect. The liniment, which also contained camphor and rosemary oil, remained popular into the mid-twentieth century. Known colloquially as 'opodeldoc' it was commonly purchased from the chemist to mix with glycerine for applying to chilblains. As soap sometimes formed part of the mass used to make pills, it is not possible to say if it was present for any therapeutic reason in the four prescriptions in the casebook where soap was present. Any laxative property that soap possessed would have been of value where a constipating drug was also present, for example opium for James Clark (p. 87) and iron for James Fane (p. 118).

Sodium was used in medicine as one of its salts – carbonate, chloride or sulphate. The latter was a very common and useful purgative. Because of its nauseous taste it was not prescribed very often (twice only by Stutter), although it was said that adding a small quantity of lemon juice or cream of tartar would make it more acceptable. Known as Glauber's Salts,[230] it was a much-used domestic remedy which retained popularity well into the twentieth century. The carbonates, more especially the bicarbonate, were in general use as an antacid in dyspepsia and acidity of the stomach, 'bicarbonate of soda' being kept in virtually every household for self-medication. Sodium chloride or common salt was rarely given by mouth, but one or two tablespoonfuls of salt dissolved in a pint of warm water made the common domestic enema. The solution was also used as a fomentation to sprained and bruised areas. Susan Plumbe (p. 70), gargled with a solution of two teaspoonfuls of salt in eight ounces of water, the basic formula that survived as a remedy colds and sore throats for over one hundred years.

Strychnine, the alkaloid present in nux vomica (see above, pp. 144–5) is a potent poison, described in the *London Pharmacopœia* of 1836 as 'one of the most virulent furnished by the vegetable kingdom'.[231] It was given in a dose of from one sixteenth to one eighth of a grain. The latter dose was said to be sufficient to kill a dog whilst 'a quarter of a grain produces a decided effect upon a man'.[232] Two young patients of Stutter, Matilda Rumble (p. 30) and Elizabeth Payne (p. 112), aged eleven and twelve respectively, were both prescribed pills of strychnine; the dose for the younger was one eighteenth of a grain and for the twelve-year-old, one twentieth of a grain. These doses are quite high when one considers that later in the century the adult dose of strychnine was put at from one thirtieth to one twelfth of a grain.[233] Strychnine was also used to relieve heartburn, nausea and flatulence and occasionally added to purgative pills because it was thought to 'improve the tone of the muscular wall of the intestines, thus relieving constipation'.[234] Stutter added strychnine to the laxative pills of colocynth he prescribed for Caroline Wayfield (p. 137). During the nineteenth century and continuing into the twentieth, strychnine was seen as a good tonic that improved the appetite to a marked degree. A proprietary tonic, with a very small amount of strychnine in the formula, continued to be marketed into the second half of the twentieth century and was described as 'A palatable and efficient tonic'.[235]

Sulphur, the brimstone that Mrs Squeers mixed with treacle for the boys of

230 Glauber, Johann Rudolf (1604–70), a German chemist who, about 1625, discovered sodium sulphate, the substance that became well known as 'Glauber's salt'. He made his living selling patent medicines and used the salt to treat almost any complaint.
231 *Translation*, p. 119.
232 *Translation*, p. 118.
233 *Guide*, p. 216.
234 *Guide*, p. 215.
235 *Extra*, p. 412.

Dotheboys Hall in *Nicholas Nickleby*, has a long history as a household laxative. Its properties were well recognised in medical practice, the *London Dispensatory* stating that 'From the gentleness of its operation on the bowels, it is one of the best means of keeping them lax in haemorrhoidal affections.'[236] It was also thought that sulphur induced sweating, making it a useful drug in chronic rheumatism, catarrh, gout, rickets and asthma. Applied externally it was a specific in cases of 'the itch' (scabies). Sulphur was not much used by Stutter, though he did augment the laxative power of senna confection for Phoebe Horrex (p. 98) by the addition of sulphur, whilst Susan Banham (p. 7) was prescribed a sulphur ointment and James Carter (p. 81) had a vapour bath of sulphur.

Dilute **Sulphuric Acid** was used in fevers, for dyspepsia and some skin conditions as well as in a gargle for quinsy.[237] Stutter prescribed it thrice only, each time with infusion of rose, but there is nothing in the casebook to suggest the reason for his prescriptions. Cullum had comments to make about its use: 'your Mother takes ten drops of what used to be called the Elixir of Vitriol, ... but I believe the Acidum Sulphuricum dilutum is used for the same, tho' I think the acidum sulphuricum aromaticum[238] is preferable, whichever you can procure, let it be pleasantly acid & not too sharp. Observe when you make use of the acid that you keep a common coarse cloth to wipe your mouth, as the acid will rot our Cambric Handkerchiefs.'[239]

A sweetened dilute solution of **Tartaric Acid** was recommended as a 'cooling and agreeable drink in fevers and other diseases' and when added to a solution of sodium carbonate 'it forms a good substitute for soda water'.[240] See Effervescing mixtures, pp. 152–3 above.

In the early 1900s **Vinegar** was produced chiefly from malt, whilst Acetic Acid came from the distillation of wood. Vinegar contained about 4 per cent acetic acid and its medical properties and uses were the same. It was reputedly a remedy for scurvy and for counteracting the effects of overdoses of narcotic poisons. Externally, lotions were used in burns, bruises and sprains, and when diluted with water was considered to be the best lotion for removing small particles of lime from the eyes.[241] Vinegar was commonly used in sick rooms as a fumigant. In 1764 Dr Norford visited a patient in Bury St Edmunds and found 'the room was so disagreeable, we were obliged, several times to sprinkle it with hot vinegar against the most intolerable stench'.[242] Other than as an ingredient of oxymel of squills,[243] Stutter only made use of vinegar twice. It was used as a vehicle in which to dissolve strychnine for Susan Jackson (p. 11), and Leah Cross (p. 42) was given vinegar of cantharides as a lotion to apply to her stomach.

236 *London*, p. 595.
237 *Ibid.*
238 Aromatic sulphuric acid; the addition of cinnamon and ginger made the acid more pleasant to take.
239 Cullum, no. 34.
240 *London*, p. 669.
241 *London*, p. 136.
242 W. Norford, *A Letter to Dr Sharpin*, Bury St Edmunds, 1764: SROB 313.
243 Made by gently boiling together honey, vinegar and squills.

BIBLIOGRAPHY

Bonner, T.N., *Becoming a Physician*, Oxford, 1995.

Bright, P., *Dr Richard Bright 1789–1858*, London, 1983.

British Pharmaceutical Codex, London, 1934.

Brock, R.C., *The Life and Work of Astley Cooper*, Edinburgh and London, 1952.

Buchan, W., *Domestic Medicine*, London, 1769.

Burn, H., and Withell, E.R., *Whitla's Materia Medica and Therapeutics*, London, 1943.

Bynum, W.F., and Porter, R. (eds), *Companion Encyclopaedia of the History of Medicine*, London, 1993.

Cameron, H.C., *Mr Guy's Hospital*, London, 1954.

Christison, R., *Dr Christinson's Dispensatory*, London, 1835.

Clarke, A., *An Essay on Warm, Cold and Vapour Bathing*, London, 1819.

Coleman, V., *The Story of Medicine*, London,1985.

Crosse, M., *A Surgeon in the Early Nineteenth Century*, Edinburgh and London, 1968.

Dewhurst, K., *Willis's Oxford Casebook 1650–1652*, London, 1981.

Dormandy, T., *The White Death: A History of Tuberculosis*, London, 1999.

Eliot, G., *Middlemarch*, first published in 1871, reprinted in London, 1994.

Ellis, R.H. (ed.), *The Case Books of Dr John Snow*, Medical History Supplement 14, London, 1994

Farquharson, R., *A Guide to Therapeutics*, London, 1877.

Harper-Bill, C., Rawcliffe, C. and Wilson, R.G. (eds), *East Anglia's History*, Woodbridge, 2002.

Harter, J., *Images of Medicine*, New York, 1991.

Hunting, P., *A History of the Society of Apothecaries*, London, 1998.

Hunting, P., *The History of the Royal Society of Medicine*, London, 2002.

Jackson, R., *Doctors and Diseases in the Roman Empire*, London, 1988.

Johnson, A. (ed.), *The Diary of Thomas Giordani Wright, Newcastle Doctor 1826–1829*, Woodbridge, 2001.

Lane, J., *A Social History of Medicine*, London, 2001.

Lane, J., *Apprenticeship in England 1600–1914*, London, 1996.

Lane, J., *The Making of the English Patient*, Stroud, 2000.

Loudon, I., *Medical Care and the General Practitioner 1750–1850*, Oxford, 1986.

Loudon, I., *The Tragedy of Childbed Fever*, Oxford, 2000.

Martindale, W., *The Extra Pharmacopœia*, 22nd edn, vol. II, London, 1943.

Martindale, W., *The Extra Pharmacopœia*, 23rd edn, vol. I, London, 1941.

Martindale, W., *The Extra Pharmacopœia*, 24th edn, vol. I, London, 1958.

Newall C., Anderson, L. and Phillipson, D., *Herbal Medicines: A Guide for Heath-care Professionals*, London,1996.

Osler, W., *The Principles and Practice of Medicine*, New York, 1892.

Paget, S., *Memoirs and Letters of Sir James Paget, edited by one of his sons*, London, 1901.

Pereira, J., *Elements of Materia Medica*, London, 1849.

Phillips, R., *A Translation of the Pharmacopœia of the Royal College of Physicians of London, 1836*, London, 1848.

Porter, R., *Bodies Politic*, London, 2001.

Porter, R., *Disease, Medicine and Society in England, 1580–1860*, Cambridge, 1987.

Porter, R., *The Greatest Benefit to Mankind*, London, 1997.

Potterton, D., *Culpeper's Colour Herbal*, Slough, 1983.

Reece, R., *The Medical Guide*, London, 1814.

Shepherd, J.A., *A History of The Liverpool Medical Institution*, Liverpool, 1979.

Steggall, J.H., *A Real History of a Suffolk Man*, London, 1857.

Stockwell, C., *A History of Plants and Healing*, London, 1988.

The Family Physician, by Physicians and Surgeons of the principal London hospitals, London, 1887.

The Life of George Crabbe by his Son, first published 1834, London, 1947.

Thomson, A.T., *A Conspectus of the Pharmacopœias*, London, 1820.

Thomson, A.T., *The London Dispensatory*, London, 1830.

Tröhler, U., *To Improve the Evidence of Medicine*, Edinburgh, 2000.

Tweeney, C., and Hughes, L., *Chamber's Technical Dictionary*, London, 1940.

Vaughan, P., *Doctors' Commons: a short history of the British Medical Association*, London, 1959.

Wallis, T.E., *Textbook of Pharmacognosy*, London, 1946.

Wear, A., *Knowledge and Practice in English Medicine, 1550–1680*, Cambridge, 2000.

Articles

Shepherd, J.A., 'William Jeaffreson (1790–1865): Surgical Pioneer', *British Medical Journal*, 6 Nov. 1965, pp. 1119–20.

van Zwanenberg, D., 'The Training and Careers of those Apprenticed to Apothecaries in Suffolk 1815–1858', *Medical History* 27, 1983, 139–150.

Turk, J.L., and Allen, E., 'Bleeding and Cupping', *Annals of the Royal College of Surgeons of England* 65, 1983.

The following three indexes cover (1) Persons and Places, (2) General and Medical Subjects, and (3) Pharmaceutical Materials and Methods. Roman numerals refer to the two Introductions (eg. xxiii), bold arabic numerals refer to Stutter's original pagination in the main text (eg. **23**), and normal arabic numbers refer to the five Appendices (eg. 23). Each block of numbers is separated by a semi-colon, to acknowledge unavoidable overlapping. An asterisk is used where a page contains more than one reference (eg. 23*), while 'n' signifies a footnote on the relevant page (eg. 23n).

INDEX OF PEOPLE AND PLACES

Aberdeen Royal Infirmary, 98
Adams, Sir Wm, 127
Addenbrooke's Hospital, xxx
Addison, Thomas (1793–1860), physician of Guy's Hospital, 122
Africa, 148n
Aldeburgh, Suffolk, 93*
Alexander, Dr, of Liverpool, 124
Allbutt, Clifford (1836–1925), 119
Ann, maidservant to Sir T.G. Cullum, 133
Arbon, Nurse, xvii; 99, 100
Armstrong, The Revd, 132
Arnold, James, xxiv; **15**; 110, 139, 156
Atkins, Kezia, xxiv; **66–7**; 140, 146n, 147, 151
Auckland, New Zealand, 105
Auenbrugger, Leopold (1722–1809), 120
Australia, 105*
Babington, William (1756–1833), physician of Guy's Hospital, London, 108*
Bacton, Suffolk, xv; 103
Badingham, Suffolk, 103
Bahamas, 141
Bailey, Henry Woodruffe, 102
Baker, Frances, xxiv, xxvii; **100–6**; 113, 133, 156
Balls, James, xxxi
Banham, Susan, xxiv; **7**; 108, 148, 154, 155, 157, 159
Barnardiston, Sophia, xxxix; 141, 150, 150n, 157
Barrell, Susan, xv; 98
Barron & Co, **1n**
Bartlet, Alexander, 97
Bayly, Thomas (1750–1834), surgeon of Stowmarket, xiv; 93
Bayne, Dr, xxii, xxx, **3**, **5**, **8**, **9**, **11**; 90, 102, 112, 124
Beck, Dr, 155
Bedingfield, James (1787–1860), surgeon of Stowmarket, 102
Bell, Charles, of the Windmill School of Anatomy, 93
Bell, John, his elaboratory, xxxiv
Bellamy, Mrs, xxn
Benedictine monk, a, 151
Bird, Dr Golding (1814–54), Guy's physician and early exponent of electrical therapy, 124

Bird, Morris, xxiv; **9**; 128
Blake, Lady, 135
Boerhaave, Hermann (1668–1734), Dutch physician of Leiden, 118
Bombay, India 157
Borough Hospitals (Guy's & St Thomas's), 96
Boswell, James, 149
Botesdale, Suffolk, 103
Boyton Hall, Great Finborough, Suffolk, 93
Brame, George, xxiv; **84–5**; 138, 148, 155
Brazil, 143
Bree, Charles Robert Bree (1811–86), surgeon of Stowmarket, 103
Brewin, Mrs, xxn
Bright, Richard (1789–1858), Guy's physician, 120
Brighton Dispensary, 95
Bristol Royal Infirmary, xxxvi
Bristol, Lord, 101
Britain, 142, 147
British Ambassador to Turkey, 115
British Museum, Natural History Department, 119
Brockeden, William, xxxvii
Broussais, F.J.V. (1772–1838), of Paris, 122
Brooke House, *see* Wickhambrook
Brown, Robert, 119
Bryant, Sarah, xxiv, xxvi; **96–7**; 113, 149
Buckle, nurse, xvii; her pay in 1840, 99
Bullass, Mary Emily, xxiv; **33**
Bunbury, Major, 105
Bungay, Suffolk, 97
Burke, Edmund, 93
Burman, Samuel, xxiv; **76–7**; 113, 141, 154, 155
Bury St Edmunds, Suffolk, xiii, xx; **122**; 95*, 96, 98, 101, 104, 105, 111, 121, 126, 135, 143, 146, 155, 159
    Angel Hotel, xx; 98
    Northgate Street, 105
    population in 1841, xvi,
    School, 93, 95*
    Six Bells, 101
    spital houses, Risbygate St, xviii
    Young Men's Institute, 95
    see also Suffolk General Hospital
Byford, E., nurse of Ixworth, 92

Calcutta, India, 94
Cambodia, 140
Cambridge, xiv, xxx, 105
    Corpus Christi, 103
    St Catherine's, 102
    Trinity College, 91
Camell, Robert, surgeon of Bungay, Suffolk, 97
Canham, Elizabeth, xxiv; **26**; 110, 152
Carter, Isaac, xxiv, xxvi; **28**; 109, 156
Carter, James, xxiv; **80**; 151, 159
Catton, George (–1829) house apothecary and
    surgeon 1827–8, xxi
    brief biography, 91
Caventou, Joseph, French chemist, 129n; *see*
    Pelletier
Cawnpore, India, 105
Chambers, Anna, 92
Channell, George, xxiv; **72–3**
Charlotte, Queen, 148n
Chedburgh, Suffolk, xxxii
China, 140, 147
Chinery, Edward, 105
Chinery, John, xxiv; **38**; 110, 133, 139, 154
Chinery, Mr, surgeon, 92
Chinery, Samuel, xxiv; **35–6**; 135, 141, 145, 147,
    151, 152
Christison, Dr, 149, 149n
Clark, James, xviii, xxi; **86**; 114, 148, 158
Clarke, Caroline, xxiv, xxx; **24**; 107, 132, 146
Clayton, Anna Maria, 104
Clayton, Benjamin Lane (–1819), surgeon of
    Norton, xv; brief biography, 91–2
Cobbold, Revd Richard of Wortham, Suffolk,
    author of *Margaret Catchpole*, 103
Cocksedge, Anne, 101
Cocksedge, John, xxiv; **82**
Coe, Thomas, 95
Collins, Mrs, xxn
Collyer, Nathaniel, 105
Columbus, 116
Colvile, Revd, xxx; 127–8
Cook, Mary, xxiv, xxxiii; **102**; 141, 142
Cooper, Mrs, xxn
Cooper, Sir Astley (1768–1841), famous Guy's
    surgeon, 94
Copping, Ann, xxiv; **62–3**; 137, 146n, 152
Corder, William, 94
Corpus Christi College, Cambridge, 103
Costerton, Mr, surgeon of Great Yarmouth, 99, 122
Cousins, Maria, xxiv; **32**; 108, 132
Crabbe, John (1754–1832), poet, xv; brief
    biography, 92–3
Creed, George, (1799–1868) JP, surgeon, Suffolk
    General Hospital, xxxi;
    brief biography, 93
Cronin, Mrs, xxn*
Cross, Leah, xxiv; **41–2**; 120n; 137, 143, 146,
    149, 153, 155, 159
Crosse, John Green (1790–1850), surgeon of
    Norwich, xiv; brief biography, 93–4
Cuba, 141
Cullum, Lady, 127

Cullum, Mrs, wife of the Revd T.G. Cullum, 132,
    156*
Cullum, Sir Thomas Gery (1741–1831), an
    aristocratic surgeon of Bury St Edmunds, 98n,
    101, 126–7*, 132, 133, 138, 143, 149n, 156*,
    156n*, 159, 159n
Cullum, The Revd Sir Thomas Gery, 101
Culpeper, Nicholas (1616–54), medical writer,
    144n, 147, 148n, 150, 152n
Cyprus, 137n
Dalton, Mr John, jnr (1803–59), surgeon, xxxi; 94*
Dalton, Mr John, sen (1771–1844), surgeon, 94
Danville, Kentucky, *see* Ephraim McDowell, 96
Day, Robert, 105
Death, Mary, xxv, xxvi; **114–15**; 109–10, 156*
Denny, Mr, 97
Dioscorides, 135
Dotheboy's Hall (*Nicholas Nickleby*), 159
Dover, Thomas (1660–1742), 143n
Downey, William, xxv; **8**; 106, 116, 156
Downing St, Westminster, 127
Dublin, 93, 105
Dunthorn, Dr J. (1791–1856), of Wickhambrook,
    xvi; 107*
    brief biography, 94
East Anglia, 111
East Suffolk Hospital, Ipswich, xvii; 98
Edinburgh, xiv, 119, 148n
Edwards, Caroline, 97
Egypt, 137n
England, brewing industry in, 143
    Victorian, 113
Erlingen, Germany, 94
Europe, 141, 142, 144, 148, 153
Fane, James, xxv, xxvi; **118**; 158
Finland, 147*
Flempton, Suffolk, xiii
Florida, 141
Ford, Sarah, xxv; **78–9**
Fordyce, Sir William (1724–92), 148n
Framlingham, Suffolk, xxiii, 96–97
France, 154
    French, 103, 116
Freeman, Spencer (1804–83), surgeon of
    Stowmarket, 103
Frost, Mr, of Hawkedon Hall, Suffolk, xxxii
Fuller, Harry (1835–1900), House Surgeon to the
    hospital, xv
    brief biography, 95
Gall, Abraham, chemist and druggist, 127
Galvani, Luigi (1737–98), 124
Gedding, Suffolk, 97*, 103
Gee, Samuel Jones (1839–1911), 145n
Gladwell, Robert, xxv; **45**; 116–17*, 146
Glasgow, 148n
Glauber, Johann Rudolf (1604–70), 158n
Goodchild, Mrs, Matron, xx
Great Ashfield, Suffolk, 103, 104
Great Finborough, Suffolk, xiv; 93
Great Yarmouth, Norfolk, 99, 122
Greene, Mr, **30**
Grew, Dr, 155

Hake, Dr, physician, xxii; 99, 102
  brief biography, 95
Halford, Sir Henry, 138, 157, 157n
Hamilton, William, surgeon of Ipswich, xvi
Hammond, Charles Chambers, 92
Hansen, Armaeur (1841–1912), 111
Hanslip, Isaac, xxxi
Haywood, Sarah, xxv; **1**; 146
Heidelburg, Germany, University of, 94
Helmont, van, Johannes Baptista (1579–1644), 122
Hervey, Lord, 101
Hinnell, George John (1823–99), 98– 99
Hodgkin, Joseph Fiott, 92
Hoffman, Erich (1868–1905), 116
Horrex, Phoebe, xxv, xxvi; **98–9**, 136, 159
Hoskins, W.G., historian, xi
Hubbard, Mr, xxxii
Hubbard, George Prettyman (1822–72), brief
  biography of, 95
Hughes, Dr Marshall, physician of Guy's
  Hospital, 111–12, 113
Hunston, Suffolk, 98
Hunter, William (1718–83), 148n
Ichikawa, Japanese research worker, 100
Ickworth House, 101
India, 107, 138, 144, 148n
  Fifteenth Madras Regiment, 103
  Indiaman (ship), 103
  Indian Medical Service, 105
  Medical and Chirurgical Society of Bombay,
    94
  Medical and Chirurgical Society of Calcutta,
    94
Ingatestone, Essex, 116
Ingham, Suffolk, xxxi
Ingram, Mrs, of Chedburgh, Suffolk, xxxii
Ipswich, Suffolk
  East Suffolk Hospital, xvii, 98
  Ipswich Journal, xvi; 107
  Mechanics Institute, 95
  School, 97
Isaacson, Esther, xxv; **60–1**; 153
Italy, Livorno, 105
  Lucca, 105
  Naples, 116
  Padua, 136
  Pisa, 105*
Jackson, Dr Alexander Russell, xxii; **118**; 146
  brief biography of, 95–6
Jackson, Susan, xxv; **11**; 141n, 159
Jamaica, 141
James, Dr Robert (1705–76), 151n
Jardine, Henry (1820–), xxi, xxxi; brief biography,
  96
Jeaffreson, William (1790–1865), surgeon of
  Framlingham, xivn, xxiii
  brief biography, 96–7
Jenner, Edward (1749–1823), 116
Johnson, Dr Samuel, 149
Kemp, Mr John, xviii
Kentford, Suffolk, 116
Kilner, John (1820–96), surgeon, 98

King, Robert Carew (1781–1842), surgeon of
  Saxmundham, xxxiii
  brief biography of, 97
King's Lynn, Norfolk, **122**
Koch, Robert (1843–1910), 107, 112
Laennec, René Théophile Hyacinthe
  (1781–1826), **133**; 118
Lancellas, Mrs, xxn
Langham, Suffolk, 92
Latham, Dr, 149
Lawrence, Mrs, xx, xxn*
Leech, Mary, xv; 98
Leech, W., xxv; **140–1**; 141n, 146n
Leiden, Holland, 118
Lifley, Martin, xxv; **21**; 147, 153
Ling, Minter, xxv; **52**; 146, 152
Lloyd, Robert, surgeon of Ipswich, xvi
London, 107, 154*
  Apothecaries Hall, xiv, xxx; **1n**; 154
  British Museum, Natural History Department,
    119
  Broad Street pump, 107
  City Dispensary, 102
  College of Physicians, xxxvii
  Dispensatory, 137, 153, 159
  Downing Street, Westminster, 127
  Goswell Street, 96
  Guy's Hospital, xxx, xxxii; 98, 102, 105, 113
    Guy's Hospital Electrical Apartment, 108
    Guy's Hospital Reports, 108*, 111, 113*,
      124
  Harley Street, 149
  London Hospital, The, 95
  Lord Mayor of, 93
  Marylebone Infirmary, 113
  Pharmacopoeia (1746), xxxvi
  Pharmacopoeia (1836), xxxvii, xxxix; **7n**;
    129, 133, 143, 151, 153, 154, 158
  Royal Maternity Charity, 96
  Southwark, 100
  St Bartholomew's Hospital, 96, 97, 99*, 100,
    119, 145*
    St Bartholomew's Hospital Reports, 91
  St George's Hospital, xxx; 93, 94, 105, 148n
  St James' dispensary, 94
  St Thomas's Hospital, 95
  Threadneedle Street, 100
Lopham Park, 97
Louis, Pierre (1787–1872) of Paris, 122
Lydgate, Dr, fictional character in *Middlemarch*,
  118
Lymington, Hampshire, 105
Lynn, G.D., surgeon of Woodbridge, 96
Malt, William, xxv; **5**; 112, 146
Marnock, Dr, 95
Maskill, James, apothecary of Aldeburgh, 92
Mathews, Elizabeth, xxv; **49**; 146n
Mauritius, 103
McAuliffe, Mrs, xxn
McDowell, Ephraim (1771–1830), American
  surgeon, xxiii, 96
McIntyre, Mr, surgeon of Newcastle, 111

Merka, Somalia, 116
Mexican Andes, 144
Middle East, 140
Midson, Ann, 92
Mildenhall, Suffolk, **72**, 104
Mingay, James, 98
Montague, Edward, 115
Montague, Lady Mary Wortley, 115
Mornement, James (1804–27), xx–xxi*
    brief biography of, 97
Morris, Frederick, surgeon of Bungay, Suffolk,
    97
Motte, Mary, xxv; **34**, 112, 154, 157
Mudd, Barrington (1822–), pupil at the hospital,
    xxi, xxxi
    brief biography of, 97–8
Mudd, Emily, 97
Mudd, Francis David (–1835), surgeon of
    Gedding, 97
Mudd, Mrs Elizabeth, 97
Mudd, Woodward, xv; 92
    brief biography of, 98
Mulley, William, xxv; **19**; 114, 135, 142n, 151,
    152, 156
Nelson, Robert, xxv; **130**; 106, 135
Nelson, William, xxv; **22**; 106, 155
New Zealand and the South Seas, 103, 105
New York, University of, 94
Newham, Samuel (1820–67), xx
    brief biography of, 98–9
Newmarket, Suffolk, 102
Nicander of Colophon, 125
Nice, France, 101
Nightingale, Florence (1820–1920), 109
Norford, Dr, 159, 159n
North America, 148
Norton, Suffolk, xiii, xv; 92, 98*
    Stanton House, xvn
Norwich, 93
    cathedral, 94
    · Norfolk and Norwich Hospital, 93, 102
Nourse, Edward, 100*
Nunn, Isaac, xxv; **37**
Nunn, John, chemist and druggist, Bury St
    Edmunds, 132n, 135n, 138
Orris, Abraham, xxv; **17**; 114, 134, 140*, 144,
    148, 151, 154, 157
Osler, Sir William (1849–1919), 105, 122
Oxford, xiv
Page, John, surgeon of Woodbridge, xv; 92
Paget, Sir James (1814–99), surgeon of St
    Bartholomew's Hospital, President of the
    Royal College of Surgeons, xv, 91, 119, 122
    brief biography, 99
Paignton, Devon, 105
Pakenham, Suffolk, 102
Pakistan, 107
Paris, France, 93, 101, 118
Pasteur, Louis (1822–95), 109
Pawsey, Elizabeth, xxv; **50**
Payne, Elizabeth, xxv; **112–13**; 108, 158
Peck, Mr, surgeon at Newmarket, 102

Pelletier, Joseph, French chemist, 129n; *see*
    Caventou
Pentney, Nurse, xvii; 99–100
Plumbe, Susan, xxv, xxvii; **68–71**; 139, 148, 154,
    158
Pott, Miss, Percival's daughter, xvi
Pott, Percival (1714–88), surgeon at St
    Bartholomew's Hospital, London, xvi
    brief biography of, 100
Pratt, Hannah, xxv; **126–7**; 115, 141n
Probart, Agnes, married Walter Scott, 101
Probart, Colonel Francis, son of Dr F.G. Probart,
    101
Probart, Francis George (1782–1861), consultant
    physician, xix, xixn, xxii, xviii; 95, 101*, 102,
    143
    brief biography of, 101–2
Pupils, xxi
Pyman, Francis Charles (1805–38), House
    Apothecary 1828–33, xvi; 101
    brief biography of, 101
Queensland, Australia, 105
Racine, U.S.A., 95
Rainey, Sophia Catherine, 101
Rands, Anne, xxv; **13**; 146, 155
Ranking, Dr, physician, xxii; 95
    brief biography of, 102
Rattlesden, Suffolk, 103*
Reeve, Susan, xxv; **108–12**; 112, 141
Riva-Rocci, Scipione (1863–97), 120
Ross, Dr Andrew, xxii; 102
Royal College of Surgeons (of England), 93
Royal Infirmary, Aberdeen, 98
Royal Maternity Charity, 96
Ruddock, Thomas, xxv; **88–9**; 136
Rumble, Matilda, xxv; **30**; 108, 132, 149, 158
Rutland, duke of, 93
Sabine, Mr, **9**
Savage, James, xxv; **3**
Savory, Thomas, chemist, founder of Savory and
    Moore, 152, 152n
Saxmundham, Suffolk, xxiii; 97*
Scarfe, William, woodsman of Thorpe Morieux,
    94
Scarff, Harriet, xxv, xxx; **128–9**
Schaudinn, Fritz (1871–1906), 116
Scheele, Karl Wilhelm (1742–86), Swedish
    chemist, 153, 153n
Scott, John, xxv; **74–5**; 109, 114, 140
Scott, Samuel, xxv; **104**
Scott, Thomas, xxv; **110–11**
Scott, Walter, MD, 101
Seneca Indians, 148
Serturner, Fredreich, German chemist, 129n
Sharpe, James, xxv; **134–5**; 151, 153
Sharpe, John, xxv; **138–9**
Sharpe, Susan, xxv; **64–5**
Sharpin, Dr, 159n
Shepherd, William, xxv; **93**; 134, 136
Simmonds, John, John Bell's assistant; xxxiv
Sindell, Matthew, xxv, xxvii; **122–3**; 150
Smith, Charlotte, xxv; **54**

Smith, John (–1802), surgeon of Wickhambrook, 92
Smith, Mr, surgeon of Clare, xviii
Smith, Nurse, xvii, 99
Snow, John (1813–58), medical practitioner of
     London, 107
Snow, Mrs, xxn
South America, 136, 141, 148
Spain, 136, 137n
     Spaniards, 141, 144
     Spanish, 116
Sparham, Widow, 98
Squeers, Mrs, 158
Sri Lanka, 137
St Catherine's College, Cambridge, 102
Stedman, Foster, xxxii; 102
Stedman, Mr, 92
Steggall, John Heigham (1789–1881) surgeon of
     Rattlesden, curate of Great Ashfield, xiv, xivn
     brief biography of, 103–4
Steggles, Frances, xxvi; **124–5**; 141, 151
Stoke by Clare, Suffolk, 96
Stone, George, 98
Stowmarket, Suffolk, xiv
Sturgeon, Jonathon, xxvi; **120**; 148
Stutter, William Gaskoin (1815–87), xi, xii, xiii,
     xvi, xxxii; 94, 105
Suffolk General Hospital, xii*, xvi, xvii, xviin;
     93, 95, 98, 102, 109, 116, 120, 125
Suffolk branch of the Provincial Medical and
     Surgical Association, 95, 101, 102
Suffolk Medical Benevolent Society, xv; 94, 98 n,
     101
Suffolk Medical Book Club, 98, 101
Surrey Dispensary, 113
Sutton, Daniel (1735–1819), surgeon of
     Ingatestone, Essex, 116
Sutton, Robert (1707–88), surgeon of Kentford,
     116
Sydenham, Thomas (1624–89), 106, 107–8
Syria, 149n
Talbot, George, xxvi; **40**; 110, 139
Taylor, Henry, 99
Teasdale, Mr, chemist, 125
Thetford, Norfolk, 102
Thingoe Union, 104
Thomson, Anthony Todd (1778–1849), 136, 145*
Thorsby, Lincolnshire, 101
Thurlow, Lord, of Great Ashfield, Suffolk, 103
Thurston, Suffolk, 92
Tibet, 147
Todd, Jane, 96
Tonga Islands, 105*
Tonga, king of, 105

Treasy, John, of Brettenham, 94
Trinity College, Dublin, 105
Turkey, 115
Tweed, David, xxvi; **116–17**; 148, 151
Vacca, Dr, 132
van Helmont, Johannes Baptista (1579–1644),
     122
Victoria, Queen, 99
Vienna, Austria, 119
Volta, Alessandro (1745–1827), 124
Wade, Mary, xxvi; **43**; 148, 157
Wales, Mrs, 104
Walsham le Willows, Suffolk, 103*
Ward, Mr William, xii; 104
Warren, Mr Nathaniel, the Secretary, xxi, xxxii
Warren, Susan, xxvi, xxvii; **47–8**; 108, 126, 133,
     139*, 140, 145, 149*
Wayfield, Caroline, xxvi; **136–7**; 135, 147, 158
Welch, Susan, xxvi; **56–9**; 138, 141, 149, 153*
Westhorpe, Suffolk, 103
White, Reverend, **5**
White, William Middleton (1813–76), surgeon of
     Gedding, 97, 103
Wickham Market, Suffolk, 96
Wickhambrook, Suffolk, xi, xv, xvi
     Brooke House, xi
     practice joined by Stutter in 1842, xxxii; 94
Wilkinson, William, xxvi; **106–7**
Willingham, Mary, xxvi, xxxvii; **132–3**; 113
Willis, Dr Thomas, 135
Withering, Dr William (1741–99), 139
Witnesham, Suffolk, 97
Woodbridge, Suffolk, 92
Woodroffe, Mrs Ann, matron, xvi, xx; 104
Wollaston, William, 154*
Worledge, James, of Ingham, xxxi
Wright, Thomas Giordani, apprentice surgeon of
     Newcastle, 111
Wright, William Middleton, surgeon of Gedding,
     103
Wyverstone, Suffolk, 103*
Yamagiwa, Japanese research worker, 100
Young, Augustus, 105
Young, Benjamin Clayton, 105
Young, Frederick John (1828–1908), 105
Young, Henry Charles (–1906), 105
Young, James Hammond (1823–1905), 105
Young, Plowman, surgeon of Norton and Bury St
     Edmunds, xvi, xviii; 92
     brief biography of, 104–5
Young, William Chambers (1822–86), 105
Yoxford, Suffolk, 97

INDEX OF GENERAL AND MEDICAL SUBJECTS

abdomen, cavity of, xxii
    circumference of, measurement of, **47***, **48***,
        56*
    pain in, **62**
abscesses, xxv, xxii; **13**
account books, Dr Probart's, xix
acetabulum (part of the hip joint), **60**
acupuncture, 117
age of patients, xxvi
albumen, albuminuria, 118; *see* urine testing
amenorrhoea, **1**, **62**, **66**, **78**, **108**, **124**, **128**; 124,
    135
amputations, xxii, xxiii; 103
anaemia, xxv, xxx; **33**, **50**, **62**, **64**, **66**, **128**, **136**;
    155
    discussion of, 106
    Addisonian, 106
anasarca (oedema), **62**
aorta, dissecting aneurysm of, 102
    aortic valve, 115
apoplexy, 151
Apothecaries Act (1815), xiv; 103; *see also* LSA
apothecary's measures, xxxiii
apprentices, training of, xiv–xvi; 92, 93, 98–9,
    104, 105
arabian medicine, 148
ascites (fluid in the abdominal cavity), **62**
asthma, 153, 157, 159
auscultation using stethoscope, 118
autobiography (of John Steggall), 103
baker's boy, xxviii, **72**
Barron & Co, **1n**
basketmaker, xxviii; **9***
bastardy charges, xv
battery, 124
baths, xvii
beaver, North American, 129; *see* Pharmaceutical
    Index *sub* Castor
bedsores, prevention of, xxix
beer, xix, xxix*; **5***, **7**, **9**, **40**, **45**, **65**, **69**, **73**, **109**,
    117, **118***, **129**, **131**, **133**, **137**
beta-haemolytic streptococcus, Lancefield
    Group A, 115
bitter apple, *see* Pharmaceutical Index *sub*
    Colocynth
blacksmith, **140**
bladder, stones in, xiv, xivn; 97
    catheterisation of, xxii, xxxii
bleeding, xxix; 120, 130; *see* venesection
    from the lungs, 155
blistering, xxvi; **9**; 111, 114, 130
blood pressure, *see* measurement of blood
    pressure

bloodstains, forensic tests for, 142
blood-taking, **9**; 122
Board Meetings of the Governors, *see* under
    hospital
boils, **54**
brewing industry, 143
British Medical Journal, 156
broken leg, 93
bronchitis, xxv; 83; **131**
    discussion of, 106
bruises, 155, 157, 159
bruit, **128***, **128n**
bubo post ulcus venerum (gland in the groin
    following venereal ulcer), xxv; **8**; 116
    discussion of, 106
Buchan's Domestic Medicine (1769), 114
burns, 155, 159
Bury and Norwich Post, xviin, xxvii, xxiv
cambric handkerchiefs, 159
cancer, xvii; 106, 113
    head of the pancreas, **82**
    open cancers, 146
    ovary, xxvii; **47**
    scrotum, 100
    stomach, **82**
cantharides plaster, *see* Pharmaceutical Index
carotid murmurs (sounds heard in the carotid
    arteries when listening with a stethoscope),
    64, **128**
carpenter, xxviii
casebook, description of, xi*
casualties, xxii
catamenia (menstrual discharge), **64**
cataplasm, *see* poultice
cataract operations, 142
catarrh, 159
catheterisation, *see* bladder catheterisation
cavity, lung, *see* pulmonary tuberculosis
chest, inflammation of, 151
    percussion of, 120
chancre (of primary syphilis), 106
chapel, xviii
chilblains, **122**; 154
child monster, 92
children, admission policy of, xvii
chimney sweeps, *see* cancer of the scrotum
chlorosis (the green sickness), xxiv, xxx; **24**; 135,
    155
    discussion of, 106–7; *see also* anaemia
cholera epidemic (1832), xvii
cholera, xvii, xviii, xxv; 94, 155
    discussion of, 107*

chorea, xxiv, xxv; 16, 17; **30**, **32**, **122***; 102, 124, 151
    discussion of, 107–8
Christison's Dispensatory (2nd ed., 1835), 149, 149n
Christmas gratuity, 99
clyster, *see* enema
cochleare, spoonful, xxxiv
colic, 137, 141, 142
    flatulent colic, 141, 147
Commission on Medical Education, 1834, 93
common cold, 151, colds, 153, 158
common diet, *see* diet, common
common place book of Sir T. G. Cullum, 149n
complaints, xxxi
congius, pint, xxxiv
conjunctivitis, 112
constipation, 148, 157, 158
consultants, *see* hospital, consultants to the
consumption, *see* pulmonary tuberculosis
cooks, xvii
country lore, 122
cowpox, 116*
cucurbitula (cupping vessel), *see* cupping
cupping, xxix; 122
    dry, description of, 123–4
    wet, **9**, **21**, **24**, **35**, **60n**, **84**, **114**, **115**, **139**, **141**; 107, 110, 114
        description of, 123
cyathus (liquid measure), 12n
deaths in hospital, xxiv, xxx
decoction(s), xxxiv; *see* Pharmaceutical Index
delirium tremens, **86**
dessertspoonful (*c. modicum*), xxxiv
diabetes, **100**; 120, 143
diarrhoea, 144, 145, 152, 154, 155, 156
    infantile, in teething, 152
diaries, Dr Probart's, xixn
diet, common, **7**, **13**, **15**, **17**, **19**, **21**, **28**, **51**, **52**, **55**, **57**, **61**, **65**, **73**, **79**, **106**, **108**, **109***, **111**, **113**, **115**, **117**, **123**, **125**, **127**, **128**, **129**, **131**, **135**, **139**, **140**
    full, **9**, **45**, **65**, **69**, **73**, **75**, **102**
    light or low, **9**, **115**, **117**, **127**, **131**, **135**, **137**, **139**
digestion, **66**
dislocations, reduction of, xxii
dispensary, xiii, xvii
    Brighton Dispensary, 95
dermatologists, 108
drachm, *drachma*, definition of, xxxiii
draught, **13**, laxative, **28**; *see* Pharmaceutical Index
drop(s), xxxiv
dropsy, xvii; 126, 138, 139, 143, 145, 149
drug bill, xxx
drugs, anticonvulsant, 117
    antidepressant, 117
dry cupping, *see* cupping
dysentery, 143, 144*, 145, 155
dyspepsia, **52**, **100**; 136, 141, 146, 147, 155, 156, 157, 158*, 159
ear infections, 111

East India Company, 96, 102
Eastern Provincial Medical and Surgical Association, 96
eczema, xxiv; **7**, **34**
    discussion of, 108, 157
egophony, aegophony, **100***
Egyptians, ancient, 147
    Egyptian physicians, 149
electrical therapy, 124
Elements of the Practice of Medicine (1839), xxix
emplaster, xxix
    of Lytta, xxix, 117
encephalitis, 111
enema, **42**; 124
enlarged glands, 154
enlarged heart, **15**, **38**; 156
epigastrium, the upper part of the stomach, **62**
    epigastric region, **82**, **96**
epilepsy, epilepsia, xxv, xxvi, xxix; **106**; 135
    discussion of, 108
epistaxis, **60***
Epsom salts, *see* Pharmaceutical Index
erysipelas, xxi, xxii
    discussion of, 109
erythema multiforme, 50, 114
    discussion of, 109
eschar, **122***, **122n**
ether, 102, *see also* hospital, first operation under ether
examination for licence to practice, *see* LSA
examining patients, xxvi–viii
experiment with frog's legs, 124
extracts, xxxiv; *see* Pharmaceutical Index
eyes, removing particles of lime from, 159
fainting fits, **66**
Family Physician (1887), 110
Fehling's test, 120
Fellow of the New York College of Physicians and Surgeons, 94
Fellow of the Royal College of Surgeons *see* FRCS
fever, fevers, **19**, **24**, **54**, **78**, **96**, **108**, **130**, **132**, **134**, **138**; 91, 105, 126, 127, 130, 135, 143, 144, 145, 153, 157, 159
    childbed fever, xviin
    gaol fever, 136
    intermittent fever (malaria) 136
    scarlet fever, 136
finger infection, **22**
fit(s), **106**, *see* epilepsy
flatulence, 158
fluxes, 152, *see* diarrhoea
Foeffment Trust, Bury St Edmunds, vxiii
footbath, **6**
foxglove, 130, 139
FRCS (Fellow of the Royal College of Surgeons), 93, 94, 97
FRS (Fellow of the Royal Society), 99
fractures, setting of, xxii
    broken leg of John Green Crosse, 93
    compound, xxii
    due to riding on waggons, xxii

fractured left ankle, **108**
fractures of leg sustained at funeral, 92
French Academy of Medicine, 109
Friendly Societies and Box Clubs, xvii
frogs, used in assay of digitalis, 139; experiments
    with legs of frogs, 124
full diet, *see* diet, full
gall bladder, gall stones, **78**; 138
galvanic troughs; xxx, *see* galvanism
galvanism, xxx; 108*, 124
garden, xxviii
    seeds for, xxviii
gas, coal, xvii
gastralgia, xxiv; **26**; 110
gastric ulcer, *see* peptic ulcer
germ theory, 109
Glauber's Salts, 155, 158
gout, **80**, **116**; 126, 141, 142, 143, 154, 159
grain, *granum*, definition of, xxxiii
groceries, xxviii
Greek and Roman Medicine, 142; Greeks and
    Romans, 147
Guy's Hospital Pharmacopoeia, xxxvi
Guy's Hospital Reports, 108*, 111, 113*, 124
haematemesis (vomiting blood), **62**
haematomas, post operative, 125
haemorrhoids, *see* piles
hair, stimulating the growth of, 147
hare lip, xxii
headache, **112**
heart disease, **40**, 102
    heart valves, damage to, 115
    rheumatic, with a leaky mitral valve, **68**
heartburn, *see* dyspepsia
hepatitis, xxiv, xxv; **28**
    discussion of, 109–10
    chronic, **74**, **114**, **115**; 157
herpes labialis, **74n**; 109, herpetic eruptions, 140
hiccough, 137
Hirudo medicalis, *see* leeches
history taking, xxvi
hives, *see* urticaria
honey, *see* Pharmaceutical Index
hops, *see* Pharmaceutical Index
horses, xxn; 153
    on horseback, xx
hospital, xvii, xviiin; 93, 95, 96, 98, 102*, 109,
    111, 112, 116, 120, 125
    admission policy, xvii–xviii
        admission and discharge days, xviii
        admission details, xxiv, xxxii
    Annual Reports, xxii, xxiv, xxx, xxviiin, xxx,
        xxxn, xxxin
    Board Meetings of the Governors
        general, xx
        special, xii
    chapel, xviii
    Committee, 95, 99, 100, 104*, 128
        committee meetings, xii, xix, xxxi*,
            xxxvi, xxxi*
    consultants, xix, xviii
        resignations, xxii

poor note-keeping, xxxi
deaths in, xxiv, xxx
diet, xxviii–xxix
duty doctors, xix
    surgeon of the week, **104**
first operation under ether, 95, 101
house apothecary, xxi; 97, 102, 104
    his hours, xxii
housemaid, xvii
matron, xx, xxx, 104
    mealtimes with matron, xx, xxxii
Medical Committee, 127
    minute books of Committee and Board
        Meetings, xii, xviin*, xxiin*, xxixn*,
        xxxn*, xxxin*, xxxiin, 111
    drug sub-committee of, xxx
plans of, xviin
porter (at hospital), xvii
Secretary, xxi, xxxii
    Assistant Secretary, xxi
    Dispenser and Secretary, xxxii; 95
staff, appointments, xxi,
    election, xxii; 98
    resignations, xxxi, xxxii; 94*
    salaries, xvi–xvii, xix; 101, 104
subscribers, xviii, xxx
    subscription, level of, xviiin
visiting committee, xxxi
    house visitors, xxxi
    visiting times, xxix
hydrometer, 120
hypertrophy of heart (or hypertrophia cordis),
    xxiv; 154
    discussion of, 110
    see also enlarged heart
hypertrophy of the right side (of heart), xxvi; **40**;
    110
hypochondriasis, 132
hypochondrium, right, **78**, **84**, 110
hysteria, **1**, **3**, **66**, **136***; 135, 142, 148, 155
    discussion of, 110
impetigo, 112
Indian Medical Service, 105
infected finger, xxv
inflammation (of skin), 155
influenza, 151
infusum, infusion, xxxiii, xxxiv; *see*
    Pharmaceutical Index
internal bleeding, 155
Inventum novum (1761), by Leopold Aubrugger,
    120
Ipswich Journal, xvi; 107
Ipswich Mechanics Institute, 95
iron filings in wine, 106
issue, 125
itch, the, *see* scabies
Jacksonian prize, Royal College of Surgeons, 93
James' fever powders, 151
jaundice (?obstructive), **114**; 110, 138, jaundiced,
    114; 109
Jesuit's bark, *see* Pharmaceutical Index *sub*
    Cinchona

Journal of the Provincial Medical and Surgical Association (1836), 102
Kendal or Lancaster Black Drop, 145
kidneys, **48**
kitchen girl, xvii
labourer, xxviii
Lancet, The, xxn; 102, 122, 145
Lark, River, xxviiin
laryngitis, 135
laundry maid, xvii
leeches, medical, xxix*, xxx; **13, 22, 32, 45*, 56, 57, 66, 67, 68*, 71*, 82*, 100*, 101, 110, 111, 132**; 112, 117, 125, 129
    discussion of, 125
leg ulcers, chronic, xvii
leprosy, or Hansen's disease, xviii; 111
leucophlegmatic (having a dropsical tendency), **66**
leucorrhoea, xxiv, **26, 98**; 110
light diet, *see* diet, light
Linnean Society, 101
Lithotomy, xxiii(n)
    instruments, xxiii,
    lithotomist, 93
    lithotrite, 96
liver complaints,
    use of vapour baths in, 126,
    use of dandelion in, 138
local newspapers, xii
locum tenens, xii
London College of Physicians, xxxvii
London Dispensatory, 137, 153, 159
London Pharmacopoeia (1746), xxxvi
London Pharmacopoeia (1836), xxxvii, xxxix; **7n**; 129, 133, 143, 151, 153, 151, 154, 158
LSA, Licenciate of The Society of Apothecaries, xiv; 94, 95, 98, 102
malpractice, 103
market day, Bury St Edmunds, xviii
mass, pill mass, **1n***; *see* Pharmaceutical Index
maternity cases, xvii
MD (Doctor of Medicine), 91, 93, 94, 95, 101, 102, 105
measles, xxviii, **108***; 136
    discussion of, 111–12*
measurement of,
    blood pressure, 119–20
    body temperature, 118–1
    circumference of abdomen, xxvii; **47*, 48*, 56***
    circumference of chest, xxvii; **100***
meat, xxviii; **45*, 52, 53, 65*, 67***
Medical Book Club, xix
    quarterly meetings and AGM, xx
Medical Register, 1858, xiv
Medical Repository, 145n
medical students, *see* pupils
Member of the Royal College of Surgeons, *see* MRCS
Member of the Medical and Chirurgical Society of Bombay, 94
Member of the Medical and Chirurgical Society of Calcutta, 94

menorrhagia, **100**
microscope, microscopy, 119
Middlemarch, by George Eliot, 118
minimum, minim, xxxiv; *see* Pharmaceutical Index
miscal line, the middle line of the sternum, **68**
mitral valve, a valve on the left side of the heart, **68**; 115
money worries, xxx
monster (child), 92
MRCS (Member of the Royal College of Surgeons), xiv; 93, 94*, 96, 98, 99, 102
Mycobacterium leprae, *see* leprosy
nates, **122n**
National Formulary (1960), 145
nausea and flatulence, 153, 158
naval recruit, 105
nephritis, 120
neuralgic affliction of V (fifth cranial nerve), *see* Trigeminal neuralgia
nightly perspirations (or sweats), **96**, 113
nurses, salaries of, *see* hospital staff, salaries of
obstetric case, xxxii
octaria, pint, xxxiv; *see* Pharmaceutical Index *sub* soap liniment
operations, for cataracts, 142
operating theatres, 109
opodeldoc, 158; *see* Pharmaeutical Index
opthalmia scrofulosa, xxv; **34**; 112, 154
osteomyelitis, 103
ounce, *uncial*, definition of, xxxiii; *see* Pharmaceutical Index
outpatients, numbers of, xxii
    visiting statistics, xxii, attended in their own homes xxxi
ovariotomy, xxiii, 96, 97; *see* Ephraim Mc Dowell and William Jeaffreson
ovary, ovaries, disease of, xxvi; tumour of, xxvii, 108; *see* cancer of ovary
Paget's disease, of the breast, 99
    of the bones, 99
palpation, 113, 118
palpitations, **68, 136**; 154
paracentesis abdominis, xxvii; **47**; 125–6
paralysis, 124
paraplegia, paraplegic, xxv; **5**; 112
Parkinson's disease, 154
partridges, xi*
patients, ages of, xxvi
    class and physical condition, xxvii
    complaints of, xxxi
    lengths of stay, xxvi
    occupations and marital status, xxviii
pectoriloquy, **132*, 132n**
penicillin, 115
peptic ulcer, **52, 62**
percussion, xxvii; **78, 96, 110**; 113, discussion of, 120
pericarditis, 125, 125n
peritoneal cavity, **56**
peritonitis, chronic, xxix; **133**; *see* tuberculosis, abdominal

Pharmaceutical Historian, 145n
Pharmacopoeias, *see* Pharmaceutical Index
pharyngitis, 115
phlebotomy, *see* venesection
phthisis, xxiv, xxviii; *see* pulmonary tuberculosis, 112–3
physicians, training of, xiv
  reluctance to visit outpatients in their own homes, xxxi
piles, 141, 159
pink disease, 156, 156n
placebo, **3**
plasters (common, adhesive, anodyne and blistering), 126
  poor man's plaster, 146
  see also Pharmaceutical Index
pneumonia, xxiv, xxvi; **86**; 99, 111, 113–4, 122, 124, 148
Poor Law Reform Act, 1834, xvii
pork chop, **36**
porter (drink), **26, 26n, 40, 45, 50, 51, 51n, 52, 53, 64, 65*, 75**
Pott's disease of the spine, 100
Pott's fracture, 100
Pott's gangrene, 100
Pott's peculiar tumour, 100
poultice, 122; *see* Pharmaceutical Index
pound, *libra*, definition of, xxxiii; *see* Pharmaceutical Index
PRCS (President of the Royal College of Surgeons), 99
precordium (area of the chest in front of the heart), **68, 108**
prescription writing, xxxiii
Principles and Practice of Medicine, by Sir William Osler, London (1892), 106, 115, 122
Provence rose, 147
psoriasis, xxv, **7, 17**; 144, 148, 151, 157
  discussion of, 114
pulmonary tuberculosis (phthisis), xvii, xxi, xxiv, xxvii, xxviii, xxix*; **76, 96, 100, 108, 132**; 105, 112–3, 138, 153, 154, 155
pupils, xxi; mortality of, 91
purging, xxix, **9, 11n, 60**; 130
purpura urticans, **74**
  purpura and urticaria, xxv; **74**; 114, 140
pyrosis, **82***
quinsy, 135, 151, 159
râle(s), **132*, 132n**
recipe (take), xxxiii, **1n**
rectal examination, xxviii
renal failure, 106; renal disease, 120
rheumatic fever, **72, 84, 110, 140**; 107
  rheumatic fever and rheumatic heart disease, **68**
  discussion of, 114–5
rheumatism, xxv; **9, 19*, 35, 43, 54, 72, 80, 114, 115, 116, 126, 140, 141**; 124, 130, 141, 142, 143, 145, 146, 148, 151*, 154, 159
  discussion of, 114
rheumatoid arthritis, **126**; 115
  arthritis deformans, 115

rickets, **98**; 159
Rosetta stone, xi
Royal College of Surgeons, 93
rye bread, 140; *see* Pharmaceutical Index *sub* Ergot
salivation, excessive, **114**; 109
salicylic acid, 108
scabies, **9, 80**
  scabies, the itch, 115, 128, 159
scarifier, scarificator, 123*
scarlet fever, *see* fevers
scrobiculum cordis, **52**
scrotum, *see* cancer of
scruple, *scrupulus*, definition of, xxxiii
scurvy, 159
seasickness, 141
secretary, dispenser and, xxxii
Seidleitz powders, 152; *see* Pharmaceutical Index
Serjeant Surgeon Extraordinary to Queen Victoria, 99
servants, xix
  service, in, xxviii
seton, 126
shingles, 117
shoemaker, xxviii
sickness and vomiting, 146
skin, 114
  skin complaints, 124
  skin diseases, 141, 148*, 154, 157, 159
smallpox, xvii, xviii; 115–6
  eradication programme, 116
  vaccination of the poor (1835), xviii
  vaccination made compulsory, 116
  variolation in , 115
  treatment, 136
snakebite, 148
Society of Apothecaries, xiv
Sophia Barnardiston's Notebook, 141, 157
sore throats, 158
Spanish flies (Lytta), 126, 129; *see* Pharmaceutical Index *sub* Cantharides
specific gravity, *see* urine testing
speech impediment, xxvi
sphygmomanometer, 120
Spirochaeta pallida, see *Treponima pallida*
spital houses, Risbygate St, Bury St Edmunds, xviii
sprains, 155, 157, 159
statistics, xxiv
  in phthisis, 113
St Bartholomew's Hospital Reports, 91
steam bath(s), 127*
stethoscope(s), xxvii; **132n**; 113, 118; *see* People and Places Index *sub* Laennec
stomach conditions, 138
stomach cramps, 137
Stutter's resignation, xxxii
Suffolk branch of the Provincial Medical and Surgical Association, 95, 101, 102
Suffolk Medical Benevolent Society, xv; 94, 98n, 101
Suffolk Medical Book Club, 98, 101

sulphur, 108
    vapour baths, xxx; 127–8
surgeons, their capabilities, xxii
    British, 116
    earnings of, 94, 116
    London, 96
    poor note keeping by, xxiii, xxxi
surgery, xxii;
    cardiac, 115
surgical emergencies, xvii
    wards, 109
swollen joints, 154
syphilis, discussion of, 116, 154, 156–7*; *see* bubo
syrups, xxxiv; *see* Pharmaceutical Index
tablespoonful (*c.amplum* or *magnum*), xxxiv
tape-worms, 149
teaching hospital, xiii
teaspoonful (*minimum* or *parvum*), xxxiv; *see* Pharmaceutical Index
teeth, loss of, xxvi, 109; *see* salivation, excessive
teething, 156*
temperature, *see* measurement of body temperature
terminal care, xxix*
    hospital admission policy for, xxx
tetanus, treated with tobacco smoke enemas, 124
    treated with ether, 102
thermometer, *see* measurement of body temperature
threadworms, 149
tic douloureux, *see* trigeminal neuralgia
tinctures, xxxiv*; *see* Pharmaceutical Index
tobacco smoke, enemas, *see* tetanus
    tobacco smoking, 106
tonsillitis, 115, 151
tonsils, 141
toothache, 137, 153
Transactions of the Provincial Medical and Surgical Association (1837), xxiii
treatments, xxix–xxx
Treponema pallida, 116
Trichinella spiralis, 119
tricuspid valve, 115
trigeminal neuralgia, xxv; **45**; 26, 116–7
trocar, 126
tuberculosis of the spine, 100; *see also* pulmonary tuberculosis
tuberculosis, xxi;105, 106, 113
    abdominal, **132**

    see also pulmonary tuberculosis
tumour of ovary, *see* cancer of ovary
typhoid, 136, 155
ulcerated legs, **54**
University of New York College of Physicians, 94
urinary complaints, 144
urine testing, 120
    specific gravity and albumen, xxvi; **24**, **40**, **41***, **47**
urinometer, *see* hydrometer
urticaria (nettle rash), 50
    discussion of, 114
vaccination, 116; *see* smallpox
vaginal examinations, xxviii
vapour baths, **18***, **18n**; 126–8
    sulphur vapour baths, xxx
variolation, 115–6; *see* smallpox
vegetables, xxviii*; **7**
venereal disease, xvii; **8**, 141, 148, 156, ulcer, 156; *see* bubo, syphilis
venesection, xxix; **15**, **15n**, **21**, **38***, **40***, **48**, **60**, **61**, **84***, **100**, **101**, **108**, **109**, **114**, **139**; 111, 113*, 114, 124
    discussion of, 121
veterinary medicine, xxxvii, 153
    veterinary pharmacy, xxxvii
vinegars, xxxiv; *see* Pharmaceutical Index
visiting and account books (Stutter's), xi, xxxiin
    visits (home), xxxii
vitamin A, xivn
waggons, fractured limbs from riding on, xxii
washerwoman, servant to, xxviii*
washing machine, xxxi
water closets, xvii
water retention, **80**
waterman, xxviii*; **122***
water pillows, xxix
wet cupping, *see* cupping
whooping cough, 97, 153
willow bark, 130
wine, xxix*, **118***; *see also* Pharmaceutical Index
World Health Organisation, 116
worms, 130, 151
wounds, suturing of, xxii
X Rays, 113
Young Men's Institute, Bury St Edmunds, 95
Zambesi, forests of, 133

INDEX OF PHARMACEUTICAL MATERIALS AND METHODS

Acacia, **19**, **30**, **42**, **48**, **66**, **67**, **69**, **82**, **91**, **97**, **108**, **109**, **127**, **139**, **141**; 131; discussion of, 132
  mucilage, 132
Acetic acid, **19n**; 149, 159
alcohol, 153
alkaline mixture, **70**
alkaloids, 129, 130
Aloes, **1**, **24***, **30**, **32***, **49***, **50**, **51**, **67**, **78**, **79**, **124**, **125***, **128**, **129**, **136**, **137**; 132, 137; discussion of, 132
Alum, **122**, **123**; 153
Aluminium, 150
  lotion, **123**, **123n**; 150
Ammonia; discussion of, 150–1
  foetid spirit, **32**, **67**, **67n**, **109**, **136**, **136**, **137**
  liniment, **80**, **81**, **136**, **137**; 147, 151
  sal volatile, 150–1
  solution, **67**, **136**, **137**
  spirit of, **21**, **66**, **89***, **93**, **99**, **115**
  with potassium iodide, 154
Ammonium acetate, **5**, **19**, **33**, **35**, **84**, **85**, **96**, **97**, **120**, **132**, **133**
  bicarbonate, **67**, **85**
analgesic liniment, **62**
anthraquinones, active principles of Senna, 148–9
Antimony, **19**, **36**, **38**, **53**, **54**, **55**, **59**, **71**, **77**, **87**, **93**, **100**, **101**, **102**, **103**, **106**, **108**, **112** **115**, **116**, **124**, **125**, **134**, **135**, **138**, **139**; 112*, 113*, 138, 146, 151; discussion of, 151
antiseptic, 19th-century definition, **123n**
Antimonial Powder (Dr James's Powder), 151
aperient, domestic, **68**
  draught, **21**, **71**, **122**, **123**
  mixture, **67**, **68**, **98**, **99**, **116**
  pills, **59**, **66**, **67**, **84**, **85**, **89**, **91**, **98**, **99**, **103**, **104**, **105**, **139**
  powder, **68**, **106**, **107**, **113**
Aromatic confection, **115***, **133**
Arrowroot, **137**
Arsenic, **17**; 108, 156; discussion of, 151–2
  organic compounds, 156
Asafoetida, **3**, **32**, **41**, **49**, **66**, **136**; 135; discussion of, 132
Aspirin, 130,144
Atropine, 130
Bark, Peruvian, Jesuit's, *see* Cinchona bark
barley, decoction of, **30n**, **30**
  water, 129
beaver, North American, source of the drug castor, 129
Beecham's pills, xxxvii
beer, *see* General & Medical Subjects
Bismuth, **26**, **52**, **53**; discussion of, 152
Bitter apple, *see* Colocynth

Black Drop, *see* Opium
blistering, xxxix, **9**, **45**, **78**, **84**, **93**, **98**, **96**, **136**, **138**; 134
Blue Pill, 156*; *see also* mercury pill
bolus, xxxvi
breadcrumbs, **11**, **30**, **113**, **114**
  used in making pills, **11**n
British National Formulary (1960), 145
Broom tops, **47**, **48**, **100**, **101**; 149; discussion of, 133
Burgundy Pitch, *see* Pitch
Calomel, **60**, **68***, **74**, **100**, **108**, **112**, **124**, **126**, **134**; 113, 137, 138, 138n, 141, 144, 156
  in infant teeth powders, 156; *see also* mercurous chloride
Calcium Carbonate, *see* Chalk
Calumba, **19**, **20**, **26**, **35**, **37**, **38**, **68**: discussion of, 133
Camphor; discussion of, 133–4,
  injection, 134
  julep, xxxvi, 133, 133n
  liniment, **9**, **66**, **67**, **71**, **79**, **108**, **109**, **110**, **111**; 134, 147
  mixture, xxx, xxxvi; **1**, **3**, **13**, **15**, **19**, **21**, **22**, **24**, **33**, **35**, **38**, **40**, **48**, **50**, **51**, **66**, **67**, **69**, **70**, **71**, **77**, **85**, **89**, **91**, **93**, **97**, **99**, **108**, **109**, **117**, **120**, **123**, **125**, **127**, **129**, **130**, **131**, **133**, **136**, **137**, **141**
  price of, 137
  tincture, **109**, **109n**, **130**, **137**, **141**; 134, 147
Camphorated Oil, *see* Camphor liniment
Cantharides, xxix; **5***, **9**, **18n**, **18**, **35**, **40**, **41**, **42**, **45**, **66**, **71**, **77**, **78**, **79**, **85**, **91**, **93**, **99**, **100**, **109**, **131**; 129; discussion of, 134
  adverse effects, 134
  cerate, xxxix
  fatal poisoning by, 134
  internal use, **18n**
  plasters, xxxix; **5**, **9**, **40**, **45**, **66**, **71**, **79**, **85**, **91**, **93**, **99**, **105**, **109**, **131**
cantharidin, 134n
Capsicum, **19**, **35**, **36**, **38**; discussion of, 135
  gargle, 135
  poultice, 135
carbon dioxide, in effervescent mixtures, **40**; 152
Caraway, 148
Cardamom, 148
Cascarilla, **130**, **131**; discussion of, 135
Castor oil, **1***, **30***, **66**, **67***, **82***, **84**, **85***, **93**, **97**, **100**, **101**, **108**, **132**, **133**, **136***, **137**; 112, 149; discussion of, 135–6
Castor, **136**, **137**, **137n**; 129, 130*, 132; discussion of, 135
  used in cure of henbane poisoning, 135

cerates, xxxix; *see also* ointments and plasters
Chalk, **20**, **62**, **63**, **114**, **115**, **122**, **123**, **132**, **133***; 112, 145; discussion of, 152
Chamomile, **17**; 144
Cherry laurel leaves, source of hydrocyanic acid, 130, 153
Chillies, *see* Capsicum
Chiretta, **66**, **67**, **88**, **89**, **93**, **98***, **99**; discussion of, 136
Cinchona, **11**, **19**, **70**, **99**, **129**; discussion of, 136–7; *see also* Quinine
bark, 136
Cinnamon, **41**, **49**, **63**, **115**; discussion of, 137
medical essence of, 137
Citric acid, discussion of, 152
Codeine, 130, 145
Colchicine, xxix; 130, 137*; see also* Colchicum
Colchicum, **19**, **22**, **40**, **49**, **80**, **81**, **108**, **109**, **110**, **111**, **116**, **117**, **120**, **126**, **127**, **140**; discussion of, 137
acetic extract, **19n**
Colocynth, **1***, **7**, **17**, **19**, **21**, **40**, **41**, **49**, **57**, **69**, **70**, **74**, **75**, **80**, **81**, **101**, **108**, **109**, **110**, **111**, **116**, **117**, **120**, **122**, **123**, **124**, **125**, **126**, **127**, **128**, **134**, **135**, **136**, **137**; 130, 138, 142, 156, 158; discussion of, 137–8
confection, **9**, **19**, **35**, **36**, **40**, **115**, **133**
of rue, 147
of senna, **9**, **67**, **96**, **97**, **98**, **99**, **112**, **136**, **137**
of sulphur, **99**
preparation of, xxxvii
use of in pill-making, **35n**
conserves, xxxix; *see also* confection, electuary
counter-irritant, **52**, **68**, **114**, **124**, **134**; 134, 138, 149, 151
plaster, **130**; 151
cream of tartar, **57n**
Creta, *see* Chalk
Croton oil, **56**, **57**, **59**; 130, 138; discussion of, 138
Cucumber, wild, *see* Elaterium
Dandelion, discussion of, 138
extract, **84**, **85**
decoctions,
Chamomile, 144
Elm bark, **17**, **18**; 140
Mallow, **17n**; 139
devil's dung, *see* Asafoetida
diet, *see* General & Medical Subjects
Digitalis, xxix; **5**, **15***, **21**, **38**, **40**, **41**, **47**, **48**, **56**, **59**, **68**, **69**, **93***, **111**, **118**; 130, 133, 141, 149, 154, 156; discussion of, 139
use of live frogs in assay of, 139
digitoxin, 130; *see also* Digitalis
digoxin, 130, 139; *see also* Digitalis
Dover's powder, **54**; 143, 143n, 144, 145
with aspirin, 144
draught, xxxiii, xxxvn; 132, 146, 152, 157, 159
ear, blistering plaster applied to, **45**
effervescent mixtures, **17**, **17n**, **35**, **40**, **59**, **59n**, **63**, **69**, **101***; 159; discussion of, 152–3
use in 20th century, 153

Elaterium, **40**, **47***, **47n**, **56**, **57**, **59**; discussion of, 139
Elderflowers, **17**, **18**; discussion of, 139–40
electuary, **56**, **57**, **66**, **67**, **91**, **98**, **99**
preparation of, xxxvii
Elixir of Vitriol, *see* Sulphuric Acid
Elm Bark, discussion of, 140
decoction, **17**, **18**
embrocations, xl
emetic, 143, 145, 151
emulsion, **109**
enema,
common, **41**, **42**, 42n
domestic, **68**, **71**
Epsom Salts, *see* Magnesium sulphate
Ergot, **74**, **75**, **75n**, **102**, **103**; discussion of, 140
Ergotamine, 140; *see also* Ergot
Ether, 130; discussion of, 153; *see also* Nitrous Ether, Sulphuric Ether
extracts,
preparation of, xxxv
used in pills, xxxv
eye drops, xl
ferri, Ferrous, *see* iron
fever,
mixture, **24**, **131**, **138**, 139
powder (Dr James's), 151
flowers of sulphur, **99n**
fomentation, 144
of mallow, **17**
sodium chloride, 158
foxglove,
purple, 130, 139
white, 130; *see also* Digitalis
Galbanum,
pills, **1***, **32**, **35**, **38**, **41**, **66***, **67**, **78**, **79**
plaster, **67**, **91**, **93**, **98**, **99**
Gamboge, **47**, **57**; discussion of, 140–1
gargle, xl; **70**
of capsicum, 135
of sulphuric acid, 159
with honey as ingredient, 143
Gee's Linctus, 145
Gentian, **26**, **36**, **47**, **66**, **85**, **98**, **99**, **125**, **137**; 136, 138, 145; discussion of, 141
Ginger, **36**, **57**, **102**, **103**, **112**, **113**, **123**, **125**; 148; discussion of, 141
Glauber's Salts, *see* Sodium Sulphate
glycosides, 130
grey powder, **133n**; *see also* mercury with chalk
Guaiacum, **11**, **19**, **126**, **127**, **140**, **141**
discussion of, 141–2
Hemlock, **76**, **77***, **102**, **103**; discussion of, 142
Henbane, **9**, **21**, **40**, **41***, **49**, **59**, **69***, **71**, **82**, **93**, **96**, **97**, **118**, **123**, **125**, **130**, **131**, **135**, **139**; 138; discussion of, 142–3
home remedies,
acacia, for inflammation of bladder and kidneys, 132
aloes, for constipation, 132
camphorated oil, for rheumatism, etc, 134
gentian, as a tonic, 141

ginger, for irritation of piles, 141
henbane, for tooth-ache, 143
nitrous ether spirit and alum for tooth-ache, 153
rye, yeast and almond oil poultice for gout, xxxix
Seidlitz powders for hang-over, 153
senna, as household laxative, 148
sulphur, as household laxative, 159
Honey, **41**; 145, 129, 149; discussion of, 143
honey bee, 129
Hops, **26, 26n, 43, 45, 53**; 135, 146, 152; discussion of, 143
humulus lupulus, 143n; *see also* Hops
hydragogue, 139n
Hydrocyanic acid, 7, **17, 18, 40, 40n, 42, 52, 53*, 68, 69, 77, 82, 96, 97, 124, 125, 136, 137**; 130, 140; discussion of, 153–4
sales of (in 1820), 154
hyoscine, *see* Henbane
Hyoscyamus, *see* Henbane
Iodides,
of iron, **43, 47**
of mercury, **8, 43**
of potassium, **19*, 35*, 38*, 43, 116***
Iodine, **22, 34, 47, 66, 104, 105**; 112, 130, 153, 154; discussion of, 153–4; *see also* iodides
tincture for home first-aid, 154
Ipecacuanha, 1, **19, 20, 35, 37, 54, 55, 57, 66, 68, 70, 85, 88, 89, 91, 93, 113, 114, 115, 120, 122, 123, 130, 133**; 112*; discussion of, 143–4
Iron, 1, **33, 43, 63, 64, 68, 70*, 74, 78, 96, 124, 128**; 108, 141, 146; discussion of, 155
deficiency, **24**
mixture of, xxx; **1, 24, 33, 38, 54, 55, 65, 67, 68, 69, 97, 125, 129, 136**; 107, 146, 155, 155n
nitrate, **122, 123**; 155
oxide, **45, 67, 97**
persesquinitrate, **123n**; 155
pills, of, **32, 41, 49, 50, 51, 62, 63, 66, 67, 70, 74, 75, 79, 97, 118, 125, 129, 137**; 155, 155n
tartrate, **41, 57, 63, 70*, 125**
Jalap, **6, 24, 47*, 57*, 60, 61, 62, 68, 71, 109, 112, 113**; discussion of, 144
julep, xxxvi, 133n
Juniper, **101**
Langdale's Essence, *see* Cinnamon
Laudanum, *see* Opium
Lead, 138; discussion of, 155
for external use, xxix, xl; **7, 13, 17, 22, 109**; 117, 126, 155, 155
for internal use, **77, 84**
lemon as source of citric acid, 152
lemonade, 152
leeches, medical, xxix*, xxx; **13, 22, 32, 45*, 56, 57, 66, 67, 68*, 71*, 82*, 100*, 101, 110, 111, 132**; 112, 117, 125, 129
liniments, preparation of, xxxix, xl
Liquorice powder, **36**
Lupulus humulus, **26n**; 143n; *see also* Hops

Lytta, 108, 117; *see also* Cantharides
Magnesia, **1*, 41, 84, 85, 114**; 156
Magnesium, discussion of, 155–6
carbonate, **115, 125, 127**; 110, 155
oxide, 155
sulphate, **9, 17, 37, 73, 84, 85, 93, 98, 99, 100,**101, **109, 113, 114, 115, 116, 117, 120**; 109, 147,155
mallow, common, **17**; discussion of, 144, 144n
marsh mallow, 144n
Meadow Saffron, *see* Colchicum
medicine chest, 150
Mercuric chloride, **10, 18, 18n**
Mercury, xxix, **1, 7, 9, 15, 17, 18, 21, 24, 28, 37, 38, 40, 47, 48, 49, 55, 56, 68, 74, 84, 100, 108, 111, 113, 114, 120, 122, 122, 124, 126, 134**; 116, 130, 138, 141, 144, 145, 146, 147, 148, 149, 152, 157; discussion of, 156–7
adverse effect on gums and teeth, **100**; 109, 156
iodide pills, **8**, 156
liniments, **57, 68, 71**; 157
ointments, **1, 43**; 148, 157
pills, **1, 8, 15, 21, 28, 37, 38, 47, 59, 71, 115, 120, 123**; 109, 157
preparation of, **1n**
salivation, 156–7
submuriate of, **1n**
teething powders, 156
with chalk, **1, 1n, 35, 55, 84, 85, 133n**; 152
Mercurous chloride, **1*, 7, 9, 17, 19, 24, 35, 40, 40n, 41, 57, 59, 60, 61, 68, 69, 71, 74, 75, 100, 101, 108, 109, 112, 113, 117, 124, 125, 126, 134, 135**; 144, 156
milk, **41, 115, 133, 139**
mixtures, preparation of, xxxv
Morphine, **13, 33*, 45, 50, 71, 76, 77, 84, 85, 93, 96, 97, 136, 137**; 115, 129, 130, 139, 145, 146
Myrrh, **33, 136**
narcotic, **76, 102**
Nitric acid, xxix, **8, 17, 40, 45, 53*, 77**; 153; discussion of, 157
lotion, xl
Nitrous ether spirit, **15*, 21, 37, 40, 41, 47, 59, 60, 61, 68, 69, 70, 96, 97, 101, 120*, 123, 132, 133, 135**; 150, 153
Nux Vomica, **36**; discussion of, 144–5; *see also* Strychnine
ointments, preparation of, xxxix
Opium, xxix; **19, 35, 47, 48, 49, 54, 59, 63*, 67, 68, 69, 70, 71, 86, 87, 89, 101, 114, 115, 122, 130, 132, 133, 140, 141**; 113, 129, 134, 137, 142*, 143, 146, 152, 157; discussion of, 145–6
poppy, 129, 146
opodeldoc, *see* soap liniment
Orange, discussion of, 146
infusion, **11, 125**; 146
syrup, **1, 5, 17, 35**
tincture, **35, 99, 129**
Oxymel,
of Squill, **48, 97, 109**; 143, 149, 159
preparation of, xxv, 143

pain,
  griping, **41**
  in abdomen, **62, 82, 114, 132, 134**
  in back, **60, 61, 128**
  in chest, **100**
  in foot, **60, 108**
  in head, **60, 64, 68, 100, 124**
  in joints, **98, 126, 140**
  in knee, **140**
  in legs, **52**
  in loins, **64, 98**
  in region of heart, **68**
  in shoulder and neck, **114, 122**
  in side, **66, 68, 78, 96, 114**
  in stomach, **124**
  liniment to relieve, **49**
  morphine to relieve, **50**
  of blister, **45**
  rheumatic, **116, 126**
paregoric (compound tincture of camphor), **109n**
Peppermint water, **1, 41, 67, 85**; 149
Persesquinitrate of iron, *see* Iron
pharmacopoeias,
  Bristol Royal Infirmary, xxxvi
  Guy's Hospital, xxxvi
  London, xxxvi, xxxvii, xxxix; **7n**; 129, 133,
    143, 151, 153, 154, 158
  St George's Hospital, xxxvi
  Suffolk General Hospital, xxx, xxxvi
  University College Hospital, xxxvi
pills,
  Beecham's, xxxvii
  preparation of, xxxvi
    mercury pills, **1n**
    pill mass, xxxvi
    pill rolling, xxxvi
    ready prepared mass, xxxvi
    use of breadcrumbs, **7n**
    use of pestle and mortar, xxxvi
    varnishing, xxxvi,
placebo, **3**
plaster, **5, 24, 35**
  adhesive, 126
  anodyne, 126
  blistering, **9, 45, 68, 75, 84, 93, 98; 100**; 126
  common, 126
  of antimony, **35, 36, 100, 102, 103, 106**; 151
  of cantharides, xxxix; **5, 9, 35, 40, 45, 66, 67,
    71, 85, 91, 93, 99, 100, 105, 107, 131**
  of galbanum, **66, 67, 93, 98, 91, 99**
  of mustard, xxxix
  of pitch, **24, 38, 53**; 126, 146
plasters, preparation of, xxxix
    spreading, xxxix
    use of plaster iron, xxxix
pork chop, **36, 88**
poor man's plaster, *see* pitch plaster
porter (beer), *see* General & Medical Subjects
Potassium,
  acetate, **47*, 48, 100, 101**
  arsenite, **17**
  bicarbonate, **17, 40, 43, 45**; 157

bromide, 144
  iodide, **19, 38, 43, 45, 116, 117**; 154
  nitrate, **5, 15, 19, 21, 40, 41, 54, 55, 59, 60,
    68, 71, 78, 79, 84, 85, 93, 108, 109, 125,
    134, 135, 139**; 153
  solution, **7, 24, 67**; 157
  sulphate, **17**
  sulphuret of, **17, 17n**
  tartrate, **17, 47, 48, 57, 88, 89, 93*, 125**
Poppy syrup, **22, 66, 91**; 144; discussion of,
  146–7
poultices, xxxix, **13, 68, 71, 115, 122, 123**; 122
  domestic,
    barley meal, xxxix
    bread and milk, xxxix
    capsicum, 135
    mashed turnip, xxxix
    kaolin, xxxix
    remedy for gout, xxxix
    yeast, **122, 123**
  powders, preparation of, xxxvii
  prescriptions, writing, xxxiii
  prussic acid, *see* hydrocyanic acid
Quinine, xxix, **19, 45, 72, 74, 102***; 108, 139,
  141; discussion of, 136–7
  price of, 137
  sulphates, **5, 13, 19, 36, 73, 75, 93, 103, 113,
    123**; 136, 146, 147
  rhizome, 141n
Rhubarb, **24, 28, 38, 54, 54n, 55, 68, 69, 84, 85,
  102, 103, 109, 112, 113**; 141; discussion of,
  147
rice, **115, 133, 139**
Rose petals, discussion of, 147
  confection of, xxxvii; **19, 36**
  decoction, 132
  infusion, **5, 9, 13, 19, 21, 36, 72, 73, 75, 93,
    100, 102, 103, 106, 110, 111, 113, 123**;
    159
  water, 150
Rosemary **137**; 147; discussion of, 147
Rue, **36**; discussion of, 147
Saffron, **117, 117n**; discussion of, 147–8
Salicin, 130
salivation, 156; *see also* Mercury
Sal volatile, *see* Ammonia
Sarsaparilla, **7, 8, 17, 18, 43, 45**; 157; discussion
  of, 148
Scammony, **68, 69, 120**; 137; discussion of, 148
seaweed, source of iodine, 130
Seidlitz powders, **53n**; 152–3
Senega, **84, 85, 86, 87**; discussion of, 148
Senna, xxxvii; **1*, 66, 67, 74, 75, 91, 96, 97, 98,
  99, 112, 136, 137**; 130, 155, 159; discussion
  of, 148
  confection of, 148n
Silver nitrate, xl; **17, 34**; 108, 112, 155, 157;
  discussion of, 157
  caustic pencils, 157
sinapism, xxxix
Soap, discussion of, 157–8
  in pills, **43n, 43, 85, 87, 118**

liniment, **49**, **63**, **67**, **126**, **127**, **140**, **141**;
157–8
Spanish, **85**
Soda water, 152
Sodium, discussion of, 158
bicarbonate, **1**, **21**, **26**, **28**, **32***, **35**, **57**, **85**, **93**,
102, **103**, **109**, **112**; 138, 141, 153
carbonate, **33**, **35**, **69**; 152, 159
chloride, xl; **70**, 158
sulphate, **17**, **26**, **28**; 158
smelling salts, *see* Ammonia
Spanish beetle, fly, 129; *see also* Cantharides
Sparteine, 133; *see also* Broom Tops
Spearmint water, **15**; 146
Squill, **15**, **37**, **40**, **47**, **48**, **56**, **59**, **96**, **97**, **102**, **103**,
108, **109**; 145, 149, 156; discussion of, 149
St John's wort, 150
Strychnine, **9**, **11**, **30**, **112**, **113**, **136**, **137**; 145,
159*; discussion of, 158; *see also* Nux Vomica
weighing small amounts of, **11n**
Sulphur, **17**; discussion of, 158–9
confection, **99**
electuary, **99**
fumigation, **9**
ointment, xxxix; **7**, 108, 159
vapour bath, xxx; **19**, **80**, **81**; 128, 159; *see
also* appendix IV, pp. 126–8
Sulphuric acid, **36**, **100**, **102**, **103**, **106**; 130, 147,
153; discussion of, 159
aromatic, 159
Elixir of Vitriol, 159
spirit of, **67**
Sulphuric ether spirit, **41**, **66**, **67**; 153
sweating, promoting, **19**
sweet spirit of nitre, *see* nitrous ether spirit
Syrup, **5**, **8**, **11**, **19**
of Orange, **1**, **5**, **17**, **35**
of Poppy, **21**, **66**, **67**; 144
tablets,
Brockenden's patent for shaping pills,
lozenges and black lead, xxxvii
manufacture of, xxxvii
tartar emetic, *see* Antimony
Tartaric acid, **17**, **35**, **40**, **69**, **76**; 153; discussion
of, 159
price of, 137
tinctures, preparation of, xxxiv, xxxv
maceration, xxxv

percolation, xxxv
tonics, **6**, **11**, **13**, **19**, **66**, **19**, **32**, **66**, **72**, **88**, **98**;
112, 151, 152
arsenic, **17n**
bitter, **72**, **88**, **98**
nerve, **30**
Turpentine, **30**, **33**, **41**, **42**; 143, 146, 149;
discussion of, 149
liniment of, **41**, **132**, **133**; 149–50
Valerian, xxx; **1***, **5**, **33**, **51**; discussion of, 150
vapour baths, **19n**
vegetables, **1**, **7**
Vinegar, xxxv; **11**; discussion of, 159
distilled, **11**
of Cantharides, **42**; 159
of Squill, xxxv; 149
vitriol, elixir of, *see* Sulphuric Acid
water, pure, **33**, **40**, **45**, **53**, **69**
weights and measures,
of apothecary,
drachm, xxxiii, xxxiv
drop, xxxiv; **52n**
gallon, xxxiv
grain, xxxiii
minim, xxxiv
ounce, xxxiii–iv
pint, xxxiv
pound, xxxiii, xxxiv
scruple, xxxiii
symbols, xxxiii, xxxiv
of household,
dessertspoonful, xxxiv
glass, **20n**
tablespoonful, xxxiv
teaspoonful, xxxiv
white liniment, *see* Turpentine
willow bark, 130; *see also* Aspirin
Wines,
antimony, **19**; 112, 151
colchicum, **23**, **120**
ipecachuanha, **67**, **70**, **85**, **89**, **131**; 144
preparation of, xxxv
Yeast poultice, **122**, **123n**
yellow wax (beeswax), 126
Zinc ointment, **17**
Zinc sulphate, **122**, **123n**; 108*